DATE DUE

		4-29-09	
			Demco

SAFETY AND ETHICS IN HEALTHCARE

to those who suffer needlessly

Safety and Ethics in Healthcare
A Guide to Getting it Right

BILL RUNCIMAN

ALAN MERRY

MERRILYN WALTON

ASHGATE

Published by
Ashgate Publishing Limited
Gower House
Croft Road
Aldershot
Hampshire GU11 3HR
England

Ashgate Publishing Company
Suite 420
101 Cherry Street
Burlington, VT 05401-4405
USA

Ashgate website: http://www.ashgate.com

British Library Cataloguing in Publication Data
Runciman, Bill
  Safety and ethics in healthcare : a guide to getting it
  right
  1. Medical errors - Prevention 2. Medical ethics 3. Medical
  policy 4. Health facilities - Safety measures 5. Medical
  care - Quality control
  I. Title II. Merry, Alan III. Walton, Merrilyn
  362.1'068

Library of Congress Cataloging-in-Publication Data
Runciman, Bill.
  Safety and ethics in healthcare : a guide to getting it right / by Bill Runciman, Alan Merry, and Merrilyn Walton.
       p. cm.
  Includes index.
  ISBN: 978-0-7546-4435-4 (hardback)
  ISBN: 978-0-7546-4437-8 (pbk.) 1. Medical ethics. 2. Clinical medicine--Decision making. 3. Medical errors. 4. Health services accessibility. I. Merry, Alan. II. Walton, Merrilyn. III. Title.
  [DNLM: 1. Medical Errors. 2. Quality of Health Care--ethics. 3. Safety Management--ethics. WB 100 R939s 2007]

  R725.S244 2007
  174.2--dc22

                                                                          2006031461

ISBN: 978-0-7546-4435-4 (HBK)
ISBN: 978-0-7546-4437-8 (PBK)

Printed and bound in Great Britain by TJ International Ltd, Padstow, Cornwall.

Contents

PART 4: PREVENTING THINGS FROM GOING WRONG

APPENDICES

List of Boxes

List of Tables

List of Figures

Foreword

It has become customary to link the start of our present widespread concern with patient safety to the Institute of Medicine's influential report, *To Err is Human: Building a Safer Health System*. And, indeed, the 1999-2000 period was a watershed for the patient safety movement. The year 2000 saw the beginning of a flurry of high-level statements from government agencies in various countries that broadcast the extent of the harm caused by medical errors and systemic deficiencies. But the operative word here is 'broadcast'. These high-impact publications did not so much break new ground as bring to prominence research evidence and epidemiological findings that had been in the public domain for well over a decade.

One of the many reasons why this book is so very significant is that its clinician-authors, Professor Bill Runciman and Professor Alan Merry, have been carrying out innovative studies in anaesthetic safety (*inter alia*) over the past 20 years or so. They are among the true pioneers of the patient safety movement and this long exposure to the conceptual and methodological problems besetting this field makes itself apparent in this book. Few authors could write with such knowledge and authority as that displayed here.

Some years ago, I heard a newly appointed director of safety announce that safety management was not rocket science. And he was absolutely right. Rocket science is trivial compared to the complexities and difficulties that confront those charged with assuring that their operational risks are *kept as low as reasonably practicable* (the ALARP principle) while *still staying in business* (the ASSIB principle). ALARP without ASSIB would be relatively easy; it is trying to achieve both of these things at the same time that is so hard.

Even in highly standardized and largely automated domains such as commercial aviation and nuclear power generation, managing safety is a difficult and constant challenge. But healthcare has very few of these mitigating features. Its activities and equipment are highly diverse, its products are delivered in a close and personal fashion and their recipients are vulnerable and needy people (see Chapter 5).

If safety management anywhere is intrinsically complex, ensuring patient safety is especially so, not least because the necessity of managing it is not always apparent. If your core business is to heal the sick and repair the injured, then it is not unreasonable to assume that patient safety is simply a naturally emergent property of these therapeutic processes. But it is not. It is something that needs to be trained for and managed, just like any other medical activity. Recognizing this and acknowledging that healthcare professionals are fallible and will commit harmful errors are the first steps along this path.

Making an error, even one with damaging consequences, rarely equates to incompetence – it simply confirms the maker's humanity. The capacity to go wrong is an inerasable part of being human: we cannot change the human condition, but we can change the conditions under which human beings work. This is the first rule of error management, a process that lies at the heart of effective safety management.

Prerequisites for engaging in any demanding activity, but especially the struggle for improved patient safety, are conceptual frameworks – 'road maps' that set out, clearly and simply, the 'geography' of the task. And herein lies one of the considerable merits of this book. Chapter 1 presents a comprehensive and comprehensible representation of the major dimensions of quality in healthcare in which the major goals – acceptability, effectiveness, efficiency, safety, timeliness, and the like – are mapped on to the various layers of the health system: the patient, the clinician, the team, the organization, and so on. A second model provides a framework for classifying patient safety information – and it is here that the extensive experience of the authors makes its mark. Together, these two schemes integrate and make sense of the enormous volume of material that could otherwise be overwhelming. They define the 'woods' that would be so easy to lose sight of when confronted with so many diverse 'trees'.

Adverse events in any complex hazardous enterprise are rarely the result of single causes, either human or technical. They mostly arise from the (often diabolical) conjunction of many contributing factors originating at different levels of the system. Analyses that assign these contributions to separate categories (i.e., human error, workplace deficiencies, organizational conditions, and the like) produce numbers that, while convenient to manipulate, distort the very essence of event aetiology, namely the complexly interactive nature of their causation. These properties are best caught by stories and case studies. Narratives rather than numbers are the primary data of the safety sciences. Don't get me wrong – numbers have their place, but not when they add up to little more than vacuous clerking.

The risk associated with a particular event is commonly defined as the product of its likelihood and severity. But, as Carl Macrae[1] argued very recently, such an assessment gives little or no indication of the true nature of the threat posed by this or similar events. What is important is not the actual outcome of any one event, but what the consequences could have been had it combined with other factors – each possibly inconsequential by itself – to breach the organizational defences and barriers. Event narratives play a vital referential role in assessing the organizational risks of these 'could-have-beens'. A crucial stock-in-trade for those making these judgements is a head full of varied case studies. Ideally, these stories should also include serious organizational accidents in healthcare institutions. For the moment, however, these accounts are relatively few and far between, though such reports are gradually finding their way into the public domain – see the seminal analysis of a vincristine tragedy by Toft.[2]

One of the many strengths of this book is that it is richly studded with case studies drawn from a wide variety of activities and specialties. These along with the integrating frameworks, the penetrating analyses of the present healthcare system, the extensive coverage of research and the in-depth consideration of the ethical issues make up what must be the most comprehensive toolkit currently available. In short, the book has – in Ron Westrum's[3] elegant phrase – *requisite imagination*. It will, I am sure, be a landmark publication.

James Reason

Notes

1. Macrae, C.J. (2006), 'Assessing Organizational Risk Resilience: Assessing, Managing and Learning from Flight Safety Incident Reports', University of East Anglia, School of Environmental Sciences: PhD Thesis.
2. Toft, B. (2001), 'External Enquiry into the Adverse Incident that Occurred at Queen's Medical Centre, Nottingham, 4th January 2001', London: Department of Health.
3. Westrum, R. (1991), *Technologies and Society: The Shaping of People and Things*, Belmont CA: Wadsworth Publishing Company.

Preface

The vast majority of humans have a spontaneous urge to help their fellow beings when they are in trouble. Attempts to alleviate pain, sickness and suffering are evident from the beginnings of recorded history. A considerable number of people systematically set out to help their fellow humans by training for roles in healthcare. Our overwhelming experience has been that almost all of these people, all over the world, are highly motivated to help those afflicted by disease and injury.

Healthcare has become progressively more refined over the centuries and now constitutes a vast health 'industry'. There have been huge advances over the last 150–200 years with the development of safe, effective anaesthesia and pain relief, asepsis and modern surgery, antibiotics, immunization, new drugs and diagnostic techniques, and a far better understanding of the scientific basis of medicine, culminating in advances such as organ transplantation, molecular engineering and nanotechnology.

However, increasingly, this road is not an easy one to travel for those delivering the care. As more and more people survive into old age, the burden of caring for them becomes greater and greater. Although it is now possible to alleviate many of the afflictions that beset mankind, no society can afford to pay for all the healthcare that is now available or technically possible. People working in healthcare increasingly have to do more with less. Rationing takes many forms, mostly covert, and the less privileged in most societies end up struggling to get their proper share of the available healthcare dollar. All too often, those in the front-line have to deal with the consequences of this 'rationing by default'.

All involved in healthcare want to be able to do the right thing at the right time, in the right way, for the right people – those who will most benefit from the available resources. All too often, though, people who train in healthcare in order to devote themselves to providing care and comfort for their fellow human beings find themselves rushed off their feet simply doing the basic tasks and completing all the paperwork. Healthcare professionals find themselves placing frail, sick people in ever lengthening queues, sometimes asking them to wait for hours in the middle of the night under uncomfortable and even unsafe conditions. Worst of all, people find themselves working under conditions they would rather avoid in which the safety margin for those they are caring for has been greatly diminished. We are all aware that under these conditions the chance of making a mistake which can seriously harm or even lead to the death of a patient is greatly increased. What can we do about this? How can one be sure that one is doing the right thing when faced with having to practice an uncertain science on vulnerable patients in a complex system under ever-changing conditions? When does one cross the invisible line from reasonable to irresponsible or unethical behaviour by tolerating conditions or tacitly accepting practices which may be regarded as unacceptable, even though one may have little immediate control over them?

This book is a guide to getting it right for healthcare professionals. It is about:

- doing the right thing – appropriate and based on best evidence, but acceptable to the recipient;
- in the right way – in a way that is safe, effective and efficient;
- at the right time – when it is needed or most effective; and
- for the right people – those who will benefit most from the proper use of the available resources (which implies equitable access to care).

These are the dimensions of quality in healthcare, and although some are in conflict (equitable access and efficiency, for example), adherence to ethical practice and professional behaviour will help guide healthcare practitioners through the minefield of often conflicting priorities.

The World Health Organization has defined health as 'a state of complete physical, mental and social well-being and not merely the absence of disease or infirmity'. We must try to ensure that appropriate efforts are directed towards preventing illness and injury as well as providing care when people have been hurt or have become unwell. We must also try to ensure that a powerful few do not selectively consume limited healthcare resources at the expense of the vulnerable and disenfranchised.

The Layout of the Book

This book has four parts. The first is about healthcare today, the things that are wrong with it, and how some of these have come to be. In Chapter 1, the dimensions of quality in healthcare are considered together with a consideration of different approaches to funding for the various layers of healthcare. How resources are distributed, and how they might be, both within and between nations, is touched upon, together with the uncertainty about what may be considered the best healthcare and the variations in care that result. In Chapter 2 we outline the risks associated with healthcare and the nature of iatrogenic harm, referring in some detail to the large studies which have documented this to be a public health problem on a scale that rivals the road toll. In Chapter 3 we consider factors which contribute to making the system dysfunctional – its haphazard evolution, its hierarchies, its competing agendas, and its poor organization. In Chapter 4 we discuss the unfortunate human propensity for naming, blaming and shaming when things go wrong, and how the tort system has contributed to the blame cycle, while failing to adequately compensate those harmed or prevent the same problems from happening again.

The second part of this book is about the basic principles which need to be understood if the safety and quality of healthcare is to be improved. Chapter 5 is about getting an understanding of the nature of human error and how errors differ from violations, about complex systems, and about the factors that predispose to error and influence outcomes within complex systems. This is fundamental to any attempt to reduce iatrogenic harm or to make the regulation of healthcare more effective. In Chapter 6 we discuss the concept of evidence-based medicine, and the interpretation of the results of medical research. To do this requires a consideration of the problems of fraud in research and of misleading marketing. Chapter 7 is about ethics, professional behaviour and regulation.

The third part of this book is about what to do when things go wrong and how to respond when a patient has been harmed. In Chapter 8 we identify the victims of iatrogenic harm: the patient, primarily, but also the healthcare worker involved in causing that harm. Each needs to be cared for. Open disclosure is essential – getting the facts into the open so that people know what has happened and so that action can be taken to prevent the recurrence of a similar problem. In Chapter 9 we consider methods for preventing similar problems from recurring, preferably *before* a major disaster occurs. Incident reporting is dealt with together with root cause analysis. Having identified a problem, something needs to be done about it. The first step of this is to understand what really went wrong, and this requires looking beyond the 'smoking gun' and identifying the systemic factors which predisposed to an accident in the first place.

The fourth part of this book is about preventing iatrogenic harm and improving quality of practice. In Chapter 10 we focus on how to get the best out of the people involved in healthcare, including the patient. The challenge is to exploit to the maximum what people are good at, and make the best of the valuable resource that they represent. In Chapter 11, we consider the system and how to improve it. This involves gathering information, assembling evidence, identifying risks and problems, making the right decisions and then preventing things from going wrong when carrying them out. This requires optimizing the design of equipment and processes, and enhancing the early detection of and response to problems when they do occur. Finally, in Chapter 12, we consider where we should be going next, and what the attributes of an ideal system might be.

Terminology

It will be evident from the title of this book and the language used so far that we have chosen to use 'generic' terms for those involved in healthcare. We have chosen to talk about patients rather than clients or consumers, although we recognize that a healthy pregnant woman, a child undergoing immunization or an adolescent seeking counselling may not be regarded as patients. The term healthcare professionals embraces doctors (physicians), nurses and practitioners of para-medical disciplines (pharmacists, physiotherapists, occupational therapists, biomedical engineers, and others). We use the term clinician to refer to those involved directly with the interactions between patients and the healthcare system.

List of Abbreviations

ACC	Accident Compensation Commission
ACLS	Advanced Cardiovascular Life Support
AIDS	Acquired Immune Deficiency Syndrome
AIMS	Advanced Incident Management System
APSF	Australian Patient Safety Foundation
ARR	Absolute Risk Reduction
AS/NZS4360	Australia/New Zealand Risk Management Standard
AU$	Australian Dollars
AvMA	Action Against Medical Accidents
CPD	Continuing Professional Development
CPR	Cardiopulmonary Resuscitation
CT	Computerized Tomography
DALY	Disability Adjusted Life Year
DRG	Diagnostic Related Group
DVD	Digital Video Disc
EBM	Evidence-based Medicine
EMST	Emergency Management of Severe Trauma
ENT	Ear, Nose and Throat
FMEA	Failure Mode Effects Analysis
FNA	Fine Needle Aspiration
GDP	Gross Domestic Product
GP	General Practitioner
HDC	Healthcare Disability Commission
HIV	Human Immunodeficiency Virus
HRO	High Reliability Organization
HRT	Hormone Replacement Therapy
ICD	International Classification of Diseases
ICMJE	International Committee of Medical Journal Editors
ICU	Intensive Care Unit
IHD	Ischaemic Heart Disease
IT	Information Technology
JCAHO	Joint Commission on Accreditation of Healthcare Organizations
MET	Medical Emergency Team
NAT	Nucleic Acid Testing
NCPS	National Centre for Patient Safety
NHS	National Health Service
NNH	Number Needed to Harm
NNT	Number Needed to Treat
OR	Odds Ratio
PDCA	Plan, Do, Check, Act

PDSA	Plan, Do, Study, Act
PET	Positron Emission Tomography
PIN	Personal Identification Number
PSO	Patient Safety Officer
QALY	Quality Adjusted Life Year
RCA	Root Cause Analysis
RCT	Randomized Controlled Trial
RR	Relative Risk
SAC	Severity Assessment Code
SSM	Soft Systems Methodology
STPRA	Socio Technical Probabilistic Risk Analysis
UK	United Kingdom
USA	United States of America
US$	United States Dollars
VA	Veterans Administration
VAP	Ventilator Associated Pneumonia
WAPS	World Alliance for Patient Safety
WHO	World Health Organization

Acknowledgements

It is of course impossible to list the thousands of people who have contributed to our understanding of the issues outlined in this book. They include our clinical and administrative colleagues and mentors, the many patients (with their relatives, friends and carers) we have been privileged to learn from, and those from other disciplines into whose domains we have wandered, and been welcomed.

We have drawn heavily on the work of pioneers in the field of patient safety – Jim Bagian, David Bates, Don Berwick, Troyan Brennan, Jeff Cooper, Nick (Joachim) Gravenstein, Don Harper-Mills, Bob Helmreich, Hal Kaplan, Lucien Leape, Alan Maynard, Don Norman, Charles Perrow, Jeep Pierce, Jens Rasmussen, Jim Reason, John Senders and Tjerk van der Schaaf. Chapter 5 owes several passages to Jim Reason who wrote a chapter for a multi-author book which, in the end, was not completed, and generously offered the material to us for this book. However, he should not be held accountable for any misconceptions we might have transmitted.

Bruce Barraclough, Ursula Beckmann, Jim Battles, Noel Cass, Kaye Challinger, Lyn Currie, Jan Davies, David Gaba, Ross Holland, Cliff Hughes, Anthony Ilsley, Dorothy Jones, Pat Mackay, Sandy McCall-Smith, John Mainland, Craig Morgan, Richard Morris, Maureen Robinson, Libby Roughead, David Studdert, Fiona Tito, Bob Webb, Johanna Westbrook, Rod Westhorpe, John Williamson and John Zelcer have been influential colleagues.

We would like to thank those who reviewed the entire book and made constructive suggestions – Jeffrey Braithwaite, Michael Edmonds, Michelle McKinnon, Peter Malycha, Villis Marshall, Sally Merry, Stavros Prineas and Amanda Rischbieth. We also thank those who provided advice in their areas of special expertise – David Galler, David Merry, Ron Paterson, Glen Salkeld, Mary Seddon and Craig Webster.

We would also like to thank those who have waded through more drafts than they (and we) would care to remember – Penny Boyce, Sarah Hartnett, Dianne Grieve and Debbie Beaumont. A special thanks to Klee Benveniste who has tracked down many thousands of references and original manuscripts, and meticulously checked those which have been included.

Finally, we thank our families and friends for their support and forbearance in the face of the many disruptions to their lives by way of the logistical demands of writing and the numerous telephone calls at inconvenient hours, necessitated by the aversion to e-mail of one of the authors.

About the Authors

Bill (WB) Runciman MBBCh, FANZCA, FJFICM, FHKCA, FRCA, PhD

Bill Runciman is Professor of Anaesthesia and Intensive Care at the University of Adelaide and Head of the Department of Anaesthesia and Intensive Care at the Royal Adelaide Hospital. He founded the Australian Patient Safety Foundation in 1988, and is the current President. He has been a member of task forces which produced world patient safety standards for both Anaesthesia and Intensive Care. He was Chairman of the Safety and Quality of Practice Committee of the World Federation of Societies of Anaesthesiologists from 1992 to 2000. He has been a member of the Australian Council for Safety and Quality in Healthcare and of the Australian Health Information Council, and is joint co-ordinator of groups developing research tools and an International Patient Safety Classification for the World Alliance for Patient Safety of the World Health Organization.

Alan (AF) Merry MB ChB, FANZCA, FFPMANZCA

Alan Merry is Professor of Anaesthesiology at the University of Auckland. He chairs the Quality and Safety Committee of the World Federation of Societies of Anaesthesiologists. He is a Councillor of the Australian and New Zealand College of Anaesthetists, chairs the College's Quality and Safety Committee, and has chaired its New Zealand National Committee. He co-chaired the New Zealand Medical Law Reform Group and has been president of the Auckland Medico-Legal Society. He is co-author of the books *Errors, Medicine and the Law* (with Alexander McCall Smith; Cambridge University Press, 2001) and *Essential Perioperative Transoesophageal Echocardiography* (with David Sidebotham and Malcolm Legget; Butterworth-Heinemann, 2003).

Merrilyn Walton BA, BSW, MSW, PhD

Merrilyn Walton is an Associate Professor in the Faculty of Medicine at the University of Sydney. She chairs the Personal and Professional Development Theme and teaches students and clinicians about ethical practice, quality and safety. Her interests include enhancing the training environment for medical students and doctors and advocating for patients to be fully engaged in health care at every level. She was the founding Commissioner for the NSW Health Care Complaints Commission (1993–2000), and is a board member of the NSW Institute for Medical Education and Training and chairs its Prevocational Training Council.

Chapter 1

Setting the Stage: An Overview of Healthcare

Why Safety?

Avoidable harm caused by the process of healthcare itself, rather than by an underlying injury or disease, is called *iatrogenic harm*, and has been recognized since the time of Hippocrates, 2,400 years ago.[1] However, it is only in the last decade that the extent of this harm has been widely appreciated. Recent data from studies in which investigators systematically searched medical records for instances of preventable harm to patients have established iatrogenic harm as one of the top four or five public health problems in the developed world; only cardiovascular disease, cancer, infection, smoking and mental health problems have a greater impact on society (Table 1.1[2-9]). Many authorities were surprised to the point of disbelief when it was found that 10 per cent of admissions to acute-care hospitals are associated with an *adverse event* (an incident that results in harm to a patient),[5] and that the number of deaths associated with these events exceeds the road toll.[7]

Table 1.1 A selection of important causes of death world-wide[2]

Cause of Death	No of Deaths per Day
Lack of clean water and basic healthcare (children)[3]	30,000
Smoking [4]	14,000
Iatrogenic harm – acute care[5]	10,000
HIV/AIDS[6]	8,000
Road traffic accidents[7]	3,000
Natural disasters (earthquakes, tsunamis, floods, hurricanes)[8]	100
Terrorism[9]	20

Why was the scale of this problem not recognized sooner? One reason is that most of these adverse events had been given innocuous-sounding labels, such as 'complication', 'misadventure' and 'sequela' and had, over the years, become accepted as part of the usual pattern of clinical medicine. Also, many who work in healthcare recognize that they are applying an imperfect science to sick people, frequently under less than ideal conditions, and so have tended to accept as inevitable that things can and do go wrong. These problems were, for many years, viewed as part of the price to be paid for the great benefits of modern healthcare.[10]

Iatrogenic disasters involving death or major harm to a patient were regarded as isolated events 'deeply unfortunate and best forgotten'.[11] Because these events occurred one at a time and had been given a variety of labels, with no uniform system for collecting them, they had never been put together and counted. Occurring singly, they do not have the same public impact as disasters such as airline crashes in which several hundred people may die at one time. In fact, traveling in an airplane is far safer than being a patient in hospital (see Tables 2.1 and 2.2).

This book covers all aspects of quality in healthcare (Figure 1.1), but the emphasis is on safety. Safety has social value in that it reduces the uncertainty of interactions between healthcare professionals and patients and reduces the risk and cost of healthcare. Some authorities view safety as separate from quality in healthcare. This makes little sense; safety comes at a cost, and the benefit 'purchased' must be weighed against opportunities lost in other dimensions of quality in healthcare. However, the term 'safety and quality' has been used in recent years to place emphasis on the element of safety in the belief that this aspect of quality has often been neglected. It is hard to argue that a healthcare system could be of high quality unless it was also acceptably safe, and very safe healthcare facilities would be of little value unless they also provided effective treatments to those who need them.

It is important to keep the primary goal of healthcare in mind, namely the improvement of health. Health has been defined by the World Health Organization (WHO) as: 'a state of complete physical, mental and social well-being and not merely the absence of disease or infirmity'.[12] One can identify three approaches to healthcare: the treatment of illness; the prevention of illness; and the promotion of health. The third of these goes well beyond the first two, and provides insight into what it means to fail patients. There is more to patient safety than simply the elimination of error or the avoidance of direct harm. We would argue that any avoidable failure to achieve the WHO definition of health, whether through error, violation, over treatment, under treatment or inappropriate treatment, constitutes harm to patients.

Safety has been defined as 'freedom from hazard' where hazard is 'a circumstance or agent that can lead to harm, damage or loss' (see definitions in Appendix I). Safety is inversely related to risk: safety increases as risk is reduced to an acceptable level. Acceptability of risk in healthcare relates to a balance between the potential for harm, the likelihood of doing good, and the choices available at the time. In healthcare there is often risk in doing nothing. Social context is very important in determining priorities in healthcare. For some services the balance between risks and benefits leaves no room for any compromize on safety. Heart lung transplantation is a good example of a procedure in which the net benefit of a whole programme may be small even when things go well, and the balance can be shifted from positive to negative by a few preventable adverse events. If heart lung transplantation is to be undertaken at all, the imperative to do so safely is very high (see Box 1.1). On the other hand, there are situations in which patients' immediate needs offset the requirement for a high level of safety. For example, after the 2004 Boxing Day tsunami, the demand for basic, life-saving healthcare was overwhelming.[13] Although safety remained important, certain compromises were justified simply so that services could be provided at all. Under such circumstances an anaesthetic without sophisticated monitoring may be better than no anaesthetic at all.[14]

Why Ethics?

There is a minefield of often conflicting considerations that has to be navigated in the everyday work of a healthcare professional (see Table 7.1). Politicians put pressure on administrators, administrators put pressure on managers, and managers and patients (and their families) make demands of frontline clinicians. These pressures and demands are sometimes difficult to reconcile. The basic premise of this book is that healthcare professionals have a duty to do the right thing, *as defined from the perspective of their patients*. Unfortunately, it is not always easy to determine what the right thing is. The clinical aspects of a situation may be far from clear, and the issue may be further complicated by the values and beliefs of patients, healthcare workers and the society in which they interact. Some healthcare professionals believe it is their duty to do everything possible to advance the cause of *their particular* patients, and some place their own beliefs ahead of the desires and needs of patients (see page 164). Sometimes what is right for one patient can only be provided at the expense of a large number of other patients (see page 12). For example, always giving broad spectrum antibiotics to *your* patients is likely to facilitate the breeding of 'super bugs' for which there is no effective treatment, and may actually harm others.

Good communication is all-important in managing this type of conflict, at the level of individuals and at the level of the community in which the individuals live, work and depend on each other. Open and frank discussion between health professionals and their patients (and their patients' friends, relatives and carers), their colleagues, and the community at large helps resolve difficult questions about appropriateness in healthcare. The healthcare system exists for the benefit of patients. We need continually to ask 'Would I be happy if this were happening to me or one of my loved ones?' Given that resources are finite and often fall short of expectations, the answer may at times be 'No', at least for some patients. In effect this represents a conflict between a 'common good' view of health economics, and the principle of duty to individuals. Because a resource spent on one patient cannot be used on another, a sound ethical framework will be helpful in identifying the right thing to do (see Chapter 7 for further discussion of these issues).

The Dimensions of Quality in Healthcare

The tragic case of Jessica Santillan (Box 1.1) sets the scene for a book on safety and ethics in healthcare. Was this operation (and more particularly the second operation) appropriate in the first place, given the shortage of organs in the United

States and (more fundamentally) the difficulties in accessing basic healthcare experienced by many of this country's citizens?

Box 1.1 A death at Duke[15]

In February 2003, at Duke University Medical Centre, Jessica Santillan (who was 17) died after undergoing heart-lung transplantation because of a simple mistake. The circumstances of this case were particularly poignant. Her family and the wider community had gone to extraordinary lengths to make her operation possible. Jessica had been brought to the United States by her father, a truck driver from Guadalajara, Mexico, to seek treatment for her condition. She suffered from a severe congenital heart problem, and was disabled to the extent that she fainted on any exertion. The only treatment for her condition was a heart-lung transplant. Her family begged in the streets to raise funds for Jessica's procedure, until a North Carolina businessman adopted her cause. Money was then raised by a grass-roots foundation by building houses with donated materials and selling them.

On the evening preceding the operation, there were considerable logistical difficulties in obtaining the organs. They were eventually implanted, but, after a short time it became apparent that they were not functioning well. The transplant coordinator then called to inform the team that the transplanted organs were incompatible: Jessica's blood type was O and the donor's was A. Jessica spent two weeks in intensive care, critically ill. She underwent a second heart-lung transplant, but to no avail. On 22 February she was pronounced brain dead, and life-support was withdrawn.

During this period there was a full disclosure of the facts by Duke University Medical Centre. The chief executive officer admitted publicly that an error had been made. A chronology of the events was posted on a web site. Public apologies were made. Subsequently, a root cause analysis (see Chapter 9) was undertaken, and changes instituted into transplant procedures at Duke, with a view to reducing the likelihood of recurrence of this type of tragic event.

Was this an example of the good use of healthcare resources? How did things go wrong? How was such a basic requirement – to check the compatibility of the blood groups – overlooked by such highly skilled, highly motivated and well intentioned professionals? Should anyone be blamed? How can errors of this sort be avoided? Was the hospital's response appropriate? Should litigation follow? Should the family be compensated? In short, Jessica's story raises questions not only about safety and ethics, but also about how countries should provide the best return on their investment into the health of their people across all the dimensions and layers of healthcare (Figure 1.1).

Unfortunately, despite excellent intentions and many outstanding successes, healthcare too often falls short of acceptable standards. It may be unsafe, inefficient, ineffective, provided too late or not at all, unevenly distributed across populations, and provided with little regard to cultural or societal sensitivities; legitimacy is sometimes debatable and the allocation of funds patchy and irrational.

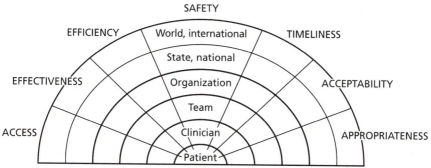

Figure 1.1 The dimensions of quality and organizational layers of healthcare[16]

Access

Access reflects the degree to which people can obtain the healthcare they need. Barriers to access are often financial, but they may be physical (after the New Orleans hurricane for example), or even cultural or religious. Unequal access results in inequity and inequality – inequity is the degree to which distribution of healthcare amongst the members of a population is less than just and fair, and inequality refers to differences in the healthcare received by individuals. It is obvious that some people in the world have access to as much healthcare as they would like, while others have none at all. This variation is most apparent at the international level. Different countries expend different amounts on healthcare. In general, countries spend more if they have more (Figure 1.3). However, access to healthcare in some countries is as much influenced by how healthcare is allocated as by how much is available or affordable. The USA, for example, spends huge amounts on healthcare, but 45 million of its citizens do not have access to basic care.[17] In Australia, indigenous people receive notoriously poor healthcare, and have a life expectancy of only 58 years, compared with 80 years for the rest of the population.[18] Patients with mental health problems also have a high mortality rate from all kinds of diseases.[19]

Efficacy and Effectiveness

Efficacy is the ability of a healthcare measure to bring about an improvement in health. Effectiveness is the degree to which attainable improvements in healthcare are actually attained. An efficacious treatment may not be effective at the level of a population or even an individual. For example, the use of a special mask and machine for 'continuous positive airway pressure' can effectively manage sleep apnea and prevent its complications, but is only effective in some patients because many people abandon this treatment on account of the associated noise and discomfort.

Should scarce funds be directed to treatments of unproven efficacy just because they are fashionable? The terms 'complementary' or 'alternative' medicine mean medicine for which efficacy has not been proven: once efficacy has been proven for a substance or treatment, it becomes mainstream medicine.[20] It is difficult to justify the use of alternative medicine funded by the public purse in situations where there are limits on resources. Nevertheless, the intensity of consumer demand may be high, and this may explain the widespread use of acupuncture (for example) for indications unsupported by evidence. It is astonishing that these unproven uses of acupuncture have been adopted by many medically qualified practitioners, taught in courses run by reputable universities, and supported financially by some governments. Many mainstream therapies are similarly unsupported by convincing scientific data. Should the demands of individuals or groups consume funds which might be better spent, say, on further improving childhood immunization?

Efficiency

Efficiency (strictly, technical efficiency; allocative efficiency is dealt with under appropriateness) refers to the relationship between the cost of healthcare and its effectiveness and safety. Increasing efficiency could imply reducing expenditure without reducing safety or effectiveness, or increasing effectiveness and safety for a given level of expenditure. Providing appropriate care in the best way also increases efficiency. It has been shown that nurses may spend up to an hour per shift compensating for system deficiencies and for the errors of their colleagues.[21] This is clearly inefficient.

Safety

Safety is the inverse of risk (the subject of Chapter 2). Risk might be increased by making the wrong plans, or by not carrying them out as planned. It can be reduced by better designs, practices, and systems. However, safety comes at a cost, which must be weighed against the potential human and economic costs of the risk in question. Perceptions of risk, and therefore of what constitutes an appropriate degree of safety, vary considerably. As discussed on pages 31–36, the level of risk that is acceptable depends on the context. It may be worth accepting considerable risk if the potential benefits are great.

Timeliness

Efficacious treatments need to be applied to the right people for the right indications at the right time if they are to be effective. Timeliness refers to the relationship between the timing of an intervention and its effectiveness. Immunization is no good if given too late to prevent the disease. If a hip replacement is undertaken two years after the patient has become completely incapacitated, that patient will have lost two years of potential benefit; in addition, his or her disability may have become entrenched because of prolonged immobility, and the chance for a good result may be considerably reduced. Coronary artery surgery may prolong life, if undertaken in the presence of the correct indications, by preventing myocardial infarction – but only if it is undertaken before the infarction occurs.

Acceptability

Acceptability is the extent to which the wishes, desires, expectations, cultural norms and religious beliefs of patients and their families are met. Acceptability encompasses (amongst other things) the ease with which healthcare can be accessed, the relationship between patients and their healthcare providers, the attributes and amenities of healthcare facilities (such as the extent to which privacy can be provided), respect for the individual's cultural and religious beliefs, and the degree to which the perceptions of patients and society about risks, priorities and equity are met.

The provision of acceptable care may lead to conflicts in relation to other elements of quality in healthcare. How much should be spent on erythropoietin for a Jehovah's Witness, when the use of blood transfusion is standard therapy, cheaper, and could prevent an intensive care admission? Should such a religious group be asked to pay the difference? When should cosmetic plastic surgical procedures be funded from the public purse?

Appropriateness

To be appropriate, care must be acceptable, but appropriate care, in a world of finite resources, must also be that which is most effective for the available resources, at least for publicly funded care.. This dimension, allied to 'allocative efficiency', is very poorly developed, as manifested by variations in the provision of healthcare which are not driven by any obvious demographic characteristics or logistical constraints.

In 1982, John Wennberg published data highlighting the variability in prostate surgery and hysterectomy across the USA and suggested that this variability was due to differences in practice between providers of healthcare rather than to differences between groups of patients.[22] More recently, his group published a series of healthcare atlases which document major variations in many aspects of healthcare between regions and even between institutions in the same region.[23] This variation exceeds anything that could be explained by the types of cases involved or economic differences between areas. For example, the variation in angioplasty and stenting between regions in the USA was 18-fold; for carotid endarterectomy it was 8-fold; and for vena cava filter placement, 26-fold. Variation of this type appears to be the rule, even in the most advanced healthcare systems in the world. This is clear evidence of substantial levels of inappropriate healthcare. McGlynn and co-workers also showed evidence of under and over-treatment, with a random sample of the US population receiving appropriate healthcare just over half the time (see Figure 1.2).[24]

Condition

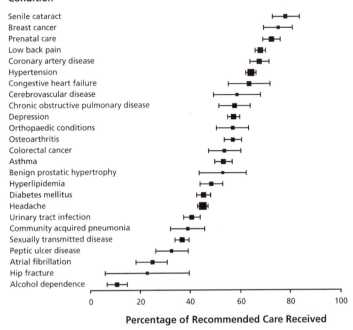

Percentage of Recommended Care Received

Figure 1.2 Adherence to quality indicators according to condition, adapted
from McGlynn et al.[23] (The areas of the boxes reflect the number of
times eligibility for a quality indicator was met for a particular
condition, and the bars show the 95 per cent confidence intervals).

Failing to provide a patient with appropriate treatment is not good. Providing
an unnecessary or inappropriate treatment is also undesirable, even if it is provided
flawlessly, because of the opportunity costs implied in this waste of resource
(inefficiency). From the safety perspective, the patient is placed in double jeopardy
because risk is increased both by subjecting him or her to a wrong or inappropriate
plan, and by the possibility of that plan not being carried out properly.

Reaching the right people is very important in optimizing the return on
investment in healthcare. Immunizing one person is of little value to society;
immunizing the majority of a population has the potential not only to protect those
immunized, but also to protect those who for whatever reason are not immunized,
because of the phenomenon known as herd immunity. This raises an interesting
ethical question over the moral position of those who opt out of the (low but real)
risks of being immunized but benefit by courtesy of their fellow citizens who do
accept that risk. The appropriateness of such opting out can only be evaluated in a
wider social and political context, taking into account the weights one places on
community responsibility and individual autonomy.

There is also a relationship between the effect size of a treatment and the underlying risk of the condition treated, which affects appropriateness. The provision of statins to a group of people at low risk of coronary events will provide little benefit; this is most easily understood in the extreme case – there is no point in giving these drugs to children (for instance) because their risk of coronary disease is negligible. Selecting patients known to be at high risk will provide a much greater return on the investment, and also a better balance between the risks of these drugs and their potential side effects.

Funding and the Layers of Healthcare

The amount spent on healthcare varies considerably between countries. Thus the value placed on human life, defined by the amount a country will spend to save one, varies at least 100-fold, from less than US$20,000 to US$2 million.[25] Generally, those countries with a higher gross domestic product (GDP) spend more on healthcare, but there are marked discrepancies between countries with respect to their overall expenditure on healthcare, and how funds are distributed within their boundaries. Spending more on healthcare does not necessarily improve outcomes for patients.[26] Appropriateness and efficiency will make a big difference to the return on investment, as will the distribution of funds between public health, primary, secondary and tertiary healthcare. The fact that Americans spend nearly three times as much on healthcare as New Zealanders does not mean that they are getting three times the value. Indeed, some public health indicators, such as infant mortality, are worse in the USA than New Zealand.[27,28]

The International Layer

Timely communication, co-operation and mutual support amongst the countries of the world are extremely important. The need for international surveillance and control of recently encountered diseases such as Avian influenza (bird flu) and Ebola virus and more familiar diseases such as tuberculosis and dengue fever are examples which illustrate this importance. Another such example is the need for countries to assist each other with natural disasters.

Support via aid agencies as well as assistance from governments is often forthcoming after dramatic events, such as the 2004 Boxing Day tsunami; billions of dollars were pledged and an international project funded to provide early warning of future tsunamis. The World Health Organization (WHO) plays a vital role in facilitating these co-operative activities. WHO is now also to take a lead in

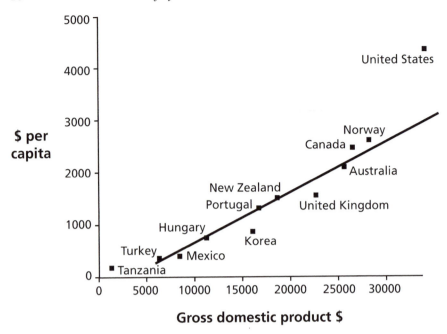

Gross domestic product $

Figure 1.3 Per capita health expenditure in relation to gross domestic product (GDP) in selected countries; $ are US$ in purchasing power parities[29, 30]

supporting and developing patient safety policies and practices globally.[31]

International commitment to alleviating the problems of the world varies greatly. International aid may be very limited if events fail to capture the public imagination. Examples are the Tianjin earthquake in China (which killed 250,000 people in 1976) and the floods in Bangladesh (which killed over 300,000 people in 1970).[32] Other major ongoing causes of widespread harm and suffering seem to go largely unnoticed by the media. At present, more than a billion people live in extreme poverty, existing on the equivalent of about US$1 per day. At this level of poverty, people (particularly children) die from malnutrition and a lack of basic healthcare. According to the United Nations fund for children (UNICEF), 11 million children die needlessly each year. If the world's poorest families had access to safe drinking water and basic healthcare, that number could be reduced by two-thirds.[33] It is encouraging that at the last meeting of 'G8' countries, it was decided to cancel foreign debt for the poorest countries in Africa.[34]

There is little consistency between countries in the provision of resources to manage global threats to the health and well-being of the human race, and little agreement on the best strategies for deploying these resources, particularly in countries with corrupt governments.[33] The United Nations has asked that wealthy countries give 0.7 per cent of their gross national income in foreign aid. At present some countries (such as Denmark, Norway and Sweden) exceed the target, while others, despite being wealthy, fall far below it. The US gives only 0.13 per cent, and Australia only 0.30 per cent, less than one-fifth of which is for health.[32,35]

Global warming has the potential to ruin the economies and encroach on the living space of many countries. The US, with less than one-twentieth of the world's population, is responsible for more than one-third of its greenhouse gas emissions, while Australia, with 0.3 per cent of the world's population, produces 1.4 per cent; both countries refused to sign the Kyoto protocol, an agreement designed to begin addressing this issue.[33]

How does war fit into the picture? In the USA, military expenditure rivals that spent on health (US\$450 billion versus US\$500 billion).[36] One third of the US military expenditure would meet the total WHO requirement for aid around the globe. This amount of aid (currently US\$160 billion) would enable the poorest countries to cut poverty by half by 2015, and eliminate it by 2025.[37]

It has been estimated that the Iraqi invasion caused 100,000 deaths more than the number expected had there not been an invasion.[38] The increased mortality has continued since then.[39] This war rates as a man-made tsunami with respect to loss of buildings, infrastructure and lives. The fact that it was initiated on the basis of false 'intelligence' about weapons that did not exist has been accepted by many with surprising equanimity. That territorial disputes and the pursuit of ideological imperatives continue to ruin the health and lives of hundreds of thousands of civilians is a sad commentary on the human condition. War is a massive public health problem, albeit that the exact extent of its direct and indirect morbidity and mortality is difficult to estimate, in part because communication systems tend to break down during periods of conflict.[40]

The State or National layer

Setting priorities Each country makes a finite amount of money available for healthcare, so this should be spent in the best possible way. One conceptually attractive way of allocating resources is by ranking healthcare interventions according to their cost per Quality Adjusted Life Year (QALY) – albeit with caveats in relation to underlying assumptions and complex ethical considerations.[41] If a 1 year old with a life expectancy of 81 years gets a life saving antibiotic and makes a full recovery from what would have been a fatal meningitis, then 80 QALYs will have been purchased for the cost of a consultation and the course of antibiotics (say \$80). Each QALY has therefore cost \$1, which is clearly value for money. In practice, adjustments are made, such as amortization of the amount and discounting QALYs over time (increasing life expectancy from one year to two is arguably more valuable than increasing it from 80 years to 81). The use of QALYs allows adjustments to be made to account for enjoyment of life. For example, if a patient who has attempted suicide is saved by an intensive care admission, but lives out his years so severely depressed that he has to be institutionalized, QALYs will be calculated at one-third the normal rate. This is based on research which has determined that people in that state would trade two-thirds of their remaining life expectancy if they could return to a normal state. This 'time trade off' technique is one way to estimate QALYs as, for example, a fraction of the utility of being completely healthy (see Table 1.2).[42] The Disability Adjusted Life Year, or DALY, is another internationally standardized unit which was developed for estimating the global burden of disease (see Chapter 12).[43,44]

Table 1.2 Utilities calculated by the 'time trade-off' technique

Health status	Utility
Completely healthy	1.00
Life with a kidney transplant	0.84
Severe physical disability from pain	0.67
Hospital dialysis	0.56
Angina, severe disability	0.50
Becoming blind or deaf and dumb	0.39
Being confined to hospital, depressed	0.33
Severe dementia, institutionalized	0.10

Existing healthcare interventions can be ranked according to their cost per QALY and improvements or additional measures can be added to this ranked list by calculating the marginal increase in cost per marginal increase in QALY. Some examples of these are given in Table 1.3.[45] A strong objection can be made to this approach; many would say that there is no ethical basis on which one person can rate the value of another's existence, and there are several major reservations with respect to equity (discriminating against the disabled and elderly for example), and to applying this approach to people from different ethnic groups to those who set the priorities.[46] On other hand, there is an ethical imperative to spend healthcare dollars as effectively as reasonably possible.

In practice, this technique is not applied across the board, but is used in selected areas. For example, in Australia, certain prescription drugs are made available to the population at heavily discounted prices. In determining which drugs should be available on this 'pharmaceutical benefits schedule', calculations of cost per QALY are made.[47]

An argument for transparent, explicit rationing by setting priorities for the healthcare that should be made available to all citizens, funded by the public purse, will be presented in Chapter 11. Although ethical and technical objections can be raised in relation to existing methods for ranking priorities in order to ration healthcare, these pale into insignificance compared to the massive disparities which currently exist (e.g. see Table 1.3 and Box 1.2), and the ease with which those with vested interests can manipulate the system for their own benefit.

The value of a procedure depends on the characteristics of the patient as well as the nature of the procedure. For example, for fixing a fractured neck of the femur in a patient with severe dementia, the cost per QALY may be 10-fold higher than for a patient whose mental faculties are intact and who is otherwise fit and well. The view of the patient cannot be discounted (although it may be difficult to establish directly), but many people would agree that they would place very

Table 1.3 The cost of healthcare interventions by QALY[45]

Intervention	Present value of extra cost per QALY gained (US$)
Pacemaker for heart block	4,000
Hip replacement	5,000
Coronary artery bypass (severe angina)	6,000
Kidney transplant	16,000
Screening for breast cancer	20,000
Heart transplant	35,000
Coronary artery bypass (mild angina)	50,000
Hospital-based haemodialysis	60,000

different values on the prolongation of their own lives in these two situations. An argument can be made that it would be worthwhile to operate on the former patient to relieve suffering and facilitate nursing, but that expensive post-operative care in a high dependency or intensive care unit would be harder to justify, particularly if, for example, this prevented a young multi-trauma patient from being cared for appropriately.

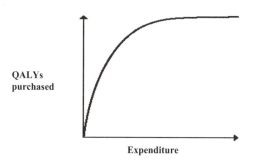

QALYs purchased

Expenditure

Figure 1.4 The relationship between QALYS purchased and expenditure

Figure 1.4 shows a conceptual relationship between the number of QALYs that may be purchased against expenditure for a range of interventions. Low cost – high value interventions lie at the bottom end or steeper part of the curve; examples would include setting a badly fractured leg or treating septicaemia associated with childbirth, whereas an example at the other end of the spectrum would be replacing an aortic valve in a 90 year old patient. The point at which the expenditure of public funds should be questioned depends on many factors, including the overall wealth of a country.[48]

In summary, QALYs provide a tool for use in evaluating the cost-effectiveness of medical treatments in defined groups of patients, but there are limitations to their use. In practice, after extensive community consultation, it has been found that some societies are prepared in principle to spend more on some sorts of diseases and interventions than on others. The state of Oregon in the USA tried to fund its healthcare in this way. Its ranking differed from that predicted by a purely technical approach.[49] One reason for this difference was the value placed by the public on life-saving interventions. There is a strong 'rule of rescue' phenomenon that seems to be a hallmark of human behaviour.[50] This is exemplified by the huge amounts of taxpayers' money regularly expended on exercises such as rescuing lone yachtsmen or women, who have deliberately taken extreme risks in ocean racing for no greater objective than sporting achievement.

Healthcare is characterized by islands of excellence in a sea of mediocrity. Health funding is no exception. For example, rational scientific processes are often used with great care in deciding which drugs to subsidize, while, at the same time and within the same countries, money is spent on other areas of healthcare in a manner that appears to be totally arbitrary and irrational (see Box 1.2).

Box 1.2 An extreme example of irrational health policy

Over 14 million dollars are spent each year on nucleic acid testing (NAT) of donor blood in Australia, a test which is able to detect Hepatitis C infection at one week rather than the up to ten weeks required by tests of sero-conversion, and Human Immunodeficiency Virus infection at 11 days rather than 22 days.[51] As only a couple of extra infected donations are found each year which would not otherwise have been detected,[52] the cost is AU$7 million per infected blood donation removed, whereas only AU$120 is spent on prevention for each death from cigarette smoking. Far greater improvements in safety would be obtained by initiatives to reduce the number of unwarranted blood transfusions (of which there are many). As many as 10,000 lives could be saved in Australia in the future if the NAT money was used on smoking prevention through programs which have been shown to work.[53]

Ideally, public health measures should be ranked alongside direct interventions when allocating funds for healthcare. It took half a century for the WHO to finally get agreement on a policy on smoking,[54] and the same difficulties are now being encountered in relation to obesity and fast food. Expenditure on diseases associated with obesity has risen ten-fold in the last 20 years and now accounts for over 12 per cent of the US health budget. Obese individuals cost the system US$1,244 per person per year more than their non-obese counterparts.[55] Up to one third of all cancer, the leading cause of death in western countries, is associated with obesity.[56]

One of the features of democratic governments is their willingness to allow undue influence of powerful lobby groups on policy. It was reported recently that the Australian Federal Cabinet blocked the introduction of their own program for increased health warnings on cigarette packets despite the fact that 20,000 Australians die each year from smoking related disease – a mortality rate in smokers 60-fold greater than that from traffic accidents.[57,58]

Models for funding healthcare One measure of a civilized society is the extent to which it cares for its disempowered and needy citizens. In some systems the financial burden for healthcare is placed primarily onto the individual, although various arrangements, such as health insurance programmes, are used to smooth the peaks and troughs of this burden. In other systems all or most of the responsibility is taken by the state or country. In most countries there is a mix between private and public funding of healthcare, although the role accepted by the state in the provision of healthcare for those who cannot pay may be small in some (see Appendix II). In parts of the USA, personal income must be one-eighth of that at the poverty line before eligibility for publicly funded healthcare cuts in.[59]

The arguments over what proportion of state funding is ideal are largely based on perceptions of social responsibility and efficiency. Different funding models have been tried, including fee for service, capitation, full state funding with no linkage between funding and the number of patients treated, and insurance-funded managed care. Each approach has its proponents and detractors. The incentives, some perverse, provided by each of these approaches, are discussed in Chapter 3 (pages 75–77). Some emphasize the right of the individual to choose (and pay for) the professionals who will provide their care, and when and where this will be done. Others place greater emphasis on equity, and argue that the state has an over-riding responsibility to ensure that the limited resource allocated provides basic care for the entire population. Advocates of private healthcare point to the market as the great regulator of quality and promoter of efficiency; facilities which are performing poorly will not be chosen by patients who have the ability to go elsewhere. Others argue that healthcare is not a commodity, and that market-based approaches create undesirable distortions in the allocation of resource. Thus commercially driven providers may tend to concentrate on elective procedural work in the not-too-ill (e.g. hip joint replacements and plastic surgery) and to neglect the 'uneconomic' aspects of medicine (such as the treatment of major trauma) and aspects of primary healthcare such as immunization and preventive medicine. In America there is evidence that not only do the poor and the uninsured suffer, but that private insurance provides poor primary care to children.[59] In a true market-driven environment preventive medicine would presumably be seen as counter-productive. Ethical questions arise about those systems which provide different levels of healthcare for people with different abilities to pay, but, in practice, most countries have a mixture of approaches (see Appendix II).

The Hospital or Organizational Layer

In the past, healthcare facilities or hospitals often received funding on the basis of what they had received historically, plus or minus an adjustment for new, defunct or redundant services. Most hospital funding, private and public, is now based on some measure of activity. Typically, this may be on the number of conditions managed and interventions undertaken, coded into diagnostic-related groups (DRGs).[60,61] On discharge or death each patient's medical record is examined by a 'coder' who allocates relevant codes from the 10,000 morbidity or mortality codes of the International Classification of Diseases (ICD) coding system. These codes are grouped into DRGs which represent certain activities thought to be homogeneous with respect to resource consumption. Funding is then based on the number of DRGs handled per year.

This approach has a number of problems. There is an acknowledged tendency for 'gaming' in which deliberate efforts are made to come up with combinations of codes which will get the greatest remuneration. Also, medical records are not always complete or clear and all relevant aspects of the patient's care may not be recorded. Often the amounts provided are adjusted for political reasons after the DRG calculations have been made. Nevertheless, the use of DRGs does represent an attempt to fund healthcare on a rational basis.

Within health services, funds are apportioned between competing services. There is great variation in how hospitals and healthcare organizations are structured and how funds are allocated within these structures. Furthermore, much interaction takes place through informal pathways, following unofficial agendas. Members of specific services within a hospital will usually manage their own affairs reasonably well, but this often involves putting their own priorities ahead of the needs of others (sometimes at the expense of the best interests of patients). Providing timely service to other teams or organizations may not be seen as worthwhile. These issues are discussed further in Chapter 3 (page 67).

Approximately 70 per cent of a hospital's budget goes to salaries, two-thirds of which are nursing salaries. The apportionment of funds between staff, services, equipment, drugs and infrastructure is often arbitrary and determined by the political influence of various competing groups. There are many incongruous effects of this unsatisfactory arrangement (see Box 1.3 for an example).

In addition to secondary or tertiary organizations or facilities, there are medical centres which are made up of groups of primary care or general practice practitioners who have co-located with allied health people such as physiotherapists and occupational therapists. Additional services such as radiology and pathology are joining these groups to provide 'one-stop' coordinated care. Public health and research facilities as well as free-standing diagnostic services and day surgeries also exist. There are advantages and disadvantages for each of these arrangements. The real challenge is coordinating the provision of healthcare to ensure the optimal use of each facility and the best overall result for patients. We are, as yet, a long way from meeting this challenge.

The Team Layer

As healthcare has increased in complexity, large numbers of specialties and sub-specialties have evolved. The actions of the many individual people directly in contact with the patient at any point in time are vitally important. To be safe and effective their actions need to be integrated, so that patient care becomes a matter of coordinated teamwork rather than a series of loosely-connected encounters. Much of healthcare now relies on interactions between and within teams, departments or units. The teams need to be supported by the organizations within which they work, and the objectives of the organizations should be congruent with those of its employees (the team players).

Box 1.3 An example of a perverse incentive

There is good evidence that central venous catheters impregnated with certain antibiotics prevent blood stream infections in a cost-effective way.[62] These blood stream infections cause prolonged hospital stay, cost money and may necessitate admission to intensive care, or even lead to death from septicaemia. In Australia, these catheters could save as many as 1,000 lives each year,[63] equivalent to more than half the road toll, yet their introduction has been slow and patchy. Why is this? First, savings do not manifest in the bottom line of a hospital budget but rather in the creation of extra capacity and hence extra throughput of patients. As hospitals are funded by activity, this results in no profit, merely more work. Second, the disposables budget for the hospital will be adversely affected, as the antibiotic impregnated catheters are considerably more expensive than the usual catheters. Blood stream infections can be rapidly fatal, and patients who die are less of a drain on resources than those who continue to live, so there is a double impost on the budget. Not only must the more expensive catheters be paid for, but care must also be provided for more survivors.

An obvious solution to this problem is for the funder (e.g. the state government or regional health authority) to pay for the catheters, because it is at this level that the overall savings will be realized. However, this simple solution appears to be beyond the capacity of most funders to implement. One wonders if there would be the same inertia if 1,000 people were dying each year as a result of a problem in a motor vehicle which could easily be corrected at the same time as saving money.

Sometimes, these teams are relatively constant. For example, a cardio-thoracic surgical team includes surgeons, anaesthetists, perfusionists, physio-therapists and others, all of whom work in much the same group every day and become familiar with each other's needs and ways of doing things. A high degree of stability in a team of this type enhances safety and efficiency. At other times different people have to work together who do not know one another. Agency or locum staff are being used increasingly because nurses and doctors are in short supply. Temporary and short-term staff are often not familiar with local protocols, charts, equipment and other members of the team. This situation must be less safe and efficient than that of a regular team whose members know each other well. Teams are discussed further in Chapter 10 (see pages 237–240). The situation can be considerably improved by developing standard operating procedures and team training so that everyone not only knows their own role, but is confident that other team members know their roles as well.

The Individual Layer

Healthcare was once delivered by a single medical practitioner who was consulted by a patient and his or her family, and who was responsible for all aspects of their care. 'Doctor-patient' relationships of this type remain important in healthcare. It is ideal for a doctor, who has a special and trusted relationship with the patient, to co-ordinate all aspects of his or her care. However, patients may have to interact with many people from different disciplines. This complexity makes healthcare difficult to organize. Breakdowns in these arrangements are the subject of Chapter 3 (see page 77, and Boxes 3.3 and 3.6).

Consider a patient whose general practitioner (GP) arranges for her to see a gastroenterologist to have an endoscopy. An operation is required after the endoscopy, so the GP, in discussion with the patient, recommends a surgeon. The surgeon then coordinates a number of other healthcare professionals to manage the various aspects of pre-, intra-, and post-operative care (e.g. a physician, an anaesthetist, a physiotherapist and so on). Each of these individuals will need to establish and maintain a relationship with the patient, and each other. This increasing complexity of healthcare demands of practitioners a range of team working, communication and other non-technical skills. Traditionally, training in these non-technical skills has been inadequate. In many traditional medical schools training in 'communication skills' centres on how doctors talk to patients and largely ignores how they talk to each other.

The Patient

A high quality healthcare system should be patient-centred. This implies that the system should be layered around the patient, who should be seen as part of the system, and as an important contributor to safety and other dimensions of quality (see Figure 1.1 and Chapter 10, pages 221–224).

As discussed above, there may be conflicts between an individual's wishes, considerations of equity and what an individual doctor may regard as appropriate (see Box 1.4). Ideally, the patient's GP will provide guidance while at the same time acting in a trustworthy way towards society as a whole. It may be difficult for patients to get information on the various options, and the personality of a doctor may be a powerful influence. Patients will sometimes unwittingly receive ineffective or unnecessarily risky care, which consumes resources that could be more effectively used elsewhere. The tragic case of Mrs. Green (Box 1.4) was not only a disaster for her and her family, and for the staff involved, but incurred substantial costs.

Strengthening the role of the patient at the centre of the system is a priority if quality and safety in healthcare is to improve. This will require patients to be better informed and to be encouraged to make decisions and be responsible for important aspects of their care. This requires a new partnership between patients and healthcare professionals. The ways in which this may be done will be discussed in Chapter 7 (pages 166–1770 and in Chapter 10 (pages 221–225).

Box 1.4 A tragic outcome from an unnecessary procedure

Mrs. Green was a middle-aged woman who had two teenage children at the time of her adverse event. She was a keen gardener. She injured her shoulder in a fall whilst playing tennis and suffered an injury to her rotator cuff. She saw two orthopaedic surgeons in different practices, several months apart, who both recommended physiotherapy and strengthening exercises. Eventually, because the arm was sore while gardening, she went to a third orthopaedic surgeon who agreed to repair the rotator cuff, but who also indicated that the procedure was only marginally indicated.

The anaesthetist suggested that she have a regional anaesthetic (an interscalene block) and sedation. However Mrs. Green, who had previously had an unsatisfactory epidural block for a caesarean section, wanted a general anaesthetic. During the procedure Mrs. Green become disconnected from the ventilator. The surgeon noted that the anaesthetist had to go under the surgical drapes in order to reconnect the breathing circuit to her endotracheal tube and commented that he was not sure that he had seen her chest moving for quite a while.

After the operation Mrs. Green failed to wake up and had worrying metabolic signs. She was admitted to an Intensive Care Unit, but did not recover. No one was sure how long she had been disconnected from the ventilator, as the vital signs that had been charted during the anaesthetic were normal. However, the anaesthetic record was severely criticized by the coroner as being incomplete and barely legible. The anaesthetist had not used a 'low pressure-disconnect alarm' which was available but not in routine use in the orthopaedic operating theatre. Pulse oximeters were also available in the hospital, but were usually used only on high-risk patients. Capnographs were available as well, but were mainly used in the neurosurgical operating theatre.

Mrs. Green had her operation one year before the use of these devices was mandated by the College of Anaesthetists. She remained in a vegetative state, and after a delay of several years, the case was settled out of court. The medical defence organization compensated the family to cover her ongoing care. She lived for several years, opening her eyes, 'tracking' moving objects and possibly recognizing some family members, but was unable to stand, dress or feed herself.

Getting it Right

This book is about providing a guide to doing the right thing in healthcare. There are a number of dimensions to quality and many layers of healthcare, and it is unlikely that we will make overall improvements by considering any one dimension or layer in isolation from the others. Huge advances have been made in the efficacy of medical treatment, and in the understanding of the basic science underpinning healthcare. Healthcare used to be safe but ineffective. It is now highly effective but potentially hazardous.[64] Risk must always be considered in relation to benefit, but the fact is that the benefits of healthcare are not reaching everyone. We are failing many, often those who most need help. Worse still, in many instances we are actively harming people with the very treatments that are intended to help them.

The story of Jessica Santillan (Box 1.1) illustrates the heights of what is now possible and the lows of our propensity to get things wrong. Meeting the needs of those who cannot afford or access healthcare (and Jessica, at the outset, was just such a person) is an urgent need in most countries today. Avoiding the risks and costs of over-treatment is also essential. The challenge is to meet the basic healthcare needs of all people, and to ensure that we do so in a manner that is as safe and ethical as local resources and circumstances allow.[65]

This is difficult for individual healthcare professionals, although every opportunity should be taken to address inequities and irrational or wasteful practices. What is within the power of individual healthcare professionals is to ensure that they consistently behave, in their everyday activities, in a manner that is safe, and understood by and acceptable to their patients. This individual behaviour will translate, collectively, into a culture change, and unsafe practices will become unacceptable.

The system has proven remarkably impervious to major changes in clinical practice since the problem of iatrogenic harm was brought to the fore in the year 2000. It is apparent that major 'above down' changes will take a long time to be reflected in everyday patient care in most jurisdictions. However, many individuals and teams have made major strides in improving professionalism and patient safety in the last five years. Healthcare, generally, continues to be a mosaic, with practices that are excellent in close juxtaposition to those that are outdated and inappropriate. There are physicians who are otherwise excellent, but who never wash their hands between examining patients. There are surgeons who are highly skilled but who do not inform their patients properly of the material risks of proposed interventions or of reasonable alternatives.

The substantial advances that have been made in healthcare lie mainly in changes driven and maintained by individuals. In order to properly harness the enormous resource represented by the healthcare workforce, we need to understand how to collect and access the necessary information, respond appropriately to things that go wrong, and develop and apply effective strategies for preventing similar problems in the future. We need to understand how the various components of the system interrelate and how the available information may be used effectively. To this end we have developed several frameworks which we will use throughout this book to underpin our recommendations for safer, better healthcare (see below).

Human error is a problem in any complex system, and ultimately lies behind much iatrogenic harm, so we must continue to develop systems which are error tolerant. However, the greatest strength of healthcare systems lies in the enormous resource represented by the individual and collective efforts of healthcare professionals supported, increasingly, by their patients.

Conceptual Frameworks

In this section we present two conceptual frameworks to illustrate the relationships between the various topics dealt with in this book. These need not be studied in detail now, but are provided for reference when aspects are dealt with in relevant parts of this book.

Framework 1 – An Integrated Framework for Quality and Risk Management

Framework 1 (Figure 1.5)[66] integrates activities related to safety and other elements of quality, risk management and quadruple-loop learning, and incorporates Framework 2 (Figure 1.6)[66] and the risk management framework shown in Figure 2.1. The main features are put into context in the legend on the facing page, and are discussed in the relevant chapters indicated in **bold** in the figure. Quadruple-loop learning will be discussed in Chapter 11 (page 271) and refers to learning and applying the lessons learnt at personal, team, national and international levels (see Box 11.9).

The top half of this figure shows the elements of a reactive response to an individual incident. The bottom half shows how aggregated information from all available sources can be used, in conjunction with a comprehensive patient safety classification, to feed a patient safety data repository (preferably a national one). This can then be used as a resource for proactively identifying, evaluating and analyzing risks in order to devise and implement corrective strategies. Some of the techniques for doing this will be discussed in Chapter 11.

Framework 2 – An Information Model for a Patient Safety Classification

This framework provides a model for deconstructing the things that go wrong in healthcare into their functional components, so that each component can be studied and addressed. It is shown in Figure 1.6, with an indication of where the various components of the framework are dealt with in this book.

Although many adverse events and incidents result from a unique conjunction of contributing factors and circumstances that may never be repeated, some of the ingredients of a particular disaster will often be common to many other incidents. There is merit in studying and addressing those contributing factors that feature regularly, using processes such as incident monitoring and root cause analysis (Chapter 9). As indicated in the framework, information from these and many other sources can then be collated using a universal classification and made available in a useful form for a patient safety data repository. If these root causes can be properly understood and designed out of the system, whole classes of problems can be prevented from happening again.

It is important to note that information should also be collected about how the impact of adverse events is minimized, and how incidents may be prevented from turning into adverse events. This information, about successful strategies, can then be used to devise preventive and corrective strategies for similar problems, preferably before patients are harmed.

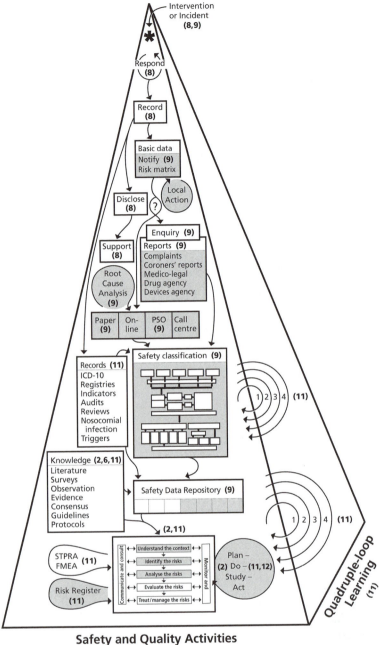

Safety and Quality Activities

Figure 1.5 An integrated framework for safety, quality and risk management in healthcare[65] with relevant chapters identified in bold numbers.

At the apex of the pyramid, an asterisk represents an *intervention* or an *incident*. The first thing to do is to *respond*, and then *record* what happened and what was done. If an incident has resulted in harm, those affected (patients, staff and their families and friends) should be informed of the facts (*disclose*) and arrangements made to look after them (*support*) (Chapter 8). The causes of the underlying diseases or injuries may be coded from the *records* on discharge or death using the International Classification of Diseases (*ICD*). Subsets of information may be extracted for *registers, indicators, audits* and *reviews* of activity, and for activities such as the surveillance and tracking of *nosocomial infection; triggers* may be used to identify certain types of problems.

For all significant or informative incidents, and especially when harm has occurred, *basic data* (what, who, when, where, risk, consequences) should be logged so that it can be passed on to the relevant people (*notify*), so that they can recommend and/or take the necessary *local action* (Chapter 9, pages 201 and Box 9.3). This process is designed to elicit sufficient information to generate a *risk matrix* or assessment to determine whether further investigation and/or remedial steps are needed (see Appendix III). If so, a process should be undertaken to determine if there is culpability *(?)*; if there is, an *enquiry* may need to be commissioned and appropriate action taken. Other processes may be invoked such as a *complaint, medico legal* or *coroners' report*, or a report to a *drug* or *device agency* (pages 45 and 201).

If the event has caused harm or a recurrence would pose a significant risk, details should be elicited, classified and stored, using a universal *patient safety classification*. Details may be elicited by a reporter via a paper report, going 'on-line', by a *PSO* (patient safety officer) or by a *call centre*; high risk incidents should be subjected to a *root cause analysis* (Chapter 9). *Knowledge* from all available sources, including the *literature, surveys* and *observation* studies, and *evidence* from all levels including *consensus* meetings, *guidelines* and *protocols* (Chapter 6) make up the patient *safety data repository*.

This information can then be used to *understand the context, identify the risks, analyze the risks*, and *evaluate the risks* in order to *treat or manage the risks* (see Figure 2.1). Risks that can be dealt with should be subjected to a quality improvement cycle (*plan-do-study-act*) and those that cannot, should be placed on a *risk register* for future attention, and accepted and/or indemnified against (page 259). *ST-PRA* (sociotechnical-probabilistic risk analysis) and *FMEA* (failure mode effects analysis) represent pro-active approaches to identifying problems and setting priorities (page 260). These activities may all contribute to *'quadruple-loop' learning* shown on the side of the pyramid (page 271). The shaded areas in Figure 1.5 represent activities which are often managed in a piecemeal manner, but which should ideally be handled using an integrated system (Chapter 9, Appendix VIII).

Contributing Factors and Hazards

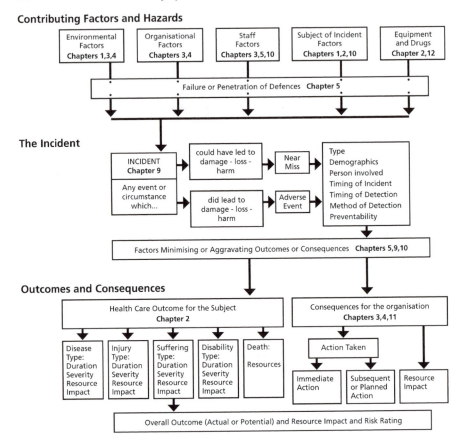

The Incident

Outcomes and Consequences

Figure 1.6 A generic reference model for deconstructing individual incidents see Appendix VIII.[67]

Notes

1   Hippocrates (400 BCE). *Of the Epidemics*, Book 1, Section II, part 5, translated by Adams, F. <http://classics.mit.edu/Hippocrates/epidemics.html> accessed 17 May 2006.

2   The top public health problems are reported in: World Health Organization (2005), *The World Health Report 2005: Make Every Mother and Child Count* (Geneva: World Health Organization) Annex Table 2: Deaths by Cause, Sex and Mortality Stratum in WHO Regions, Estimates for 2002, p. 120-5. The figures in Table 1.1 are extrapolations from the sources 3–9 cited below.

3   Anonymous (2004), *The Bulletin* (Sydney: ACP Publishing) 21 December, p. 39.

4   Estimated 2002 annual world mortality due to smoking was 5,000,000 or approximately 14,000 per day. World Health Organization (2003), *World Health Report: 2003: Shaping the Future* (Geneva: World Health Organization) p. 91.

5   An extrapolation of figures from developed countries to the rest of the world; an underestimate as iatrogenic harm to those requiring acute care but with no access to healthcare in developing countries would not be counted. See Table 2.6.

6   Steinbrook, R. (2004), 'After Bangkok – Expanding the Global Response to AIDS', *New England Journal of Medicine* 351:8, 738–42.

7   Estimated 2002 annual mortality due to road traffic accidents was 1,192,000 in WHO member countries or approximately 3,300 per day. World Health Organization (2004), *World Health Report: 2004: Changing History* (Geneva: World Health Organization) p. 124.

8   *The New Scientist*, 29 January 2005, cites 30,000 deaths per year 1994–2004 (earthquakes, floods, hurricanes). The 2004 Asian tsunami killed as many as 300,000 – this has been averaged over 50 years (16 per day) and added to the 30,000 per year (82 per day) to yield nearly 100 per day.

9   Estimated world mortality due to terrorism in 2005 was 14,602 of which 8,728 were in Iraq (an occupied country). Excluding Iraq, the mortality is 6,000 per annum or 16 per day: National Counterterrorism Center (2006), *Report on Incidents of Terrorism* <http://wits.nctc.gov/Reports.do> accessed 17 May 2006.

10   Moser, R.H. (1956), 'Diseases of Medical Progress', *New England Journal of Medicine* 255:13, 606–14.

11   Health Policy and Economic Research Unit, British Medical Association (2002), *Patient Safety and Clinical Risk* (London: British Medical Association) p. 3.

12   World Health Organization, Preamble to the Constitution of the World Health Organization as adopted by the International Health Conference, New York, 19–22 June, 1946, signed on 22 July 1946 by the representatives of 61 States (*Official Records of the World Health Organization* no. 2, p. 100) and entered into force on 7 April 1948.

13   VanRooyen, M. and Leaning, J. (2005), 'After the Tsunami – Facing the Public Health Challenges', *New England Journal of Medicine* 352:5, 435–8.

14   Paix, B.R. et al. (2005), 'Anaesthesia in a Disaster Zone: A Report on the Experience of an Australian Medical Team in Banda Aceh Following the "Boxing Day Tsunami"', *Anaesthesia and Intensive Care* 33:5, 629–34.

15   Modified from: Runciman, W.B. and Merry, A.M. (2003), 'A Tragic Death: a Time to Blame or a Time to Learn? *Quality and Safety in Health Care* 12:5, 321-2.

16   Modified from: Minister of Health (2003), *Improving Quality (IQ): A Systems Approach for the New Zealand Health and Disability Sector* (Wellington: New Zealand Ministry of Health). The contribution of Dr. Mary Seddon to the development of this diagram is acknowledged.

17   Roughly 45 million Americans have no health insurance at all. Bush, G.W. and Kerry, J.F. (2004), 'Health Care Coverage and Drug Costs – the Candidates Speak Out', *New England Journal of Medicine* 351:18, 1815–9.

18   For the period 1999–2001, life expectancy was estimated to be 56 years for indigenous males and 63 years for indigenous females (versus 77 and 82 for all Australians). Australian Institute for Health and Welfare (2004), *Australia's Health 2004* (Canberra: Australian Institute for Health and Welfare) p. 196.

19   Lawrence, D., Holman, C.D.J. and Jablensky, A.V. (2001), *Duty to Care: Preventable Physical Illness in People with Mental Illness* (Perth: Centre for Health Services Research, University of Western Australia).

20   Dawkins, R., 'Foreword', in Diamond, J. (2001), *Snake Oil and Other Preoccupations* (London: Vintage).

21   Tucker, A.L. and Edmondson, A.C. (2002), *Why Hospitals Don't Learn From Failures: Organizational and Psychological Dynamics That Inhibit System Change* (Boston: Harvard   Business   School).   <http://www.hbs.edu/research/facpubs/workingpapers/papers2/0203/03-059.pdf> accessed 18 May 2006.

22   Wennberg, J. and Gittelsohn, A. (1982), 'Variations in Medical Care Among Small Areas', *Scientific American* 246:4, 120–34.

23   *The Dartmouth Atlas of Health Care* [website] <http://www.dartmouthatlas.org> for United States national, State and specialty-specific editions of the atlases, accessed 17 May 2006.

24   McGlynn, E.A. et al. (2003), 'The Quality of Health Care Delivered to Adults in the United States', *New England Journal of Medicine* 348:26, 2635–45.

25   Pearce, F. (1995), 'Global Row Over Value of Human Life', *New Scientist* 19 August, p. 7.

26   Fisher, E.S. (2003), 'Medical Care – is More Always Better?', *New England Journal of Medicine* 349:17, 1665–7.

27   The infant mortality rate (deaths of infants aged 1 year or less per 1,000 live births) for the United States for 2004 was 6.4. Munson, M.L. and Sutton, P.D. (2005), 'Births, Marriages, Divorces and Deaths: Provisional Data for 2004', *National Vital Statistics Reports*, 53:21 (Hyattsville, Maryland: National Center for Health Statistics).

28   The infant mortality rate for New Zealand for 2004 was 5.6. Statistics New Zealand (2005), *Deaths – Summary of Latest Trends* (Wellington, New Zealand: Statistics New Zealand) <http://www.stats.govt.nz/popn-monitor/deaths/deaths-summary-of-latest-trends.htm> accessed 17 May 2006.

29   Modified from: Ministry of Health (2002), *Health Expenditure Trends in New Zealand 1980–2000* (Wellington: Ministry of Health). Purchasing power parities are rates of currency conversion that equalize the purchasing power of different countries, allowing comparisons of health spending.

30   The estimated Gross Domestic Product per capita for 2004 for Tanzania was a purchasing power parity of US$700. Central Intelligence Agency, United States (2006), *The World Factbook* [web resource] <http://www.cia.gov/cia/publications/factbook/geos/tz.html> accessed 17 May 2006.

31   World Alliance for Patient Safety [web-site] <http://www.who.int/patientsafety/en/> accessed 17 May 2006.

32   Singer, P. (2004), 'Ethic Cleansing', *The Bulletin* (Sydney: ACP Publishing) 15 December, pp. 39–42.

33   Singer, P. (2002), *One World: The Ethics of Globalization* (New Haven: Yale University Press).

34   BBC News (2005), 'Cautious Welcome for G8 Debt Deal', *BBC News*, 12 June, <http://news.bbc.co.uk/1/hi/business/4084574.stm> accessed 17 May 2006.

35   Downer, A., Minister for Foreign Affairs, Australia (2006), 'A More Effective Aid Programme'. Media release FA042/AA0617, 9 May. <http://www.foreignminister.gov.au/releases/2006/fa042_06.html> accessed 20 June 2006.

36   In 2004, the United States of America spent US$456 billion on military defence compared to US$240 billion on health and US$269 billion on Medicare. Office of Management and Budget, United States of America (2005), *Mid-Session Review: Budget of the US Government, Fiscal Year 2006* (Washington D.C: Office of Management and Budget, Executive Office of the President of the United States) p. 39 <http://www.whitehouse.gov/omb/budget/fy2006/pdf/06msr.pdf> accessed 17 May 2006.

37   Sachs, J.D. (2005), 'Can Extreme Poverty Be Eliminated?', *Scientific American* 293:3, 56–65.

38   Abad-Franch, F. (2005), 'Mortality in Iraq', *Lancet* 365:9465, 1134.

39   Civilian casualties reported in the media in the two year period 20 March 2003 to 19 March 2005 total 24,865 or 34 per day: Sloboda, J. (2005), *Iraq Body Count: a Dossier of Civilian Casualties in Iraq 2003-2005*, [web-site] <http://reports. iraqbodycount.org/a_dossier_of_civilian_casualties_2003-2005.pdf> accessed 17 May 2006.

40   Murray, C.J. et al. (2002), 'Armed Conflict as a Public Health Problem', *British Medical Journal* 324:7333, 346–9.

41   La Puma, J. and Lawlor, E.F. (1990), 'Quality-Adjusted Life-Years: Ethical Implications for Physicians and Policy Makers', *Journal of the American Medical Association* 263:21, 2917–21.

42   These are selected values from Torrance, G.W. (1987), 'Utility Approach to Measuring Health-Related Quality of Life', *Journal of Chronic Diseases* 40:6, 593–603.

43   Murray, C. J., Lopez, A.D. and Jamison, D.T. (1994), 'The Global Burden of Disease in 1990: Summary Results, Sensitivity Analysis and Future Directions', *Bulletin of the World Health Organization* 72:3, 495–509.

44   Murray, C.J.L. and Lopez, A.D. eds, (1996), *The Global Burden of Disease and Injury Series, Volume 1: A Comprehensive Assessment of Mortality and Disability From Diseases, Injuries, and Risk Factors in 1990 and Projected to 2020*, Harvard School of Public Health on behalf of the World Health Organization and the World Bank (Cambridge, Massachussetts: Harvard University Press).

45   Estimates adapted from Maynard, A. (1991). 'Developing the Health Care Market', *Economic Journal* 101:408, 1277–86.

46   Drummond, M., Torrance, G. and Mason, J. (1993), 'Cost-Effectiveness League Tables: More Harm Than Good?', *Social Science and Medicine* 37:1, 33-40.

47   George, B., Harris, A. and Mitchell, A. (1999), *Cost Effectiveness Analysis and the Consistency of Decision Making: Evidence from Pharmaceutical Reimbursement in Australia 1991–96* (Melbourne: Centre for Health Program Evaluation).

48   Eddy, D.N. (1996), *Clinical Decision Making: from Theory to Practice* (Sudbury, Massachusetts: Jones and Bartlett).

49   Oregon used a quality of well-being (QWB) scale to calculate nett benefits for health services. The nett benefit is the QWB with treatment versus the QWB without treatment, multiplied by the duration of the effect of treatment.

50   McKie, J. and Richardson, J. (2003), 'The Rule of Rescue', *Social Science and Medicine* 56:12, 2407–19.

51   Australian Red Cross Blood Service (2002), 'New National Blood Management System to Be Introduced', *MediLink* 5:3, 1–2.

52   Seed, C.R. et al. (2002), 'Assessing the Accuracy of Three Viral Risk Models in Predicting the Outcome of Implementing HIV and HCV NAT Donor Screening in Australia and the Implications for Future HBV NAT', *Transfusion* 42:10, 1365–1372.

53   Research and Evaluation Committee of the National Expert Advisory Committee on Tobacco (1999), *Australia's National Tobacco Campaign Evaluation Report*, Volume 1 and 2 (Canberra: Commonwealth Department of Health and Aged Care).

54   Da Costa e Silva, E., ed. (2003), *Policy Recommendations on Smoking Cessation and Treatment of Tobacco Dependence. Advancing Tobacco Control in the XXIst Century* (Geneva: World Health Organization).

55   New Scientist (2005), 'Ballooning US Waistlines Swell Healthcare Costs', *New Scientist* 2 July, p. 6.

56   Calle, E.E. et al. (2003), 'Overweight, Obesity, and Mortality from Cancer in a Prospectively Studied Cohort of U.S. Adults', *New England Journal of Medicine* 348:17, 1625–38.

57   Applied Economics (2003), *Cost Benefit Analysis of Proposed New Warnings on Tobacco Products* (Canberra: Commonwealth Department of Health and Ageing).

58   Ridolfo, B. and Stevenson, C. (2001), *The Quantification of Dr.ug-Caused Mortality and Morbidity in Australia, 1998*, AIHW Catalogue Number PHE 29, Dr.ug Statistics Series No. 7 (Canberra: Australian Institute of Health and Welfare).

59   Starfield, B. (2005), 'Insurance and the US Health Care System', *New England Journal of Medicine* 353:4, 418–9.

60   Commonwealth Department of Health and Family Services (1998), *Development of the Australian Refined Diagnosis Related Groups (AR-DRG) Classification Version 4* (Canberra: Commonwealth of Australia).

61   Duckett, S.J. (1998), 'Casemix Funding for Acute Hospital Inpatient Services in Australia', *Medical Journal of Australia* 169:Suppl, S17-S21.

62   Marciante, K.D. et al. (2003), 'Which Antimicrobial Impregnated Central Venous Catheter Should We Use? Modelling the Costs and Outcomes of Antimicrobial Catheter Use', *American Journal of Infection Control* 31:1, 1–8.

63   Collignon, P.J. (1994), 'Intravascular Catheter Associated Sepsis: a Common Problem. The Australian Study on Intravascular Associated Sepsis', *Medical Journal of Australia* 161:6, 374–8.

64   Schimmel, E.M. (1964), 'The Hazards of Hospitalisation', *Annals of Internal Medicine* 60, 100-10.

65   Brownson, R.C. et al. (2003), *Evidence-Based Public Health* (Oxford: Oxford University Press).

66   Adapted from Runiciman, W.B. et al. (2006), 'An Integrated Framework for Safety, Quality and Risk Management: An Information and Incident Management System based on a Universal Patient Safety Classification', *Quality and Safety in Healthcare* 15:Suppl I, i82-i90.

67   Adapted from Reason, J. by the Australian Patient Safety Foundation (2002), *Briefing Book: The Australian Incident Monitoring System* (Adelaide: Australian Patient Safety Foundation).

Chapter 2

Risk and the Harm Caused by Healthcare

Risk and Harm

Risk is inherent in all human activities. It may be defined as the chance of something happening which will have a negative impact on achieving one's objectives. Risk can be characterized as the product of its consequences and its likelihood.[1] Traditionally, concern has been focused on corporate risk (i.e. risk of financial loss or reduced productivity) or occupational risk (i.e. in healthcare, risk to those who provide the care). We are mainly concerned with clinical risk, or risk to patients. It is increased if the wrong plan is made or a plan is not carried out as intended. This manifests as harm to patients (iatrogenic harm), the obverse or 'flip-side' of which is patient safety. The harm done by healthcare will be dealt with later in this chapter. Understanding and dealing with risk allows a prospective approach to the problem of iatrogenic harm. Dealing with the aftermath of such harm and understanding what went wrong is discussed in Chapters 8 and 9, and amelioration of risk and harm in Chapters 10 to 12.

It is important to recognize that just looking at the harm side of the ledger provides a misleading and somewhat pessimistic impression of healthcare. Taking risks and accepting that some degree of harm may be unavoidable in many clinical situations is clearly appropriate when the risks are weighed against the expected benefits.

Risk

The Australian/New Zealand Risk Management Standard (AS/NZS 4360) provides a framework for managing risk (and thereby improving safety).[2] A simple outline is provided in Figure 2.1, which also shows where in this book the various components of this framework are discussed. The sources of risk lie in the various contributing factors and hazards shown at the top of Figure 1.6. In this chapter we will consider ways of expressing risk, risk perception, risk trade-offs and balancing risk against benefit. We will then consider some of the risks related to patients and to diagnostic and therapeutic interventions. Environmental and organizational risk factors, and those affecting the behaviour and performance of staff, are considered in Chapters 3–5.

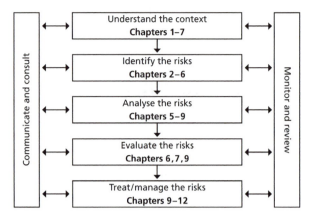

Figure 2.1 A framework for risk management[2]

Ways of Expressing Risk

Quite different impressions can be gained of how great a risk is if it is expressed in different ways. In the year after the Chernobyl nuclear power plant disaster, it was estimated that there were 3,500 additional cases of cancer in the Ukraine – which sounds bad. However, the increased risk of any individual getting cancer was increased by only 0.5 per cent, which would probably be of less concern to the average person than the previous statistic.[3]

Risk is influenced by exposure. If you never climb a tree, you are unlikely to fall out of one. In healthcare, you may be exposed to risk not only by having things go wrong when you have appropriate investigations or treatment, but also by having inappropriate healthcare or by failing to have appropriate healthcare (see page 8). In Chapter 6 we discuss decision making in relation to these issues. Making these decisions may be difficult, even if one has the right evidence, because different impressions can be obtained if the risk in relation to exposure is expressed in different ways.

Death is one unambiguous manifestation of risk, but even the risk of death will appear to differ if it is expressed in relation to different definitions of exposure (see Tables 2.1 and 2.2). If one considers death per hour of exposure to an activity, one perspective is obtained of risk. As is evident from Table 2.1, this perspective shows that flying is twice as dangerous per hour as being in traffic (but 20 times safer than being in hospital) and undergoing anaesthesia is as safe (or dangerous) as being in hospital at all. This is a tribute to the efforts of anaesthetists in safeguarding patients during complex surgical procedures, but slightly blurs the fact that mortality related to anaesthesia today tends to occur in the intensive care unit or on the ward, and seldom on the operating table. However, if one examines the number of people killed per year, one gets a quite different impression. As can be seen from Table 2.2, only 50 in 100 million people die from flying in commercial aircraft (half in aircraft that can carry less than ten passengers), whereas 15,000 are killed in road traffic accidents. This is because most people spend many more hours in traffic than in aeroplanes. Similarly, only about 100 people a year die from anaesthesia per 100 million people, whereas nearly 33,000 die in association with acute-care hospital admissions, and aortic surgery may seem not much worse than pregnancy.

Table 2.1 Death rates by exposure to various activities[3,4]

Activity	Deaths per 100 million hours of exposure
Being pregnant[4]	1
Working in a chemical factory[5]	1
Travelling by train[5]	5
Working at home[5]	8
Getting HIV from a unit of donated blood[6]	20
Being in traffic (overall, in any capacity)[5]	50
Flying in a commercial aircraft[5]	100
Undergoing anaesthesia in a developed country[7]	1,000
Being a patient in an acute-care hospital[8]	2,000
Parachute jumping[4]	20,000
Undergoing elective aortic surgery[9]	200,000
Undergoing emergency aortic surgery[10]	2,000,000

The perception of a particular risk is strongly influenced by factors other than its true magnitude. One important factor is the degree to which the risk is controllable. The average citizen is not required to get involved in parachuting and thus may avoid this particular risk (although 700 Americans die each year from being struck by falling objects, not many of these objects are people on the end of parachutes).[11] On the other hand, most of us cannot avoid considerable exposure to road traffic accidents. Risks are also generally perceived to be lower, or at least more acceptable, if they are familiar. Thus the relatively high risks of traffic, falls and smoking tend to worry people less than unusual risks, such as being killed by a shark.

It is evident from these two tables that healthcare is a risky business in comparison to travel or working in most industries, regardless of whether the risk is expressed as hours of exposure or overall number of deaths.

Risk Perception

As the perception of risk is a function of perceptions of both the nature of the hazard and of its probability, both need to be considered. Unfortunately, perceptions are subjective and differ markedly from person to person. Most human beings are inherently unable to conceptualize odds ratios of much more than 10:1. Furthermore, they will attach, both individually and at a societal level, enormous weight to manifestations of risk that they find mysterious or particularly abhorrent (e.g. from radiation or food additives).[3] Complications (such as nosocomial infection in a prosthesis, or a stroke after cardiac surgery) with which clinicians may be very familiar, and may therefore regard (perhaps wrongly) as reasonable, may be contemplated with dread by a patient. People will accept risks at least a thousand times greater if they are taken voluntarily, are known and understood, and are at least potentially controllable, even if they choose not to control them. This is one reason why, wherever possible, it is so important for patients to understand, in advance, the material risks associated with a planned procedure or investigation. Patients who find themselves in a situation they were not warned about, and therefore had no opportunity to avoid, tend to become very distressed and angry, and more likely to litigate.[4] The issue of informed consent is addressed in more detail in Chapters 6 (pages 148–152) and 7 (pages 167–170).

Table 2.2 Overall death rates from various activities

Activity	Deaths per 100 million people per year
Being pregnant[12]	150
Working in the manufacturing industry[11]	240
Travelling by train[11]	2
Drowning in the bathtub[11]	120
Getting HIV from a unit of donated blood[13]	1
Being in traffic (overall in any capacity) [11]	15,000
Flying in a commercial aircraft[11]	50
Undergoing anaesthesia[14]	100
Being a patient in an acute-care hospital[15]	33,000
Parachute jumping[16]	9
Undergoing elective abdominal aortic surgery[17]	320
Undergoing emergency abdominal aortic surgery[18]	640

Risk Perception, Behaviour and Health Policy

Perceived risk, rather than actual risk calculated by dispassionate experts, is what drives much human behaviour. This is true at the level of daily interactions between individual patients and clinicians, and also at the level of policy development by managers and politicians. A patient may undergo 'breast screening' annually whilst paying no attention to diet or exercise (activities providing up to a 100-fold greater reduction in the risk of dying)[19,20] or may decline a blood transfusion because of the risk of contracting HIV, but continue to smoke cigarettes (the difference in risk being at least 200,000-fold).[13,21]

It can be argued that policy decisions based on perceptions such as these are not only hopelessly irrational, they are also unethical, as the money wasted on tiny increments of safety for blood transfusions, for example, (many of which are unnecessary) becomes unavailable for high-yield health measures, such as promoting exercise and preventing obesity in children (see Box 1.2).

Risk Trade-offs

The situation is made yet more difficult because each available course of action may have different types of risks. Tamoxifen, a drug taken to reduce the recurrence of breast cancer, increases the risk of uterine cancer. Taking tamoxifen is statistically worthwhile because the risks of breast cancer recurrence outweigh those of uterine cancer, but might actually be harmful in a small number of people.[11] Because the risks are different in nature as well as magnitude, informed consent is particularly important. One cannot assume that a particular patient will place equal weight on two different adverse outcomes. Sometimes, a change in practice can impact different groups of patients in different ways. For example, the move to laparoscopic cholecystectomy reduced the risk of post operative respiratory complications in obese patients, but initially increased the risk of bile duct injury to all groups of patients (see page 35).

Some decisions may lead to unexpected consequences. Officials in Peru stopped chlorinating drinking water because data from the US indicated chlorine was (slightly) carcinogenic. This caused an outbreak of cholera which killed 7,000 people and afflicted over 800,000.[11]

Box 2.1 An avoidable near death experience

Joanne Adams, a 22 year old waitress, was planning a one-year overseas backpacking holiday, and decided to get a dental check-up before leaving. The dentist told her she had impacted wisdom teeth and recommended that he remove them under general anaesthesia. As this involved considerable expense Joanne discussed this with a friend who worked for a doctor. The friend brought this up at morning coffee and the doctor, who was aware that there may be little benefit but substantial costs and risks associated with the removal of asymptomatic wisdom teeth, suggested that Joanne should defer any procedure until the teeth gave trouble. However, as the dentist was a family friend, Joanne felt she had to go ahead with the procedure, which had already been booked, although the cost would delay her overseas trip. On induction of anaesthesia in a small private hospital, Joanne suffered a severe anaphylactic reaction to suxamethonium. She was most fortunate in that her difficult resuscitation was assisted by an intensive care specialist who was called urgently, and happened to be only one block away on her way to work at the time of the call for help. After a difficult resuscitation, Joanne was transferred to the intensive care unit of a teaching hospital where she required an adrenaline infusion for 18 hours and 2 days of artificial ventilation. Although she had short-term memory loss for some weeks she eventually made a full recovery.

Informed decisions should be based on best available evidence; this is not always easy to identify. This is discussed further in Chapter 6.

Risk vs Benefit – Choosing a Course of Action

In all human endeavours, the risk of taking a certain course of action must be considered in relation to the expected benefits of that course of action. It is perfectly appropriate to embark on a high-risk strategy if it is the best available option and may save a life that would otherwise certainly be lost. On the other hand, if a procedure has not been definitively shown to be effective, or is only marginally indicated, an informed patient may be well advised to avoid its risks by not having it at all (see Boxes 1.4 and 2.1). These matters are discussed further in Chapters 4 (page 94) and 6 (pages 148–152).

Patient-related Risk

Patient characteristics have a major impact on the risk of a problem occurring as well as on the outcome when something does go wrong. In the first instance, communication difficulties may arise because of problems of language, eyesight, hearing, or intellect, or because the same situations may be interpreted quite differently by people from different backgrounds and cultures. Poor communication increases risk in healthcare, and may contribute to patients becoming non-compliant or even hostile because of unresolved concerns about their illness and its implications for their family and future work prospects.

Table 2.3 The Goldman cardiac risk index[22]

Criteria	Points
History	
age greater than 70 years	5
myocardial infarct within 6 months	10
Physical examination	
cardiac gallop or jugular venous distension	11
vascular aortic stenosis	3
Electrocardiogram	
atrial dysrhythmia	7
more than 5 premature ventricular	
contractions per minute	7
General status	
$PaO_2 < 60mmHg$ or $PaCO_2 > 50mm\ Hg$	
potassium <3 or bicarbonate <20 meq/l	
urea >50 or creatinine >3mg/dl	
signs of chronic liver disease	
patient bedridden from cardiac causes	3
Operation – intraperitoneal, intrathoracic or aortic	3
Emergency procedure	4
Total possible points	**53**

The physical condition of the patient is very important in this context. In an Australian review of medical records, three-quarters of all preventable deaths occurred in patients over 65 years of age, and the chance of an adverse event resulting in death in this age group was 10 times greater than that for patients under 45.[15] Patients may be given some idea of their individual risk for certain types of problems by reference to various risk indices or scoring systems. The risk of having a heart attack or stroke in association with a non-cardiac operation is increased by several factors, the relative importance of each of which has been encapsulated in one such index, shown in Table 2.3. The patient's risk is directly related to the total number of points scored using this table. The Euroscore is another example, and allows the risk of cardiac surgery to be predicted for individual patients with reasonable accuracy.[23]

It is possible to take steps to reduce risk, and these will manifest in lower scores. For example, it is worth delaying a procedure after a myocardial infarct and making sure that heart failure and respiratory problems are optimally treated before proceeding with surgery and anaesthesia.

Investigation-related or Treatment-related Risk

There are also risks inherent in certain procedures. The risk of thromboembolism is present with any surgical procedure, but it varies considerably between procedures; it is approximately 1 per cent for a cataract operation, 10 per cent for a hip replacement, and 40 per cent for a bilateral knee replacement.[24] The risks of various complications associated with the removal of a gall bladder using a laparoscope are listed in Table 2.4.[25]

Influence of Professional Performance and Behaviour on Risk

The frequency of some very serious complications such as bile duct injury may vary greatly between different operators (from more than one in 100 to less than one in 2,000). Many surgeons do not have accurate figures for their own results, and perform most procedures too infrequently to allow reliable interpretation of any figures if they did have them. When laparoscopic cholecystectomy was first introduced there were no requirements with respect to training and competency, and bile duct injury rates doubled.[26]

It is likely that, in the future, all practitioners who do procedures will be required to keep a record of pertinent features of procedures and patients involved in their practice, and of their complications. These data may inform them and their prospective patients of their experience and complication rates (see Chapter 12). One criticism of the surgeons involved in the Bristol enquiry was that they provided the parents of the children having cardiac operations with figures reflecting the average mortality in the literature, rather than the mortality in their own hands (see Box 2.2). Variability between practitioners applies to most procedures; it is evident, for example, in the wide ranges in Table 2.4.

A difficulty in interpreting Table 2.4 is that most published figures are from large units with a high volume of work, factors which tend to reduce complication rates. Practitioners with high complication rates may not publish their figures. Those with high rates are self-evidently contributing to the burden of iatrogenic harm. For individual patients and for the funders of healthcare (ultimately the tax payers) avoidable harm caused by the healthcare process rather than an underlying disease or injury really matters. This is the subject of the rest of this chapter.

Table 2.4 Laparoscopic cholecystectomy – risks of recognized complications[25]

Complications	Frequency
Infection	
- subcutaneous	1.5%
- intra-abdominal/pelvic	0.1-1%
- systemic	0.1-1%
- port site	0.1-1%
Bleeding	
- wound	1-5%
- intra-abdominal	0.1-1%
Haematoma formation	1-5%
Injury to bowel or blood vessels	0.1-1%
Gas embolus	0.1-1%
Conversion to open operation of operative cholangiogram	1-5%
Bile duct injury	0.1-1%
Biliary drainage after duct injury	0.1-1%
Biliary stricture	<0.1%
Liver injury	0.1-1%
Bile leak/collection/fistula	0.1-1%
Jaundice	0.1-1%
Multi-organ failure	0.1-1%
Small bowel obstruction (adhesions)	0.1-1%
Paralytic ileus	50-80%
Need for colostomy/ileostomy	<0.1%
Pancreatitis/pancreatic injury/cyst/fistula	0.1-1%
Seroma formation	0.1-1%
Pneumothorax	0.1-1%
Deep venous thrombosis	0.1-1%
Pain/tenderness	
- acute (<4 weeks)	>80%
- chronic (>12 weeks)	1-5%
Wound dehiscence	0.1-1%
Portsite hernia formation	0.1-1%
Poor cosmetic result (wound)	1-5%

Box 2.2 The Bristol Enquiry[27,28]

In 1998, an enquiry was conducted into the management of children who received complex cardiac surgical services at the Bristol Royal Infirmary between 1984 and 1995. A high number of young children died (29) or were left brain-damaged (4) following open heart surgery, with mortality twice the expected rate. A whistle-blower, a cardiac anaesthetist, raised the alarm. The Enquiry produced 198 recommendations.[27] The Department of Health agreed with the majority of the recommendations which led to reforms in communication with, and representation of patients, and changes in the process of reviewing poor professional practice in England. In addition, a national sentinel event reporting system was developed and a National Director for Children's Healthcare Services was appointed, as well as a Children's Rights Director to a new position created specifically to promote the rights of children in England.[28]

The Harm Caused by Healthcare

Harm caused directly by healthcare ranges from the mundane to the catastrophic, from a small skin tear on the arm of a frail, elderly patient being helped into bed, to quadriplegia or death after the unintentional injection of an intravenous chemotherapy drug into the cerebrospinal fluid (see Box 11.1). Acts of omission may also lead to harmful outcomes, from avoidable discomfort because simple pain relief has not been provided, to death from a pulmonary embolus after a leg fracture because the routine prescription of an anti-coagulant has been overlooked (see Boxes 2.3 and 3.8). Nearly half of the healthcare delivered to patients in the USA (and most likely in other countries) is not in accordance with basic indicators (see Figure 1.2).[29] This applies to preventive measures, care for acute conditions and care for chronic conditions. As stated on pages 8 and 30, inappropriate healthcare places patients in double jeopardy from the safety perspective.

This argument may be extended to the level of the population. One may argue that at least a fraction of the disability and death arising from a failure at a societal level to properly police drink driving or to reduce smoking is preventable and should therefore be included under the general heading of iatrogenic harm. The United Kingdom, for example, lagged behind Ireland and Australia in introducing measures to reduce smoking, despite the fact that this is one of the most serious public health problems in the world.[21] At a global level, one may also argue that failure by the community of nations to ensure that children have access to safe drinking water and basic healthcare represents a failure on the part of humanity to discharge its duty with respect to the health of its global citizens (see Table 1.1).

In addition to the direct physical harm to patients described in this chapter, delays and inconveniences may also be seen as a form of harm and can at times have a significant impact on a patient's wellbeing. In addition, the loss of or damage to the infrastructure and equipment of healthcare, or possessions of patients or staff, is also important. The definition of an incident includes all types of harm (see Appendix I), and also includes harm to staff, visitors and contractors. For example, a visitor may fall on a slippery floor or a contractor suffer inadvertent exposure to radiation. However, in this chapter, we will limit our discussion to harm to patients.

There is no convenient, single source of information about iatrogenic harm. Some sources are listed in Table 2.5; these will be considered in turn, with an outline of their strengths and weaknesses. There are currently major difficulties in scoping and tracking the extent of iatrogenic harm. Even when the same definition is used for a term like 'adverse event', it may be interpreted differently by different people or in different circumstances.

Existing Knowledge

The healthcare delivered to patients should be in accordance with the best available evidence and be designed to get the greatest benefit with respect to the seven dimensions of healthcare shown in Figure 1.1. What is required is sound research, timely systematic literature reviews to collate and interpret the information from this research, and then careful consideration and evaluation of all available evidence to identify best practice. This process is called evidence based medicine, and is discussed in Chapter 6. It should be noted that it was judged that errors of omission caused more than half the harm detected by medical record review;[15] this supports the findings shown in Figure 1.2.

Medical Record Review

One way to get some idea of how many patients are harmed by healthcare is to use trained reviewers to examine medical records looking for problems which they think were caused by the healthcare process, rather than a disease or injury. A technique for this was developed in California in the mid-1970s. At that time, California's medical indemnity market was in a state of crisis, affecting both the cost and availability of insurance. In order to examine a possible alternative, the Californian Medical and Hospital Associations set up a 'medical insurance feasibility study' to determine what a 'non-fault compensation system' would cost.[30] To do this it was necessary to determine the type, frequency and severity of disabilities caused by healthcare management.

The technique developed involved the screening of randomly selected medical records by trained nurse reviewers for any of 18 specific criteria, such as unplanned admission to intensive care or return to the operating theatre. Records with one or more of these criteria were passed to trained physician reviewers, who examined them for evidence of harm to the patient, the extent to which any such harm was caused by healthcare, and the extent to which the event might have been preventable or due to negligence.

Table 2.5 Sources of information about things that go wrong in healthcare

Medical record review
Routine data collections (deaths, discharges, GP surveys)
Observational studies
Population surveys
Existing registers, reporting systems and audits for:
- morbidity and mortality
- adverse drug reactions
- equipment failure and hazards
Existing knowledge
- research
- meta-analysis
- literature reviews
- evidence-based medicine
Incident monitoring
Complaint investigations
- hospital and state
- registration boards
- complaints commissioners
Medico-legal investigations
Root cause analyses (sentinel events)
Coronial investigations
Quality improvement and accreditation activities
Results of enquiries and investigations
Literature searches for common and rare events

The Californian study involved over 20,000 records and found that 4.6 per cent of admissions were associated with a 'potentially compensable event'.[30] The next study, known as the Harvard Medical Practice Study, of over 30,000 medical records from New York State, is regarded as the 'benchmark' for all subsequent studies.[31] An *adverse event* was defined in this and subsequent studies as unintended harm arising from healthcare, which resulted in admission to hospital, prolonged hospital stay, disability at discharge or death. For examples of how events may be classified with this technique, see Box 2.3.

A summary of studies using this methodology in relation to acute-care hospitals since the early 1990s is presented in Table 2.6. About 10 per cent of admissions to acute-care hospitals were associated with an adverse event, and 1.5–2 per cent of admissions were associated with permanent disability or death in all but one study; up to half of these problems were considered preventable, although agreement between reviewers was poor for preventability. The annual number of iatrogenic deaths exceeds the road toll in all countries studied (8,000 versus less than 2,000 in Australia).

Box 2.3 Examples of medical record review adverse event classification[15]

Complication, no causation (no adverse event) – An elderly man was admitted with a fractured neck of femur, which was managed with early fixation. Three days later the patient had a gastric bleed and died from hypotension and anaemia. There was no history of such bleeding, nor any reason for having a high index of suspicion; the problem was promptly recognized and assessed. *The patient had a complication causing death, judged not to have been caused by healthcare management.*

Injury, no disability (no adverse event) – A patient with profound central nervous system impairment was hospitalized for assessment and rehabilitation, and suffered recurrent urinary tract infection in conjunction with the use of an indwelling urethral catheter. Although this required specific therapy on more than one occasion, it did not prolong hospitalization beyond what was required for the patient's underlying condition. *The patient had a complication caused by healthcare management but no resulting disability.*

Adverse event, no preventability – A 50 year old woman underwent coronary angiography for unstable angina. During the angiogram she sustained an anaphylactic reaction to the contrast, with cardiac arrest. She was resuscitated promptly, without permanent sequelae, and hospitalization was prolonged by 10 days. Evidence for prior contrast reactions was sought and not found. *The patient had a complication, suffered disability, and causation was demonstrated, so this was classified as an (unpreventable) adverse event.*

Adverse event, high preventability – A 67 year old woman underwent a laparoscopic cholecystectomy, which proceeded to an open operation. Endoscopic retrograde cholangio-pancreatography was undertaken eight days later to remove a gallstone in the common bile duct; cannulation was not possible and the procedure was aborted. Two days later the patient collapsed and died suddenly. Autopsy findings showed deep venous thrombosis and saddle pulmonary embolus. There was no evidence of thromboembolic prophylaxis. *The patient had an adverse event resulting in death, with high preventability.*

Adverse event, high preventability – A 55 year old man with a history of multiple admissions for anxiety and palpitations was admitted in 1992 with pleuritic chest pain and pneumonia. Chest x-ray revealed a 6 cm mass lesion in the basal segment of the right upper lobe. The medical record showed that the lesion had been found on a chest x-ray in 1989. There was no report of the lesion in the record; it was referred to in an outpatient note in 1989, but no follow-up or treatment had been planned or initiated. The mass was a large cell carcinoma of the lung, with mediastinal and cerebral metastases. The patient underwent a course of chemotherapy and radiotherapy but died eight months later. *The patient had an adverse event resulting in death, with high preventability.*

Adverse event, high preventability – An 87 year old woman with osteoporosis underwent open reduction and internal fixation with an Austin-Moore prosthesis and received antibiotic therapy for a urinary tract infection. Five days after the operation it was noted that the patient had developed bilateral decubitus ulcers on her heels. No pressure-area care had been documented. The ulcers required daily dressings in hospital, and dressings by a community nurse were still required at discharge. The patient's hospital stay was extended to 39 days. *The patient had an adverse event resulting in disability and prolonged hospital stay, with high preventability.*

Lucian Leape made the point that the number of iatrogenic deaths in the USA was equivalent to two jumbo jets full of passengers crashing every three days.[32] A subsequent study demonstrated that the vast majority of the iatrogenic deaths were in elderly and/or very sick patients, so few would have been alive, well and at home three months later.[33] The jumbo jet analogy thus needs to be qualified by the notion that nearly all the passengers would be in poor health and many would be in residential care.

Table 2.6 Adverse event rates from medical record reviews

Country in which the study was done	No of records studied	Adverse events % of admissions	Permanent harm and death % of admissions
Australia[15]	14,179	10.6	2.0
America[34]	14,565	~10.0[35]	2.0
Canada[36]	3,745	7.5	1.6
Denmark[37]	1,097	9.0	0.4
England[38]	1,014	11.7	1.5
New Zealand[39]	6,579	12.9	1.9

Notwithstanding this, there is general agreement that the problem of iatrogenic harm is a major one, although undue emphasis may have been placed on deaths and high profile catastrophic events. In fact, 60 per cent of the resource consumption from adverse events identified by medical record review is from mundane problems (e.g. wound infections, failure to properly investigate or treat ischemic heart disease, unsuccessful back operations, decubitus ulcers).[40] Intensive observational studies have shown that the problem is far more pervasive than that suggested by medical record review with, for example, as many as half of all surgical patients in a teaching hospital suffering an adverse event of some sort.[41] It is worth pointing out that problems arising in association with mental health services are not captured by these studies, and nor are those which arise in patients who do not end up in hospital.[42] A Canadian study showed that 23 per cent of patients followed up after discharge suffered an adverse event (see Box 2.4).[43,44]

Box 2.4   Examples of preventable adverse events after discharge from hospital[43]

- Profound hypoglycaemia necessitating readmission, which developed days after discharge in a patient treated orally with hypoglycaemics. *Preventable.*
- Acute exacerbation of congestive heart failure in a patient with severe left ventricular dysfunction for whom diltiazem was prescribed. The patient's condition was inadequately monitored after discharge. *Preventable.*
- Transient ischaemic attack with a normal international normalized ratio (INR) in a patient known to have atrial fibrillation whose anticoagulation therapy was inadequately monitored after discharge. *Preventable.*
- Profound hypoglycaemia and acute renal failure in a patient treated with an angiotensin-converting-enzyme inhibitor and diuretics. The electrolyte levels were not monitored after discharge. *Preventable.*

A rough estimate of the makeup of the overall problem of iatrogenic harm may be obtained from Table 2.7. However, lumping adverse events into such broad categories is of no use to those wishing to devise corrective strategies. To do this it is necessary to break the events up into categories which constitute meaningful clinical entities. Nearly 600 such categories were identified in the Australian medical record study alone.[15,40] Most of the categories (70 per cent) contained only one or two cases. Large-scale collections of iatrogenic problems are necessary if these individually rare but collectively important types of events are to be characterized in sufficient detail for corrective strategies to be devised.

In summary, medical record review does give some indication of the relative frequencies of the more common iatrogenic problems in acute-care hospitals, but this approach has major weaknesses. It is very expensive and logistically demanding, and yields little information about how and why the problems are occurring. It has not captured problems in mental health patients or in those who have poor access to healthcare or do not end up in hospital. To understand the factors underlying and contributing to iatrogenic harm, especially for low frequency events, additional information must be collected in the aftermath of the events. The collection of this information will be the subject of Chapter 9.

Routine Data Collection

In many countries the *causes of death and for admission to hospital* are collected after being coded using the International Classification of Diseases.[45] Some of these codes relate to problems caused by healthcare. These were examined in Australia,[46] where nearly 3,000 deaths per year were identified as being associated with adverse events. This was less than half the 8,000 estimated by the re-analysis of the Australian adverse event study.[35] Likewise, the 4.75 per cent of admissions coded as associated with an adverse event represent less than half of the 10–12 per cent estimated by medical record review.[35] There are several reasons why ICD coding has proved to be a very poor tool for identifying adverse events in the medical record.

- The emphasis in coding is on recording the underlying disease or injury, not on identifying adverse events.
- Many problems are not explicitly identified in the record as adverse events, and thus cannot be coded as such.
- There are no specific codes for many adverse events.
- Even when there are codes for drug-related adverse events, only 11–31 per cent are correctly coded.[47]

Table 2.7 Main types of adverse event identified by medical record review[48]

Problem with or failure of an operation or procedure[49]	18%
Hospital acquired infection[50]	16%
Wrong, delayed or missed – diagnosis or treatment[51]	14%
Complication of a body system[52]	11%
Hospital acquired injury[53]	8%
Medication error or problem with a drug[54]	7%
Pain, headache, nausea and vomiting, ileus, fever[55]	6%
Haemorrhage or haematoma[56]	5%
Maternal/foetal problem	3%
Thromboembolism, failure of or no prophylaxis	3%
Problem with a device, prosthesis, catheter, or cannula	2%
Unnecessary procedure	2%
Process problem (delayed admission, premature discharge)	2%
Problem from radiotherapy or chemotherapy	1%
Eye problem	1%
Miscellaneous	1%
TOTAL	**100%**

In addition, many of the adverse event codes are too non-specific to be useful for devising corrective strategies. These limitations are well recognized. Plans are in place to devise more specific codes for adverse events and to try to make the collection of adverse events more comprehensive during routine coding. This would be an efficient way of tracking progress in reducing iatrogenic harm, at least for certain types of events, if coders can be trained to categorize them.

Routine Surveys of General Practice

Routine surveys of general practice activity are regularly conducted in Australia. Those conducted over the last few years have found that an adverse event is managed at nearly one million general practice encounters each year (0.9 per cent of over 100 million encounters for a population of 20 million).[57] Complications of treatment make up 45 per cent and adverse affects of medications make up 43 per cent of the total, with postoperative complications such as infection and pain making up the bulk of the remainder.[57]

Observational Studies

Observational or ethnographic studies have been used in healthcare to estimate adverse event rates and to try to understand how and why such events occur. They involve periods of observation, and may incorporate formal or informal interviews. In one study, the adverse event rate was estimated at 46 per cent for all admissions, with 18 per cent being associated with serious injury.[41] In another, 28 per cent of patient days were associated with moderate to fatal complications and 17 per cent of admissions for longer than two days were associated with serious adverse events.[58] These figures are probably far closer to what actually happens than those from retrospective analyses. However, observational studies are expensive. It is not necessarily essential to capture all adverse events; what matters is to determine how and why they occur, and then prevent them from recurring.

Population Surveys

Telephone-based population surveys have been conducted of the experiences of healthcare of randomly selected members of the public; 6.5 per cent of Australians[59] and 6.0 per cent of Americans[60] reported experience of a medical adverse event.

Existing Registers, Reporting Systems and Audits

There have been longstanding systematic efforts to study *morbidity* and *mortality* associated with certain clinical disciplines. Where deaths are rare, attempts have been made at national collections of data (e.g. maternal deaths associated with pregnancy[61,62] and deaths associated with anaesthesia[63]). There have been major difficulties in trying to collect *all* such deaths, because of variations in reporting practices and requirements, but clusters due to certain causes have been identified and steps taken to change clinical practice. For example, maternal deaths due to aspiration of gastric contents under general anaesthesia, once a leading cause of maternal death, are now very rare because of changes to anaesthetic practice (such as greater use of regional anaesthesia, steps to prevent regurgitated gastric contents from reaching and harming the lungs during general anaesthesia, and a requirement for a defined minimum level of experience for obstetric anaesthetists).

Anaesthesia mortality appears to have halved each decade since 1960 (although the accuracy of this statement has been questioned[64]), and maternal deaths directly related to pregnancy have fallen in both the UK and Australia to less than six per 100,000 confinements. These areas, once significant causes of iatrogenic harm, currently account for less than one per cent of iatrogenic deaths.

Many disciplines and areas conduct regular *audits* of things that go wrong in order to progressively improve the standard of care. For example, surgeons in the Lothian area of Scotland recently celebrated the fiftieth anniversary of conducting regular surgical audits. Since 1994, these audits have been extended to a combined Scottish audit of surgical mortality, in which nearly 5,000 deaths are reviewed annually.[65] This process is now being adopted in Australia and New Zealand by the Royal Australasian College of Surgeons.

Audits of morbidity and mortality, including medical record review, are increasingly carried out on a regular basis in many countries at hospital or facility level, as well as department or unit level.

Adverse Drug Reaction Reporting Systems

Many countries have a central agency for collecting adverse drug reactions (reactions to drugs which are correctly prescribed and administered). The Australian collection now holds over 100,000 reports and receives a thousand reports per month. However, adverse drug reactions make up only about 5 per cent of medication incidents, with the majority being due to problems such as wrong drug, wrong dose, wrong time, wrong route, wrong patient and failure to monitor.[66]

Equipment Failures and Hazards

There are well developed mechanisms in most Western countries for soliciting reports when patients were or could have been harmed by therapeutic devices and equipment.[67,68,69] Over 100,000 such reports are now received each year in the USA, and the Emergency Care Research Institute currently holds over one million.[70] Although less than 0.3 per cent of iatrogenic deaths or episodes of serious harm is attributable to device failure,[67] it is obviously important to prevent the sale of devices such as heart valves or pacemakers with intrinsic design faults.[69] In anaesthesia and intensive care equipment use is high; in these fields less than 10 per cent of incidents are due to actual equipment failure, but nearly half are associated with problems at the interfaces between equipment and users or patients.

Until recently, there have been few national registers which allow the tracking of devices implanted in patients; the Nordic countries are an exception. There have been major problems with premature failure of certain types of artificial heart valves, of pacemakers, and of certain types of artificial joint prostheses. Efforts are underway in many countries to set up systems to ensure that devices implanted into patients are properly tracked.

Devices may be intrinsically dangerous, owing to user inter-faces which allow or induce misuse in ways that may produce serious adverse events, even though they still meet the manufacturers' specifications. Incident reporting is one of the few ways of picking up this type of problem early and alerting other clinicians and the regulatory authorities.

Incident Monitoring

Incident monitoring involves the collection of information about any event or circumstance that could have or did harm anyone, or result in loss, damage or a complaint.[71] Various forms of incident reporting have existed in healthcare facilities for many years,[72] and over the last 10 years or so some medical specialties have set up national collections.[73] Attempts are being made to move towards standardized national reporting and classification systems for things that go wrong in healthcare (see Chapters 9 and 11).[74-75]

Table 2.8 Types of incident identified by incident monitoring[76]

Type of incident	% of reports*
Falls	29
Injuries other than falls (e.g. burns, pressure injuries, physical assault, self-harm)	13
Medication errors (e.g. omission, overdose, underdose, wrong route, wrong medication)	12
Clinical process problems (e.g. wrong diagnosis, inappropriate treatment, poor care)	10
Equipment problems (e.g. unavailable, inappropriate, poor design, misuse, failure, malfunction)	8
Documentation problems (e.g. inadequate, incorrect, not completed, out of date, unclear)	8
Hazardous environment (e.g. contamination, inadequate cleaning or sterilization)	7
Inadequate resources (e.g. staff absent, unavailable, inexperienced, poor orientation)	5
Logistic problems (e.g. problems with admission, treatment, transport, response to emergency)	4
Administrative problems (e.g. inadequate supervision, lack of resource, poor management decisions)	2
Infusion problems (e.g. omission, wrong rate)	1
Infrastructure problems (e.g. power failure, insufficient beds)	1
Nutrition problems (e.g. fed when fasting, wrong food, food contaminated, problems when ordering)	1
Colloid or blood product problems (e.g. omission, underdose, overdose, storage problems)	1
Oxygen problems (e.g. omission, overdose, underdose, premature cessation, failure of supply)	1

* More than one type of incident may be assigned to a report.

Reporting 'near misses' is valuable because new problems can be identified early and much information can be obtained about how the problems present, the factors that contribute to them, and how they may be prevented, before serious harm is done to a patient (see Box 2.5).

Incident reporting cannot define the frequency of a problem, but it can provide the information needed for its prevention. For example, algorithms for the management of any crisis under anaesthesia have been checked against 4,000 anaesthesia-related incident reports.[77]

The types of events reported differ for each specialty or domain (e.g. anaesthesia,[78] intensive care,[79] emergency medicine[80]), so it is ideal to have databases for each specialty. However, if a common classification is used, these databases can be searched for problems common to all domains (see Figure 1.5).

Box 2.5 Hypoxic brain damage under anaesthesia in retreat

Inadequate ventilation and undetected oesophageal intubation used to account for hundreds of cases of litigation for brain damage and death.[81] The introduction in the late 1980s of heart-beat by heart-beat monitoring of blood oxygenation (pulse oximetry) and breath-by-breath analysis of inspired and expired gases as de-facto standards has virtually eliminated the adverse consequences of these problems. Many hundreds of incident reports relevant to these problems and the role of those monitors had a major influence on the world standards for safe anaesthesia (see Box 11.9). In recent studies of over 1,200 medico-legal claims[82] and 4,000 incidents over 5 years in Australia there was not a single case of hypoxic brain damage or death from these causes. However, problems with airway management continue to harm patients, and need attention.[83]

Complaint Investigations

Complaints are also a rich source of information about the things that are going wrong in healthcare. A preliminary survey of several hundred complaints has shown that the types of adverse event associated with complaints are very similar to those encountered in medical record reviews and incident monitoring.[42] Poor communication or rudeness on the part of staff is frequently a major contributing factor to iatrogenic harm and can cause considerable harm in their own right in the form of frustration and anger. Complaints may be lodged and handled at local, state or regional levels, as well as by professional registration boards.

Medico-legal Investigations

Medico-legal cases may also provide valuable information about the things that are going wrong in healthcare. A series of studies has been carried out by a group in the USA on anaesthesia-related closed claims,[81] and a recent study of such claims in Australia confirmed progress made in patient safety and identified areas for improvement (see Box 2.5).[82,83] Figure 2.2 shows the more common types of adverse events associated with admissions from the Australian medical record study compared with those from a sample of medico-legal claims from a large teaching hospital in Australia.[42] Certain problems which are obviously iatrogenic, such as perforation of an organ or a fracture from a fall in hospital, have a high likelihood of litigation.

However, other problems which may be lethal and which we know could have been prevented, but for which there is a less obvious cause-and-effect relationship, have a low frequency of litigation. In some of these cases patients and/or their relatives may not have been informed that the problem would most likely not have occurred had appropriate preventive measures been taken (see Boxes 3.3 and 3.8).

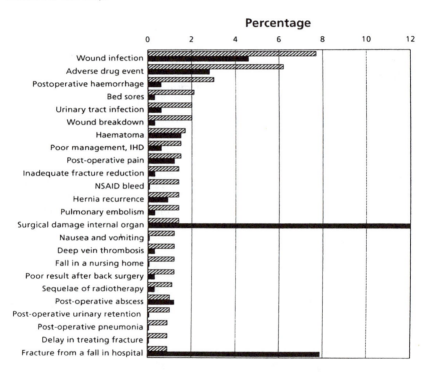

Figure 2.2   Adverse events, ranked by percentages of 2,300 events from a medical record study (light-shaded bars)**, compared with percentages of 346 medico-legal files at a tertiary referral hospital** (dark-shaded bars)[42]; IHD – Ischaemic heart disease; NSAID – Non-steroidal anti-inflammatory drug.

Root Cause Analyses and Sentinel Events

Serious adverse events with a reasonable potential for recurrence should be subjected to root cause analysis[84] (see Chapter 9). Certain serious adverse events have come to be known as sentinel events. A practical definition of a sentinel event is 'an adverse event which should never be allowed to happen'. Certain events are formally listed as sentinel events in various jurisdictions (Table 2.9). These rather bizarre collections of categories of events represent less than one in a thousand of all the types of things that can go wrong and result in death or serious physical or psychological harm. The 'catch all' category 'other catastrophic events' makes up half of all the sentinel events reported in the USA and over two-thirds of those reported in Australia.[85,86,87,88] Substantial resources are consumed by the collection at national level of information on these predefined events. Perhaps this reflects the need to be seen to be doing something apparently systematic in response to the very real human tragedies which accompany these (and a vast array of other) unfortunate incidents. This is, hopefully, a passing aberration. What is really needed is a uniformly classified national repository of all the things that go wrong in healthcare, and a properly structured system for root cause analysis of all serious adverse events, 'sentinel' or otherwise (see Chapter 9). This has recently been recognized in the USA.[89]

Table 2.9 Sentinel events on the 'official' lists

Type of adverse event	USA[85] % of 1579	Australia[86,87] % of 175
Suicide of an inpatient or within 72 hours of discharge	29	13
Surgery on the wrong patient or body part	29	47
Medication error leading to death	23	7
Rape/assault/homicide in an inpatient setting[88]	8	na
Incompatible blood transfusion	6	1
Maternal death (labour, delivery)	3	12
Infant abduction/wrong family discharge	1	-
Retained instrument after surgery	1	21
Unanticipated death of a full-term infant	-	na
Severe neonatal hyperbilirubinaemia	-	na
Prolonged fluoroscopy	-	na
Intravascular gas embolism	na	-

Coronial Investigations

Coroners have a responsibility to investigate certain deaths if the cause of death is uncertain, or thought to be due to something which should not have occurred (such as an accident or assault). In Australia, a national coroners' information system has been established by which coroners enter a minimum data set and narrative of relevant cases.[90] Accredited people can access the information. The Victorian Institute of Forensic Medicine examined 1,053 hospital deaths that were reported to the Coroner in 1999; 338 of these were further investigated as it was thought that they were associated with an adverse event. Of these, 96 were thought to have involved system failures. Extrapolating these data nationally suggests there may be about 2,000 cases per year in Australia worth closer investigation and that in about 700 cases system-based factors may be identified which contributed to the death.[42] All deaths related to adverse events should be collected and classified in the same way as other events.

Quality Improvement and Accreditation Activities

Nearly all hospitals and services maintain ongoing surveillance of certain problems. This often involves the measurement of performance in relation to defined 'indicators', such as rates of appropriate antibiotic or thrombo-embolism prophylaxis, or compliance with a range of protocols and treatment pathways. Such activities in a number of prescribed areas may be required for accreditation of a hospital or facility (see page 263).

One would expect that low rates of compliance with established principles of best practice would be associated with more adverse events. It is often easier to measure a 'process indicator' such as the percentage of patients receiving the right antibiotic prophylaxis at the right time, than an outcome such as a wound infection which may only manifest after discharge.

Results of Enquiries and Investigations

Much attention has been drawn to inadequate practices at certain institutions, or by certain individuals, through enquiries or investigations which have been triggered by particular tragedies, or by 'whistle-blowers' who have drawn attention to dangerous or unacceptable conditions or practices (see Boxes 2.2 and 7.8). Detailed discussion of these is beyond the scope of this chapter.

The Cost of Harm Done by Healthcare

Before the year 2000, the *direct financial costs* of iatrogenic harm in the US were estimated at around US$20 billion per year, those in Australia at AU$2 billion per year, and those in the UK at around £2 billion. This worked out roughly to one US dollar per week for every man, woman and child in each of these countries, and accounts for approximately five per cent of the cost of healthcare.[42]

Indirect financial costs account for at least the same amount again in loss of earnings and costs of ongoing care. The tort system costs at least an additional 1–2 per cent of the amount spent on healthcare in Australia and the UK, and possibly more in the US; 60 per cent of this is consumed by costs of the legal system and does not find its way to those being compensated.[42]

Human costs The emphasis on financial losses often distracts from the enormous human cost of things that go wrong in healthcare (see Chapter 8). These relate not only to those directly harmed, but also to their families and friends. Being involved in an event which leads to iatrogenic harm can also be a permanent life-altering event for healthcare professionals (see Boxes 4.2 and 4.5).

Summary

More than half the harm caused by healthcare results from a failure to deliver appropriate care or deciding on courses of action which are inappropriate; the rest is caused by poor basic care or investigations and interventions going wrong.

There is currently little directly relevant information about the risks of proposed investigations or interventions for individual patients in the hands of individual teams or healthcare professionals. Healthcare professionals will have to continue to do their best to help their patients make reasonable risk-benefit and risk-trade-off decisions with the current primitive information systems until some of the solutions described in Chapter 12 become available.

Harm from healthcare may be severe and have tragic consequences for all involved. It ranks prominently as a public health problem. The potential for preventing this harm exceeds that in relation to many other well-known public health problems, such as road traffic accidents.

Studies of medical records suggest that about 10 per cent of admissions to acute-care hospitals are associated with an adverse event, approximately half of these being the cause of the admission and half occurring during the admission. About one in every 50 admissions is associated with major disability or death. At least as many problems again may arise after discharge. The number of iatrogenic deaths exceeds the road toll.

One in every 100 general practice encounters involves an adverse event, and one in 15 randomly surveyed people have had experience of an adverse event. The direct costs of adverse events amount to 5 per cent of the total amount spent on healthcare, costs of litigation to a further 1–2 per cent, and indirect costs probably to another 6 per cent. Human costs to those harmed, their friends, relatives and carers, and to the health professionals involved are also very substantial and the measures to ameliorate these are currently ill-developed. Nine per cent of gross domestic product (GDP) is spent on healthcare in many Western countries (15 per cent in the USA); as much as 1 per cent of GDP is consumed by iatrogenic problems and their 'whole of life' consequences.

Root cause analysis should be undertaken to identify strategies to prevent recurrence when major harm occurs. Systematic attention should also be given to events which cause minor, transient, or delayed harm, because these are responsible for 60 per cent of the resources consumed by adverse events.

We are only now beginning to standardize terminology and refine methods of assessing the scope, nature and impact of things that go wrong in healthcare.[92] The emphasis should not be on counting problems but on improving safety. The resources are limited and should be spent on understanding how and why problems are occurring, so that preventive and corrective strategies can be devised and implemented. How to do this is the subject of Chapters 8–12.

Notes

1   Standards Australia International and Standards New Zealand (2001), *Guidelines for Managing Risk in the Healthcare Sector HB 228:2001* (Sydney: Standards Australia International).

2   Standards Australia and Standards New Zealand (1999), *Risk Management AS/NZS 4360:1999* (Strathfield, New South Wales: Standards Association of Australia).

3   Slovic P. (1987), 'Perception of Risk', *Science* 236, 280–285.

4   Based on Dutch statistics. Zelders, T. (1996), 'Patient Risks: an Underdeveloped Area', *Journal of Clinical Monitoring* 12:3, 237–41.

5   Zelders, T. (1996) above, summarized data from Kietz, T.A. (1977). 'The Risk Equations', *New Scientist*, 12 May, 320-2; Dinman, B.D. (1980), 'The Reality and Acceptance of Risk', *Journal of the American Medical Association* 244:11, 1226–8; and Pochin, E.E. (1975), 'The Acceptance of Risk', *British Medical Bulletin* 31:3, 184–90.

6   Assuming it takes one hour to transfuse one unit of blood, and there is a residual risk of one case in 5 million units transmitting HIV infection because the donor was in the 'window' period in which the infection could not be detected by current nucleic acid testing methods: Australian Red Cross Blood Service (2002), 'New National Blood Management System to Be Introduced', *MediLink* 5:3, 1–2.

7   Calculated from the number of deaths estimated to be directly attributable to anaesthesia in Australia (1 per 150,000 hours of exposure to anaesthesia). Davis, N.J. (ed.) (1999), *Anaesthesia Related Mortality in Australia 1994–1996* (Melbourne: Australian and New Zealand College of Anaesthetists).

8   Calculated from the number of deaths associated with preventable adverse events. Runciman, W.B. et al. (2000), 'A Comparison of Iatrogenic Injury Studies in Australia and the USA. II: Reviewer Behaviour and Quality of Care', *International Journal for Quality in Health Care* 12:5, 379–88.

9   Based on a 5 per cent mortality from elective abdominal aortic surgery in Western Australian cases. Semmens, J.B. et al. (1998), 'The Quality of Surgical Care Project: a Model to Evaluate Surgical Outcomes in Western Australia Using Population-Based Record Linkage', *Australian and New Zealand Journal of Surgery* 68:6, 397–403, and Semmens, J.B. et al. (1998), 'The Quality of Surgical Care Project: Benchmark Standards of Open Resection for Abdominal Aortic Aneurysms in Western Australia', *Australian and New Zealand Journal of Surgery* 68:6, 404–10.

10 Based on a 50 per cent mortality from emergency abdominal aortic aneurysm surgery in Western Australian cases, with the incremental risk being assumed to arise in the 24 hours during and after the procedure. See the two articles by Semmens et al. (1998) cited above.

11 Ropeik, D and Gray, G. (2002), *Risk: A Practical Guide for Deciding What's Really Safe and What's Really Dangerous in the World Around You* (Boston: Houghton Mifflin).

12 There were 90 maternal deaths in the triennium 1997–9 or 30 per annum in an Australian population of 18.9 million, extrapolated to approximately 150 in 100 million: Slaytor, E.K. et al. (2004), *Maternal Deaths in Australia 1997–1999* (Canberra: Australian Institute of Health and Welfare).

13 Transfusion-related AIDS deaths are a legacy of the early 1980s. This is an average for AIDS deaths by transmission category for 2000–2004 for the United States assuming a population of approximately 300 million: Centers for Disease Control and Prevention, Department of Human Services and Health (2004), 'Estimated Numbers of Deaths of Persons with AIDS, by Year of Death and Selected Characteristics, 2000–2004 – United

States'. Web-page updated February 2006. Available at: <http://www.cdc.gov/hiv/topics/surveillance/resources/reports/2004report/table7.htm> accessed 29 May 2006. In Australia prior to 1985:

> as many as 350 people in New South Wales and more than 500 Australia-wide contracted HIV through contaminated blood, blood products, organ transplants and artificial insemination by donors. In May 1985 effective universal testing of all blood products and human tissues for the HIV virus commenced throughout Australia. We are unaware of anyone in New South Wales or Australia who has acquired HIV as a result of a medical procedure after testing began.

The Hon. Elaine Nile, 'Medically Acquired AIDS Victims Compensation Bill, Second Reading', New South Wales Legislative Council *Hansard*, Article No. 6 of 19th November 1992.

14 Based on Australian figures of 130 deaths related to anaesthesia in the triennium 1997–9, or 43 per annum in a population of 18.9 million. See: Mackay, P. (ed.) (2002), Safety of Anaesthesia in Australia – A Review of Anaesthesia Related Mortality 1997–1999, Report of the Committee convened under the auspices of the Australian and New Zealand College of Anaesthetists (Melbourne: Australian and New Zealand College of Anaesthetists).

15 Wilson, R.M. et al. (1995), 'The Quality in Australian Health Care Study', *Medical Journal of Australia* 163:9, 458–71.

16 Based on 9 parachuting deaths recorded in the National Coroners Information System in 5 years from August 2000 to July 2005 in Australia in a population of approximately 20 million: extrapolated to 9 per annum in 100 million. National Coronial Information System Team (2005), 'The Benefits of the National Coroners Information System (NCIS). The World's First National Database of Coronial Information', Victorian Institute of Forensic Medicine, [web document]. Available at: <http://www.vifp.monash.edu.au/ncis/web_pages/Benefits%20of%20NCIS%20_update%20Oct%2005_.pdf> accessed 29 May 2006.

17 In 2002–03, 1,833 abdominal aortic aneurysm operations were performed in Australia: Australian Institute of Health and Welfare (2005) *Procedures for Peripheral Vascular Disease* [webpage]. Estimates based on Western Australian cases: of those who undergo elective surgery for abdominal aortic aneurysm, who represent 80 per cent of such operations, 4.4 per cent die within 30 days.: Semmens, J.B. et al. (1998), 'Population-Based Record Linkage Study of the Incidence of Abdominal Aortic Aneurysm in Western Australia in 1985–1994', *British Journal of Surgery* 85:5, 648–52. This extrapolates to 323 per 100 million population per annum.

18 Estimates based on Western Australian cases: of those who undergo emergency abdominal aortic surgery for ruptured aneurysm, who represent 20 per cent of such operations, 35 per cent die within 30 days: Semmens, J.B. et al. (1998), 'Population-Based Record Linkage Study of the Incidence of Abdominal Aortic Aneurysm in Western Australia in 1985–1994', *British Journal of Surgery* 85:5, 648–52. This extrapolates to 642 per 100 million population per annum.

19 National Breast Cancer Centre, (2004), *Early Detection of Breast Cancer – Position Statement* (Camperdown, New South Wales: National Breast Cancer Centre) <http://www.nbcc.org.au/resources/documents/EDP_earlydetectionposition0804.pdf> accessed 29 May 2006.

20 Calle, E.E. et al. (2003), 'Overweight, Obesity, and Mortality from Cancer in a Prospectively Studied Cohort of U.S. Adults', *New England Journal of Medicine* 348:17, 1625–38.
21 Estimated 2002 annual world mortality due to smoking was 5,000,000 or approximately 14,000 per day. World Health Organization (2003), *World Health Report: 2003: Shaping the Future* (Geneva: World Health Organization) p. 91.
22 Goldman, L. et al. (1977), 'Multifactorial Index of Cardiac Risk in Noncardiac Surgical Procedures', *New England Journal of Medicine* 297:16, 845–50.
23 Nashef, S.A. et al. (2002), 'Validation of European System for Cardiac Operative Risk Evaluation (EuroSCORE) in North American Cardiac Surgery', *European Journal of Cardiothoracic Surgery* 22:1, 101–5.
24 Edmonds, M.J. et al. (2004), 'Evidence-Based Risk Factors For Post-Operative Deep Vein Thrombosis', *Australian and New Zealand Journal of Surgery* 74:12, 1082–97.
25 Coventry, B. (2005), personal communication. Department of Surgery, Royal Adelaide Hospital.
26 Semmens, J.B. et al. (1998), 'The Quality of Surgical Care Project: a Model to Evaluate Surgical Outcomes in Western Australia Using Population-Based Record Linkage', *Australian and New Zealand Journal of Surgery* 68:6, 397–403.
27 Kennedy, I. (2001), *Learning from Bristol: The Report of the Public Inquiry into Children's Heart Surgery at the Bristol Royal Infirmary 1984–1995*, CM 5207 (London: The Stationery Office). Available at: <http://www.bristol-inquiry.org.uk/> accessed 29 May 2006.
28 Department of Health, United Kingdom (2002), *Learning from Bristol: The DH Response to the Report of the Public Inquiry into Children's Heart Surgery at the Bristol Royal Infirmary 1984–1995*, CM 5363 (London: The Stationery Office).
29 McGlynn, E.A. et al. (2003), 'The Quality of Health Care Delivered to Adults in the United States', *New England Journal of Medicine* 348:26, 2635–45.
30 Mills, D.H., ed. (1977), *Report on the Medical Insurance Feasibility Study* (San Francisco: Sutter Publications).
31 Brennan, T.A. et al. (1991), 'Incidents of Adverse Events and Negligence in Hospitalised Patients: Results of the Harvard Medical Practice Study I', *New England Journal of Medicine* 324:6, 370–6.
32 Leape, L.L. (1994), 'Error in Medicine', *Journal of the American Medical Association* 272:33, 1851–7.
33 Hayward, R.A. and Hofer, T.P. (2001), 'Estimating Hospital Deaths Due To Medical Errors: Preventability is in the Eye of the Reviewer', *Journal of the American Medical Association* 286:4, 415–20.
34 Thomas, M.J. et al. (1999), 'Costs of Medical Injuries in Utah and Colorado', *Inquiry* 36:3, 255–64.
35 Runciman, W.B. et al. (2000), 'A Comparison of Iatrogenic Injury Studies in Australia and the USA. II: Reviewer Behaviour and Quality of Care', *International Journal for Quality in Health Care* 12:5, 379–88. This re-analysis of the Utah-Colorado data showed that many minor, transient or delayed events shown by separate studies to have similar prevalence in the USA as Australia were apparently not counted by US reviewers.
36 Baker, G.R. et al. (2004), 'The Canadian Adverse Events Study: the Incidence of Adverse Events Among Hospital Patients in Canada', *Canadian Medical Association Journal* 17:11, 1678–86.

37 Schioler, T. et al.; Danish Adverse Event Study (2001), 'Incidence of Adverse Events in Hospitals. A Retrospective Study of Medical Records' [in Danish], *Ugeskr Laeger* 163:39, 5370–8.

38 Vincent, C., Neale, G. and Woloshynowych, M. (2001), 'Adverse Events in British Hospitals: Preliminary Retrospective Record Review', *British Medical Journal* 322:7285, 517–9.

39 Davis, P. et al. (2001), Adverse Events in New Zealand Public Hospitals: Principal Findings from a National Survey (Wellington, New Zealand: Ministry of Health).

40 Runciman, W.B., Edmonds, M. and Pradhan, M. (2002), 'Setting Priorities for Patient Safety', *Quality and Safety in Health Care* 11:3, 224–9.

41 Andrews, L.B. et al. (1997), 'An Alternative Strategy for Studying Adverse Events in Medical Care', *Lancet* 349:9048, 309–13.

42 Runciman, W.B. and Moller, J. (2001), *Iatrogenic Injury in Australia* (Adelaide: Australian Patient Safety Foundation). Available at <http://www.apsf.net.au>.

43 Forster, A.J. et al. (2004), 'Adverse Events Among Medical Patients After Discharge from Hospital', *Canadian Medical Association Journal* 170:3, 345–9.

44 Forster, A.J. et al., Ottawa Hospital Patient Safety Study (2004), 'Ottawa Hospital Patient Safety Study: Incidence and Timing of Adverse Events in Patients Admitted to a Canadian Teaching Hospital', *Canadian Medical Association Journal* 170:8, 1235–41.

45 World Health Organization (1992), International Statistical Classification of Diseases and Related Health Problems, 10th revision (Geneva: World Health Organization).

46 Hargreaves, J. (2001), *Reporting of Adverse Events in Routinely Collected Data Sets in Australia,* Australian Institute of Health and Welfare Health Division Working Paper No. 3 (Canberra: Australian Institute of Health and Welfare).

47 Roughead, E.E. (1999). 'The Nature and Extent of Drug-Related Hospitalisations in Australia', *Journal of Quality in Clinical Practice* 19:1, 19–22.

48 This represents a re-arrangement (previously unpublished) of the data in reference 40.

49 Includes breakdown/failure of repair/rejection (4 per cent); incisional/ recurrent hernia 3 per cent; poor functional or cosmetic result (3 per cent); wound breakdown (2 per cent); scar/adhesion (2 per cent); technical or mechanical failure (2 per cent); failure to reduce fracture (2 per cent) (see note 45).

50 Includes wound infection after procedure (8 per cent); urinary tract infection (3 per cent); via drain/catheter/implant/cannula (2 per cent); abscess/other post-procedural (2 per cent) (see note 45).

51 Includes management, planning, education problem (6 per cent); diagnosis delayed, not made, or wrong (6 per cent) (see note 45).

52 Includes urinary tract obstruction (3 per cent); cardiovascular – infarct, dysrhythmia (3 per cent); metabolic, fluid, electrolytes (4 per cent); neurological (stroke, nerve damage) (2 per cent) (see note 45).

53 Includes pressure sore (3 per cent); fall (2 per cent); damaged organs/blood vessels (2 per cent) (see note 45).

54 Includes side effect/toxic effect of medication (3 per cent); NSAID-related gastrointestinal bleed (2 per cent); overdose of medication (1 per cent) (see note 45).

55 Includes pain (3 per cent); nausea and vomiting (2 per cent) (see note 45).

56 Includes haemorrhage (3 per cent); haematoma (2 per cent) (see note 45).

57 Britt, H. et al. (2003), *General Practice Activity in Australia, 2002–3*, Cat. No. GEP14 (Canberra: Australian Institute of Health and Welfare).

58 Wanzel, K.R., Jamieson, C.G., Bohnen, J.M. (2000), 'Complications on a General Surgery Service: Incidents and Reporting', *Canadian Journal of Surgery* 43:2, 113–7.

59 Clark, R.B. (2004), *Healthcare and Notions of Risk* (Melbourne: Therapeutic Guidelines Limited).

60 Harris, L. and Associates (1997), *Public Opinion of Patient Safety Issues: Research Findings*, Commissioned for the National Patient Safety Foundation at the American Medical Association, September 1997.

61 The Confidential Enquiries into Maternal Deaths in the United Kingdom (2001), *Why Mothers Die 1997–1999*, RCOG Press (London: Royal College of Obstetricians and Gynaecologists).

62 Australian Institute of Health and Welfare, National Perinatal Statistics Unit (2001), *Report on Maternal Deaths in Australia 1994–96* (Canberra: Commonwealth of Australia).

63 Gibbs, N., (2006), *Safety of Anesthesia in Australia. A review of Anaesthesia Mortality 2000-2002.* (Melbourne: Australian and New Zealand College of Anaesthetists).

64 Lagasse, R.S. (2002), 'Anaesthesia Safety: Model or Myth? A Review of the Published Literature and Analysis of Current Original Data', *Anesthesiology* 97:6, 1609–17.

65 Scottish Audit of Surgical Mortality, The Royal College of Physicians and Surgeons of Glasgow, Glasgow <http://www.sasm.org.uk>.

66 Runciman, W.B. et al. (2003), 'Adverse Drug Events and Medication Errors in Australia', *International Journal for Quality in Health Care* 15:Suppl.1, i49–i59.

67 Medical Devices Agency <http://www.raps.org/2001ac/stories.22>.

68 Australian Government, Department of Health and Ageing, Therapeutic Goods Administration <http://www.tga.gov.au>.

69 Centre for Devices and Radiological Health at the United States Food and Drug Administration <http://www.fda.gov/cdrh/>.

70 ECRI, Adverse-Event and Product Defect Reporting Systems <http://www.ecri.org/Products_and_Services/Services/Product_Defect_Reporting_Systems>.

71 Shared Meanings Consultative Group, Australian Council for Safety and Quality in Health Care <http://www.safetyandquality.org>.

72 Runciman, W.B. (1996), 'Incident Monitoring', *Clinical Anaesthesiology* 10:2, 333–56.

73 Runciman, W.B. (2002), 'Lessons from the Australian Patient Safety Foundation: Setting Up a National Patient Safety Surveillance System – Is This the Right Model?', *Quality and Safety in Health Care* 11:3, 246–51.

74 United Kingdom Department of Health (2000), An Organisation with a Memory – Report of an Expert Group on Learning from Adverse Events in the NHS Chaired by the Chief Medical Officer (London: The Stationery Office).

75 Aspden, P. et al. (eds), Institute of Medicine (2004), *Patient Safety: Achieving a New Standard for Care* (Washington: The National Academies Press).

76 Australian Patient Safety Foundation, Adelaide <http://www.apsf.net.au/>.

77 Runciman, W.B., et al. (2005), 'Crisis Management during Anaesthesia: the Development of an Anaesthetic Crisis Management Manual', *Quality and Safety in Health Care* 14:3, e1.

78 Symposium (1993), 'The Australian Incident Monitoring Study', *Anaesthesia and Intensive Care* 21:5, 505–695.

79 Beckmann, U. et al. (2003), 'Evaluation of Two Methods for Quality Improvement in Intensive Care: Facilitated Incident Monitoring and Retrospective Medical Chart Review', *Critical Care Medicine* 31:4, 1006–11.

80 Vinen, J. (2000), 'Incident Monitoring in Emergency Departments: an Australian Model', *Academic Emergency Medicine*. 7:11, 1290–7.

81 Caplan, R.A. et al. (1990), 'Adverse Respiratory Events in Anaesthesia: a Closed Claims Analysis', *Anesthesiology* 72:5, 828–33.

82 Aders, A. and Aders, H. (2005), 'Anaesthesia Adverse Incident Reports: an Australian Study of 1,231 Outcomes', *Anaesthesia and Intensive Care* 33:3, 336–44.
83 Runciman, W.B. (2005), 'Iatrogenic Harm and Anaesthesia in Australia', *Anaesthesia and Intensive Care* 33:3, 297–300.
84 Bagian, J.P. et al. (2002), 'The Veterans Affairs Root Cause Analysis System in Action', *Joint Commission Journal on Quality Improvement* 28:10, 531–45.
85 Reportable Sentinel Events: Joint Commission on Accreditation of Healthcare Organizations (2002), *Sentinel Event Policy & Procedures, Updated June 2005* [web document], available at: http://www.jcaho.org/SentinelEvents/PolicyandProcedures/ se_pp.htm and latest statistics extracted from: *Sentinel Event Statistics: As of December 31, 2005* http://www.jcaho.org/SentinelEvents/Statistics/>.
86 There are eight major categories of reportable sentinel events in Australia. There were 175 for the States of New South Wales and Victoria. There were 112 sentinel events in these categories reported from public hospitals and health facilities in the State of New South Wales for the three-year period 2002–5: New South Wales Department of Health (2005), *Patient Safety and Clinical Quality Program: Second Report on Incident Management in the NSW Public Health System, 2004–2005* (North Sydney: New South Wales Department of Health) p. 11.
87 In the State of Victoria, Australia, 63 sentinel events were reported from public hospitals and health services in the eight specified categories for the two-year period 2003–2005: Rural and Regional Health and Aged Care Service Division, Victorian Government Department of Human Services (2005), *Sentinel Event Program – Annual Report 2004– 05* (Melbourne: State of Victoria, Department of Human Services) p. 14.
88 Although rape is the reportable event, the JCAHO sentinel event statistics combine rape, assault and homicide together.
89 Clinton, H.R. and Obama, B. (2006), 'Making Patient Safety the Centerpiece of Medical Liability Reform', *New England Journal of Medicine* 354:21, 2205–8.
90 National Coroners Information System (Australia), www.ncis.org.au/.
92 Runciman, W.B. et al (2006), 'An Integrated Framework for Safety, Quality and Risk Management: An Information and Incident Management System based on a Universal Patient Safety Classification', *Quality and Safety in Healthcare* 15:Suppl I, i82-i90.

Chapter 3

Healthcare: A Dysfunctional System

Millions of patients are treated every day all over the world. Most receive effective treatment and find the experience largely positive. Many patients express gratitude for having been looked after and admiration for those who cared for them. However, this gratitude is often felt in spite of disjointed and uncomfortable experiences. Sometimes, it reflects recognition of the fact that those caring for them were clearly doing their best in the face of considerable shortcomings in the system. A surprising number of people fail to get appropriate care or get inappropriate care.[1] Furthermore, particularly when there are complex problems or the patient is very sick, things can and do go wrong. Failures are more likely to occur if the best approach to the patient's problems remains uncertain, and if several clinicians from a range of disciplines are involved in dealing with them.

Inadequate resources and inadequately trained staff may compromise even basic care. To these problems we may add many more, including poor communication and availability of information, poor infrastructure, bad rostering, staff shortages and insufficient time. The sum of these malfunctions is a dysfunctional system. Morale amongst doctors, nurses and allied healthcare workers may be low, and they often feel that there is little they can do to improve matters.

In this chapter we will address the context in which healthcare is delivered (see the first line of Figure 2.1) and some of the factors which create hazards and contribute to risk (see the top section of Figure 1.6). Environmental and organizational factors are of particular relevance to this chapter; and some patient related risks were dealt with in Chapter 2 (pages 34 and 35).

Traditionally, risk management is limited to those factors that are within the control of the individuals who are trying to manage the risk. *Environmental factors* may not be under the direct control of individual healthcare professionals or of the people running the organizations, facilities and services in which they work. *Organizational factors* are within the control of those who run organizations, facilities or professional groups, but, unlike behavioural factors (see Chapter 5), they are not usually under the direct control of the individuals or teams who treat patients.

In healthcare a gulf often exists between the rhetoric of bureaucrats at the national or state level and the realities of the practice of healthcare; this has been referred to as the quality 'chasm'.[2] Similarly, within healthcare organizations there is often a gap between the administrators and the practitioners (see Box 3.1). The

---

Box 3.1 Life in the chasm

A large teaching hospital recently established a high level multi-disciplinary group to evaluate new technologies with a view to their purchase and use. A request was made to include, within the terms of reference of the expert group, an evaluation of the purchase and use of existing technologies. It was pointed out that very considerable problems were being encountered in the intensive care unit, with many near misses, with equipment such as ventilators, dialysis machines, balloon pumps and the like. Staff not credentialed to work with this equipment were having to look after patients on whom it was being used. More than 50 per cent of the intensive care nursing staff were junior and/or not critically care trained and the ratio of clinical nurse educators to staff was one sixth of that recommended by the critical care nurses association.

The official response was that 'in service' training was the responsibility of each unit. When it was pointed out that senior nurses were already working 'back to back' shifts when the unit was busy, and that it was logistically impossible to properly discharge training responsibilities, the problem was given the 'Nelsonian' blind eye by the hospital executive.

'hidden culture' of those who actually control what happens in the front line is discussed later in this chapter (also, see pages 170–172).

Much dysfunction in healthcare occurs because of problems at the interfaces between the larger system and organizations, between organizations and individuals, between different sectors of the health service and between different professional groups within hospitals.[3] Problems at one level manifest at other levels. Corrective strategies may need to address the behaviours of groups as diverse as politicians, senior administrators and clinicians. One solution is for clinicians to become involved in the management of hospitals, and this is being increasingly encouraged.[4,5] Unfortunately, the tendency is for these clinicians to be given responsibility for the delivery of healthcare but little authority or financial autonomy to empower them in the discharge of this responsibility.[6] It is not surprising that this approach adds to the sense of helplessness amongst those who actually have to deliver the healthcare.

Many healthcare workers feel trapped. They think that changing the system is too hard and have given up trying to fix it. In a study involving interns and residents in an Australian hospital the junior doctors recognized the role played by poor system design and bad work practices in the causation of errors, but they did not think these things could be changed, nor did they see which changes might be beneficial.[7]

Individuals at any level do in fact have a reasonable chance of changing those things that are within their purview, and can manage their own interactions with patients and the system so that safety is maximized and any errors or system failures are followed up (see page 233). However, it is frustrating when obvious, well documented deficiencies continue to be ignored (see Box 3.1). A fundamental problem is that hospital administrators are captive to a bureaucratic system far removed from clinical care. They are expected to come in 'on budget', and to argue for ever-more 'efficiency savings' (a euphemism for having to do the same or more work for less money). Relentless 'squeezing' actually leads to 'inefficiency costs' in terms not only of safety and quality, but of throughput (see Box 10.5).

In this chapter we will discuss factors which adversely affect system design and function (Box 3.2) and those which adversely affect the performance and behaviour of the professionals who work in the system (Box 3.4). These factors act in concert to reduce the functionality of the health system. There are many practitioners who have crafted their own immediate environments, to which many of these comments do not apply. However, in many institutions, most of the comments are all too true.

An important point in understanding the present situation is to appreciate that the healthcare system has not suddenly become dysfunctional. Many of the problems are a legacy of the haphazard evolution of healthcare over many years.

The Evolution of Healthcare

The story of the evolution of healthcare is primarily one of impressive achievements which have improved the condition of mankind. However, it is also one of frustrating failures to deliver the potential of advances in knowledge and technology by failing to introduce them systematically, with proper amelioration of the risks inherent in their introduction.

Advances in healthcare have been documented since the beginnings of recorded history. Over 250 medications of vegetable and 120 of animal origin were described by the Babylonians and the Assyrians in cuneiform script on clay tablets over 4,000 years ago.[8] Some of these, such as opium, from which morphine was extracted 200 years ago, are still in use today. Extensive medical texts were produced in Egypt, India, and China between this time and the birth of Christ. Temples of healing flourished 2,500 years ago as part of the cult of Asclepius in ancient Greece.[9] The staff of Asclepius, entwined by a single snake, has become widely adopted as the symbol of medicine. Hippocrates, thought by many to be the father of modern medicine, trained at the Asclepium on the island of Kos.

The Romans built a chain of hospitals for wounded soldiers which expanded in the middle-ages into monastic centres, where monks looked after religious followers and the poor. In England, non-profit hospitals date from the dismantling of these monastic infirmaries by King Henry VIII some 500 years ago, leaving thousands of sick and infirm without refuge. Hospitals as we now know them began to flourish about 150 years ago, when they were transformed from multi-purpose centres of charity for sheltering the sick and poor to institutions for the treatment of patients, medical research and the education of nursing and medical students. Impetus was given to these by Florence Nightingale, 'The Lady of the Lamp', who made her name during the Crimean War, after which she established the Nightingale School for Nurses in 1860.[10]

Two types of training emerged for doctors. Two hundred years ago, one could either obtain a qualification in medicine at a university to become a physician, or one could become an apprentice to a surgeon or apothecary and learn the trade from the master. Apprentices were provided opportunities to acquire manual skills, but were not expected to learn from text books.

Within the last 150 years, the discovery of modern anesthesia has been disseminated (1846),[11] Darwin propounded the theory of evolution (1858),[12] Claude Bernard founded modern physiology and described the scientific method (1858),[13] and Pasteur demonstrated that fermentation and putrification were due to micro-organisms (1864). Semmelweiss in Vienna identified the role of 'putrid particles' in the causation of puerperal fever, and introduced hand disinfection with chlorinated lime in the 1850s.[14] Lister introduced carbolic spray and the beginnings of surgical antisepsis in the 1860s, and in 1895 Roentgen published his discovery of a new type of radiation which he called 'X-rays'. The natural outcome of these advances was the development of medical specialization which occurred alongside the growth of hospitals, and which led to the evolution of the roles of the various healthcare professionals we know today. We will discuss aspects of this ongoing evolution with respect to nurses, doctors and pharmacists. A discussion of this process for the many other healthcare professionals who contribute to modern healthcare (physiotherapists, occupational therapists, dieticians, social workers, biomedical engineers and many others) is beyond the scope of this book.

Healthcare Professionals

Nurses

For over 100 years the training of nurses was hospital-based. Nurses learned on the job, under supervision, while dealing with the basic needs of patients. Since the 1970s there has been a progressive move towards a greater emphasis on the academic content of nursing training, and today many nurses are trained primarily in universities or technical institutes, with time on the wards spent in predominantly supernumerary roles, under supervision. In parallel with this change, the organization of nursing within hospitals has changed. In the past, the structure was very hierarchical. A senior nurse (the 'charge nurse') was typically in charge of the ward. Tasks were distributed on the basis of the seniority and experience of the staff. Menial tasks were seen as an appropriate part of a student nurse's training. The charge nurse supervised junior nurses and, often, junior doctors as well (perhaps informally, but usually effectively). She provided a single source for information about anything related to any of her patients. The strength of this system was that charge nurses often stayed in the same position for many years and developed high levels of expertise in their particular fields. They were a major force for coordination and safety. Today, many hospitals have moved to a much flatter system of nursing administration in which the emphasis is on individual responsibility. Patients rather than tasks are distributed, with individual nurses responsible for all aspects of any one patient's nursing care. This is said to be more holistic and equitable. In theory each nurse can know more about a smaller number of patients, and therefore take a more effective role in the management of each one. There are obviously many advantages with this approach. It has also been associated with enhanced status and expertise for nurses. On the other hand, it requires new methods of coordinating patient care, and can be problematic if the nurses are allocated patients beyond their scope of practice. With this model, peer support may be less as nurses focus solely on their own allocated patients. In addition, the increased use of agency nurses in recent years has added new problems. Patients with complex problems end up under the care of nurses with unknown skill-sets, whose competencies cannot easily be assessed, and who have little or no knowledge of local physical and functional arrangements. As the organization of doctors within hospitals has also changed over the last 20 years or so (see below), again in the context of changes to training, the net effect has been a substantially more complex interface between nursing and medical teams.

Pharmacists

Modern pharmacists have moved away from their origins in the hands-on medicine-formulating activities of the apothecaries of former times. In retail pharmacies and on hospital wards, they increasingly play a valuable role at the interface of healthcare with patients, checking the prescription and administration of drugs. To a large extent the challenges faced by pharmacists today are explicitly those of process – ensuring that prescribed medication actually completes its journey from dispensary to its target site within a patient without some form of error occurring on the way. The emphasis in training has therefore shifted from technical matters (related to the identification of plants and the preparation of drugs) to process and safety. Problems tend to occur at the interfaces between the pharmacists and those who prescribe and administer drugs (doctors, nurses, carers and the patients themselves), and administrators, who sometimes leave pharmacists out of the design of processes in which they (the pharmacists) are the experts.

Doctors

Medical students   Bedside teaching has been employed in the education of medical students for several hundred years. Today medical training involves a combination of a formal scientific curriculum with an apprenticeship under experienced clinicians.[15] Medical students are expected to participate in clinical attachments on the wards of hospitals, or in outpatient clinics. Their role is initially supernumerary, but there is usually an expectation that students will gradually begin contributing to basic tasks such as the clerking of patients, and that this contribution will increase as they become more experienced. In this way trainees learn on the job and contribute service at the same time.

Junior doctors   It became apparent that most doctors, on qualifying, would benefit from more practical experience before entering unsupervised independent practice.

For example, at Johns Hopkins Hospital in the USA it was a requirement as early as 1890 for resident physicians, surgeons and gynaecologists to have at least 18 months hospital experience before being appointed (even though these positions were unpaid at the time). In the UK, medical graduates have been required to undertake a pre-registration year as 'housemen' since 1953. Compulsory pre-registration experience was introduced in Australia as early as 1930. These house doctors or interns undertook most of the basic medical management of patients on the wards. They were expected to know all the patients under the care of their 'team' or 'firm'. They were required to work very long hours (often more than 100 per week), night and day, thereby ensuring continuity of care. In return, these long hours, often associated with heavy clinical loads, provided the opportunity to develop a high level of clinical expertise very rapidly. The trainees themselves recognized the value of this opportunity to equip themselves to enter independent practice.

Recognition by all concerned of the value of supervised training in hospitals, in combination with the development of specialization, has led to the establishment of postgraduate programmes for specialist training. The system is one of variety and complexity – there is little standardization, and little uniformity between programmes. In America, doctors at the level of specialist trainees are called residents (by the 1970s most US post graduate training programs were linked to specialist residency training); in the 'British' system they are called registrars.[16] In the British system, an emphasis on broadly-based foundations has been retained, and junior doctors are required to complete attachments in a number of different fields before starting their specialist training. The idea is to ensure basic clinical competence, and to enable specialists to recognize conditions outside their own narrow area of expertise. In the USA, the approach has been a little different. Specialization is encouraged from the earliest possible opportunity (to the extent of replacing internship with direct entry into residency). This may be more efficient in producing qualified specialist doctors (training typically takes longer in the British system), but it must of necessarily result in a loss of broadly-based basic training.

Senior doctors Apprenticeship training depends on supervision from senior doctors. Fully qualified doctors are called different things in different countries. In many countries specialist doctors may work in more than one hospital, or only part time within a hospital (the remaining time being spent in private clinics or rooms, for example). In Britain the notion of a 'consultant' became synonymous with the position of the qualified specialist, and was formalized as a grade or rank within the National Health Service. Other countries have preferred terms such as Visiting Specialist, Staff Specialist, Attending and so on to describe doctors who are no longer in training. We will adopt the term 'specialist' to mean any doctor fully trained in a medical specialty. We note that many general practitioners (or family doctors) now undergo postgraduate training equivalent to that of many specialists, but they are by definition generalists. In some areas these general practitioners have no role within hospitals, but in others they admit and care for patients in hospitals, particularly in smaller centres.

In the past, public hospital specialists held unpaid 'honorary' positions, and earned their living from their private clinics. Their obligations to the hospital included the training of medical students and the supervision of junior doctors. This arrangement was gradually put onto a more formal basis, and increasingly a remunerated one. In Britain consultants have had legal responsibility for all in-patient beds and out-patient sessions since 1948. As with nurses and junior doctors, the role of specialist doctors has continued to change with time.

Factors Which May Adversely Affect the Design and Function of the Healthcare System

There are many interacting factors that adversely affect the design and function of the healthcare system, many of which have arisen from its ad-hoc evolution (Box 3.2). Donald Berwick made famous the saying that 'every system is perfectly designed to produce the results that it does'.[17] Iatrogenic harm is the natural outcome of the way healthcare is designed and delivered. Indeed, the healthcare system has not really been designed at all, but instead has evolved haphazardly over time, and continues to do so.

Box 3.2 Factors which may adversely affect the design and function of the healthcare system

- Opaque complexity and a lack of useful data.
- Application of the machine metaphor to healthcare.
- Treatment of diseases versus promotion of health.
- Failure to deliver the right care.
- Placement of hospitals at the hub of the system.
- Specialization, compartmentalization and duplication.
- Poor coordination of care.
- Poor continuity of care.
- Conflict between training and service delivery.
- Failure to maintain standards in training hospitals.
- Conflict between clinical and corporate governance.
- Competing agendas and a clash of cultures.
- Repeated restructuring of organizations.
- Focus on the 'bottom line'.

Opaque Complexity and a Lack of Useful Data

There is no convenient, single source of information about the performance of the system, or its component sub-systems, with respect to any of the dimensions of the quality of healthcare (see Figure 1.1 and Chapter 2). The complexity of the system helps to conceal the extent of its overall malfunction. Individual staff members may only experience or observe problems once in a while, and often only perceive those that relate to their own sphere of activities. Only when the things that go wrong are collated across the whole system is the full impact on patients revealed (see pages 37–50).

This lack of relevant information[18,19] is, in part, the consequence of inadequate measurement tools.[15,20] Resistance to scrutiny of the performance of healthcare professionals is also a factor.[21,22] There is strong evidence that better health outcomes are achievable when measurement is integrated into everyday clinical practice.[23] Unfortunately, this is not often done.

Application of the Machine Metaphor to Healthcare

A mechanistic approach to fixing deficiencies in the system has been largely ineffective. The machine metaphor, which implies that a problem in one part can be easily fixed without reference to other parts, is particularly inappropriate because the health system is not static. Its components are complex, dynamic and interdependent.[24] In the imagery of Mant, healthcare is not like a bicycle, on which components can be interchanged without disruption of overall function, but like a frog. A frog does not respond well to partial dismemberment in the interests of restructuring.[25] Many who work in healthcare are aware of the problems listed in Boxes 3.2 and 3.4, but have no strategies for addressing them. It seems that few regard fixing the overall system as their responsibility, even those (notably clinicians) who may be the only people with the necessary insight into the underlying problems.

Treatment of Diseases Versus Promotion of Health

In 1948 the WHO defined health as 'a state of complete physical, mental and social well-being and not merely the absence of disease or infirmity' (see page 2).[26] Historically, healthcare evolved in a reactive mode, responding after the event to injuries and diseases. The prevention of disease and promotion of health was given low priority. It has become apparent that maintaining a good quality of life and preventing disease and disability is more cost effective than treatment. It is better to persuade people to stop smoking, exercise, eat a balanced diet, and pay attention to their blood pressure and lipid profiles than to spend huge sums managing crippling respiratory disease, heart failure, stroke and cancer. The current emphasis on the disease model of healthcare tends to reduce the focus on health and wellbeing (also see page 2), although there are some encouraging trends in the emphasis on prevention by organizations such as the National Heart Foundation in Australia.[27]

Failure to Deliver the Right Care

A study in the USA showed that care in accordance with 439 indicators (representing appropriate basic healthcare) was being delivered only 55 per cent of the time (see Figure 1.2).[1] The figure ranged from as low as 10 per cent (for the referral for counselling of problem drinkers), to as high as 80 per cent (for an appropriate response for senile cataracts). For many problems correct care was achieved about half the time. A proportion of the patients who do not receive appropriate care, or who receive inappropriate care, will come to harm. They could end up in hospital, and may even die. These patients are part of the wider problem of iatrogenic harm (see page 2 and Chapter 2).

Placement of Hospitals at the Hub of the System

Hospitals occupy the top place in the health hierarchy and teaching hospitals the pinnacle. Patients become ill or suffer injury in many places every day (and night) but often cannot be treated in a timely way or close to where they live. Many of the largest hospitals are located in the 'dead hearts' of large cities; the population they once served has long since departed. In some instances this change in demography may have been offset by the fact that central locations in cities are often well served by public transport.

The needs of the community are not always integrated optimally with the activities of the profession. Most medical and nursing training is undertaken in teaching hospitals, but much of the work required of these trainees, when qualified, is in the community, in rural areas, and in preventive medicine. Their experiences in a teaching hospital do not necessarily promote these career choices, or prepare people for them. The politics of health funding are influenced by the advocacy of those who work within the system, and if these people practise predominantly in hospitals, their advocacy may well be biased towards hospitals. Greater integration of healthcare into the community ('population based healthcare') is desirable and there are moves in this direction in many areas.[28]

Specialization, Compartmentalization and Duplication

The advent of specialties and sub-specialties benefited patients through focused research, which led to improved diagnosis and treatments. Unfortunately, specialization has also led to duplication and inefficiency. Services and staff have often been added without reference to their impact on existing services and other parts of the organization.[29]

Poor Co-ordination of Care

Healthcare today tends to function in 'silos'. Each silo might be quite efficient in its own right, but the silos often communicate poorly with each other, to the detriment of patient care. For example, a patient may require an MRI scan before a decision can be made on whether to operate, and it may take several days to fit the patient into the schedule for this. The patient may then miss the next available operating list and have to face an avoidable delay in surgery. This is a lack of *horizontal* co-ordination. Effort is now going into streamlining and co-ordinating patient care, but much remains to be done.

Poor Continuity of Care

Patients are treated in hospitals, community centres, doctors' rooms and their own homes with little consideration for the care given or delivered in the other parts of the health system. There is often a lack of *longitudinal* co-ordination of care (see Box 3.3). Patients with chronic illness are expected to manage their own medications at home, yet when they are hospitalized this responsibility is taken over by staff. The consequences of this vary, and quite a number of patients have their needed medications stopped or changed. In recent years many hospitals have improved the quality and timeliness of discharge letters, but in some cases general practitioners are not adequately informed of changes in a patient's condition or treatment (or even of the fact that their patient has been hospitalized).

Box 3.3 Rest in peace: death by oversight

Mrs. Ong was a rear-seat passenger in a vehicle involved in a high speed collision in which the driver and the front-seat passenger were killed. She suffered a badly fractured pelvis and required three months' immobilization in traction. During this period, she was put on the anticoagulant coumadin to prevent the formation of deep vein thrombosis, for which she was at risk because of her immobilization. The coumadin should have been stopped when she was able to stand up and bear weight. However, on discharge it was continued by the junior doctor who wrote the discharge letter, who had just started working in the orthopaedic ward. The general practitioner assumed that this was for a good reason, and continued prescribing coumadin and monitoring her state of coagulation.

Nine months later, while her usual general practitioner was on holiday, Mrs. Ong developed a urinary tract infection and was seen by a locum doctor, who prescribed an antibiotic. Unfortunately this interacted with the coumadin, and her coagulation system failed. Mrs. Ong collapsed with a cerebral haemorrhage. On arrival at the Emergency Department, she stopped breathing and had to be intubated and ventilated. A CT scan showed a massive bleed into her brain stem and gross swelling of her brain. The coagulation status of her blood was grossly abnormal. She satisfied the criteria for brain death and life support was duly withdrawn. This all took place in the Emergency Department and she was never formally admitted to the hospital as an in-patient. For this reason her case was never audited.

Her relatives were told that she was technically dead on arrival and that she had suffered a bleed into her brain, something which was more likely as she was on the anticoagulant coumadin. They were not told that she did not need to be on coumadin in the first place or that her coagulation status was grossly abnormal as a result of a well known drug interaction. The coroner was told that she had suffered a massive cerebral haemorrhage as a result of abnormal coagulation status nine months after a car accident, and on this basis concluded that he did not have an interest in the case.

Conflict between Training and Service Delivery

Most industries separate training from service delivery. In health the distinction is often blurred. Medical students provide little in the way of service in most western countries, but junior doctors (who are trainees) have long borne the brunt of service delivery for acute care in hospitals, particularly out of hours. Training has been the poor cousin of service delivery, and has suffered. The conflict between the training requirements of junior health professionals, particularly doctors, and the provision of 24-hour medical service was identified as a significant issue in 1988 by an Australian report and remains a major challenge for teaching hospitals.[30] Three problems were identified. First, the mix of disorders affecting patients in the major hospitals is often inappropriate for training. Second, industrial and financial pressures promote the use of rosters which are not ideal for either training or service. Interns and residents rostered at night often admit patients with little or no supervision and (because of limits on hours of work) have little opportunity to continue caring for these patients during the day, and thereby observe their progress. Third, there is often a mismatch between the number of posts required for service needs and the number required for training purposes.

The combination of training with the provision of service, even in less complex environments, is generally unsatisfactory. The dual roles of trainee and service provider give rise to significant tensions in hospitals.[31,32] Dr. Jon Cohen, the chief medical officer for New York City Hospital, acknowledged the problem when he said, 'The big culture change is (that) the institutions have to recognize and treat residents as students'.[33]

Failure to Maintain Standards in Training Hospitals

Health professionals should be trained in hospitals that maintain adequate standards of care, if they are to understand and promulgate those standards themselves. With the exception of some of the specialist colleges, there appears to be little insistence on this principle. Even when hospitals must be accredited for training, there is great reluctance to stop or withdraw this accreditation when inadequate support, supervision or conditions of work are evident. There is even less protection for interns or junior doctors whose positions are not actually in accredited training schemes. Such doctors are often ineligible for accredited positions (they may be overseas graduates on restricted working visas, for example) and there may be an element of exploitation in the arrangements used by some hospitals to cover their service loads.

Improvements in monitoring for patients undergoing anaesthesia were introduced with great reluctance by many hospitals in the late 1980s. Factors which forced their introduction included threats to withdraw accreditation of some of these hospitals for training registrars (with the consequent loss of vital manpower) and the prospect of having to tell patients, as part of informed consent before operations, that the hospital could not afford monitoring equipment to satisfy basic standards of the College of Anaesthetists. Both were instrumental in obtaining funds to meet basic standards for training and patient care.

Conflict between Clinical and Corporate Governance

Since the 1990s there have been strenuous attempts to link clinical practice and corporate management, but the relations between organizational entities within healthcare are often strained. This is partly because organizations still tend to operate in groups defined by discipline (doctors, nurses, allied health workers and administrators). These disciplines maintain different methods of education, documentation and regulation, and often have different aims. This creates parallel systems in which patient care, which ought to be the primary concern of the collective organization, becomes subservient to professional agendas. Separation of groups in this way tends to reinforce a silo mentality, and to create more discontinuity and less consistency in patient care.

Competing Agendas and a Clash of Cultures

While the system of education and training for doctors has remained relatively stable, in recent years there has been a major revolution in hospital management. Hospital managers are required to manage large complex businesses, with a very varied workforce. Clinical services are required to treat individual patients. It is in the nature of a profession to function autonomously. Many doctors are ill-prepared to work as members of large organizations. Indeed, many see themselves as working for patients, rather than for an organization. Many managers are ill-prepared for the complex ethical and practical issues that characterize healthcare. Many are less well qualified than those whose activities they are asked to manage. Other groups within healthcare may have difficulty interacting with each other and with managers, and criticism between groups is common. Other factors which may adversely affect the performance and behaviour of healthcare workers are listed in Box 3.2. These circumstances do not promote mutual respect or effective cooperation. Conflict can be reconciled if the focus is the patient. This will require moving from a system dominated by either professionals or managers to a patient centred system where patients with common problems are looked after by teams of people with a common focus (see Figure 1.1). Improved teamwork was one of the key recommendations to arise from the Bristol Inquiry.[34]

Repeated Restructuring of Organizations

An almost reflex response of politicians and senior bureaucrats to crises in healthcare has been to restructure. This commonly involves a huge bureaucratic exercise in redrawing diagrams of lines of command, producing new job descriptions, and interviewing and appointing nearly all the same people to different posts. It is possible to continue to work at the frontline without even knowing that this process is taking place. However, restructuring can also have considerable deleterious effects. Threats to job security are very bad for morale;

the normal running of the healthcare system tends to go on hold; and responses to organizational crises are compromised, because many people are busy restructuring rather than addressing problems of direct relevance to patients. There is now evidence that restructuring consumes a lot of time and may set an organization back, with no changes in efficiency, outcome or quality of care (see page 267).[35] It is to be hoped that administrators and politicians will heed this evidence.

Focus on the 'Bottom Line'

The job of a Chief Executive Officer may be at risk if the budget is overspent. Administrators at this level have the invidious task each year of having to manage hospitals full of patients who are often sicker and older than the previous year, with drugs and technology which, although usually better, are nearly always more expensive than before. Unfortunately, one of the only things that can be measured in healthcare is the amount of money spent. It sometimes seems that as the bottom line is the only thing that can be seen, it is the only thing to which attention is directed. Safety and quality is compromised in myriad ways by this approach. As we have emphasized, healthcare is often inefficient, but bureaucratic restructuring is not the answer.[35] What is needed is a focus on meeting patients' needs and ensuring that the work flow is streamlined. This topic is further discussed in Chapters 11 and 12.

Factors Which May Adversely Affect the Performance and Behaviour of Healthcare Professionals

Many systemic problems impact on the performance of individual professionals and on the interactions between individuals and groups. This means that patients are often cared for by groups of individuals who communicate with each other poorly, rather than by an integrated team working to a common plan. Again, many

---

Box 3.4   Factors which may adversely affect the performance and behaviour of healthcare professionals

- Hierarchies in healthcare – power gradients.
- Territorial behaviour – imprint or perish.
- 'Turf' disputes and professional rivalries.
- Fatigue versus continuity of care.
- Poor communication and handovers.
- Lack of supervision.
- Financial arrangements and perverse incentives.
- Dispersion of accountability and responsibility.
- Poor orientation and evaluation.
- Non-compliant behaviour.
- Poor role models.

of these problems have their origins in the way healthcare has evolved and are perpetuated in order to safeguard the vested interests of particular groups. Major reform will be needed if these problems and behaviours are to be overcome. Suggestions as to how this process may be begun are given in Chapter 11 and 12.

Hierarchies in Healthcare – Power Gradients

Doctors in training are low in the medical hierarchy and depend on supervisors for instructions and learning. Maintaining the confidence of a supervisor is paramount because this relationship can influence advancement within a career. Progression depends on reports based on informal and formal feedback and on subjective and objective assessments of competence and commitment. Complaining about conditions, identifying poor patient care, drawing attention to lack of supervision or disclosing mistakes to supervisors may have repercussions for the junior doctors involved, and for their access to ongoing training.

Territorial Behaviour – Imprint or Perish

The power gradient alluded to above and the sub-cultures developed within institutions combine to exert powerful pressures on those being inducted into the various specialties. It is not enough to remain silent about obvious deficiencies in the way that a particular unit operates. In the competitive environment of many medical specialties it is essential to create a markedly positive impression. One way of doing this is to adopt the practices, behaviours and attitudes of those who are in power within the specialty one aspires to join, in much the same way that a duckling 'imprints' its mother figure, be this a genuine mother duck or an aspiring naturalist. The net effect is to retard change and maintain the status quo.

'Turf' Disputes and Professional Rivalries

Specialization and the 'silo' mentality has led, from time to time, to disagreements about who should treat certain problems. For example, in some institutions, maxillofacial surgeons (who may have a background in dentistry), plastic surgeons, ENT surgeons and neurosurgeons (all of whom have a background in medicine) may have highly collaborative arrangements, while in others there may be competition over who should be responsible for certain cases that fall within their common scope of practice. Such competition may even manifest as protracted and acrimonious disputes over who should be allowed to use specialized equipment (for example, certain endoscopes or portable imaging devices).[36]

Fatigue Versus Continuity of Care

Traditionally the service requirements for continuity of care meant that junior doctors may have been rostered on for over 120 hours per week, with no opportunity to take leave or have a weekend off for up to six months at a time. For example, a common pattern was to work from 0800 to 1700 on day one, and then to work continuously from 0800 on day two to 1700 on day three, and then to repeat the cycle. This undoubtedly meant that they were familiar with most aspects of their patients' progress and care, but they could be exhausted at the end of a 32 or 40 hour shift, and become liable to error (see Box 3.5 and page 236). Twenty hours of continuous work has been shown to produce the same degradation of performance as a blood alcohol level of 0.05mmol/l, at which it becomes illegal to drive a car in many countries.[37,38] World-wide, hours have been progressively reduced, and now the official limit for continuous work by junior doctors is typically about 16 hours. However, with short shifts, the 'handovers' to colleagues consume a much greater fraction of the overall time available for patient care. Depending on the situation, this may take over an hour at both the beginning and the end of a shift.

Box 3.5 Fatigue can kill

Fatigue was cited as a factor in a tragic case which resulted in the death of a middle-aged family man under medical treatment in a Belfast hospital. The junior doctor looking after him had been a top student in her final year of medical school. She had worked 110 hours in the week in which the accident occurred. She injected penicillin into the wrong line, with the result that the drug was administered into the central nervous system instead of a vein, with lethal effect. She was subsequently cleared of a charge of manslaughter.[39]

Poor Communication and Handovers

Even within specialized units, continuity of care and the carrying out of plans are often compromised by inadequate handovers. Typically, the doctor or doctors who are on one shift will verbally pass on to those on the next shift aspects of care that need attention, including plans for tests, investigations or treatment. The doctor handing over may be too busy to document the details properly, and important developments and facts may be 'lost' (see Box 3.6). To make matters worse the nursing handovers usually take place at a different time, have a different format, and may communicate some of the same but also some additional information (or misinformation). One of the aspects of patient management that is usually very poorly documented is that of communication – who has said what to the patient and/or his or her friends and relatives. In reviewing medical records for adverse event studies, or as a specialist doing consultations on patients on the ward, one often has to piece together what has happened to the patient using detective work, gleaning some information from the medical record, some from the nursing notes, and some by talking to the patient.

Lack of Supervision

Inadequate teaching and supervision are constant themes in surveys of junior doctors.[40] A major Australian report which makes a direct link between safety of patients and inexperienced doctors in public hospitals was the Inquiry into

Obstetric and Gynaecological Services at King Edward Memorial Hospital (Western Australia) 1990–2000.[41] Inadequate supervision of junior medical staff by consultants was identified as a serious problem facing the hospital. It was found that unsupervised junior doctors had major responsibility for assessment and the provision of care in many complex clinical situations,[42] but did not have the necessary knowledge and experience to manage complex cases. Analysis of high-risk obstetric cases showed that errors occurred in nearly half of these.

Box 3.6 Tests (and a patient) repeatedly falling into cracks in the system

Mr. Marlborough was an elderly man with severe emphysema who was referred to the pre-anaesthetic clinic to be assessed and prepared for a hernia operation. The anaesthetist ordered a chest x-ray, as the patient was an elderly smoker, had emphysema and had recently developed a cough. He made a note that this should be looked at before the operation by another anaesthetist who was to undertake the procedure. In the event, a place became unexpectedly available as a result of a cancellation, so the patient was contacted that evening and informed that he could have the procedure the next day. When the next anaesthetist saw the patient before the operation, although the x-ray had been performed, it was still in the x-ray department awaiting reporting. This anaesthetist decided that he could proceed with a local anaesthetic and did so. The patient made an uneventful recovery, but when seen two months later for follow up by the surgeon, was still complaining of a cough. The surgical registrar ordered a chest x-ray as the patient had also complained of some weight loss. The surgical registrar then went on rotation to another clinic and when the patient came back a month later, the next surgical registrar did not pick up the story in the notes about the cough and weight loss, or the fact that two x-rays had been taken.

A month later the general practitioner wrote to the hospital asking for a copy of the x-ray reports as his patient had worsening respiratory symptoms, had lost more weight, and had already had two x-rays at the hospital. The x-ray reports were found, neatly filed in the patient's medical record. The first one identified a mass in the upper lobe of his right lung which had to be regarded as malignant until proven otherwise, and suggested a CT scan and further investigation of the mass. In the second report surprise was expressed that the mass did not appear to have been investigated, and that it had increased in size. It contained further recommendations about investigation.

Mr. Marlborough was contacted urgently and admitted to hospital. The mass turned out to be cancer of the lung, which might have been operable at the time of the original hernia procedure. However, he now had secondaries in various parts of his body, including his hip. He needed to go home to put his affairs in order, but as his hip was in danger of fracturing due to the secondary, it was decided to operate on it first. He had a cardiac arrest during this operation and died. His family was advised it was not worth seeking compensation as there were no dependents.

More than half the errors were very serious: failure to recognize a serious and unstable condition and inappropriate omission of important tasks were the two most common mistakes made by junior medical staff.[41]

The problem of poor supervision at the hospital had been acknowledged by senior clinicians in 1999 who wrote: 'Low morale at the hospital stems from years of lack of supervision and teaching. Junior staff feel unsupported and over criticized. Residents have been left to their own devices and there is simply little or no supervision for junior registrars'.[42] Junior doctors were also associated with the highest occurrence of clinical errors. Resident doctors made 76 per cent of the errors associated with high-risk cases and registrars made 65 per cent of the total number of errors.

The adage 'see one, do one, teach one', is, unfortunately, all too true in some settings (see Box 3.7). One of the authors was shown once how to insert a central venous catheter via the subclavian vein, and then produced a pneumothorax in three of the first ten patients in whom he carried out this procedure. Realizing that this was unacceptable, he sought additional instruction and returned to the dissecting room to examine the relevant anatomy. His complication rate then improved progressively, with only two pneumothoraces in the last one thousand insertions.

Box 3.7   Teaching hospitals or learning hospitals?

The term teaching hospital is reserved for hospitals with university affiliations. Features of the modern teaching hospital can be traced back to early last century when the influential Flexner Report (USA) of 1910,[43] and the Haldane Commission Report of 1911 (UK)[44] were published. Today teaching hospitals have an array of complex technology for diagnosing and treating patients and conducting research.[45] However, as is apparent from the discussion in this chapter and from the anecdote in Box 3.1, some 'teaching hospitals' may sometimes be more appropriately called 'learning hospitals'.

Financial Arrangements and Perverse Incentives

Many different remuneration methods have developed in healthcare, individually and in various combinations. The structure of the health system, government policy objectives, unions and the local culture of the medical profession all influence the mix of payment methods.

Fee-for-service Fee-for-service (FFS) has been a common payment method for doctors since the beginning of medicine and still dominates many healthcare systems. Many of the problems associated with overuse of medical services, increased risks of harm to patients and inappropriate treatments can be traced to the FFS method of payment. Arguments in favour of FFS include the maintenance of clinical autonomy and freedom of choice for patients. Arguments against it include the economic incentive to provide unnecessary or overly comprehensive services, with the concomitant increased risk of avoidable iatrogenic harm.

Salary Salaried medical officers range from the rare exception to the rule, depending on the health service, discipline, and local arrangements. In some countries the gap between salaried doctors' incomes and their FFS colleagues in the private sector is substantial, and contributes to the decreased availability of senior clinicians in public hospitals.

Given relatively low rates of pay for full and part-time salaried clinicians, those wishing to recruit and retain salaried medical officers must rely on additional non-financial incentives. These include regular and predictable on-call arrangements, the ability to take leave without one's livelihood being threatened by predatory colleagues, access to research funds and students, and time for involvement in teaching and other professional activities. Increasingly, however, additional financial incentives are also required and demanded. These range from officially sanctioning some time in the private sector through to turning a blind eye to such involvement. Private patients within public hospitals, often there to gain access to specialized care or equipment unavailable in the private sector, may be billed under a variety of arrangements for salaried medical officers to obtain additional payment from this source.

Disciplines with high FFS payments for procedures tend to be dominated by private practitioners who may or may not spend some time in the public system, whereas disciplines such as oncology and anaesthesia tend to have departments staffed largely by specialists on salaries. However, there is enormous variability with respect to these arrangements both within and between hospitals and health services.

Capitation Capitation involves a health provider delivering a range of services for an agreed number of patients for an agreed price, irrespective of the services actually delivered. This has advantages, but encourages providers to give shorter consultations, or reduce the quality or quantity of services provided in other ways. 'Managed care' is an extension of this approach, in which defined groups of patients pay set premiums for (nominally) complete healthcare, including primary and preventive aspects of that care. The notion is that the provider stands to gain by providing the optimal balance between expenditure on measures to improve health and expenditure on treatment. Choice of provider is usually lost under this type of arrangement. Utilization rates become important under capitation and are core considerations in 'managed care'. Capitation may lead to less expenditure on acute care, but, in theory at least, provides no short-term incentive to expend time and money on long-term prevention and health promotion.

Mixed methods of payment and perverse incentives It is clear that when individuals are paid from more than one source there may be tensions with respect to their allegiance to the different sources of payment. Salaried specialists may interrupt continuity of treatment of public patients to take care of private patients and visiting medical officers commonly have to try to honour their commitments to the public sector by working around their private practice commitments. Even in the NHS, some specialists may end up largely working in the private sector, whilst leaving the bulk of the clinical work in the public hospitals to trainees.

Even junior medical officers may face major tensions in this regard. Recently, out of 24 trainees in one department, only one could be induced to attend a research focus session exploring attitudes of salaried doctors. The researchers offered to schedule the sessions just before the beginning or just after the end of shifts in the public sector, to pay double the normal hourly rate for attendance and to cover taxi fares. It turned out that the major reason most of the trainees could not attend these sessions was that the public hospital roster had been constructed around their commitments to providing out of hours cover for private hospitals.

There are large disparities between the various disciplines in how much can be earned by various means. In Australia, in some disciplines with an ample demand for highly remunerative procedures, trainees and those undertaking research degrees may earn more in assistant fees in the private sector than they would if they were full-time hospital salaried specialists.

There is little research on payment methods and their relationship to quality. One Cochrane review[46] evaluated the impact of different methods of payment on clinical behaviour of primary care physicians and found that FFS compared with capitation resulted in more primary care visits to specialists and more diagnostic and curative services, but fewer hospital referrals and repeat prescriptions. However, patients were less satisfied with access to the FFS physician. This review noted that salaried and capitation payments may encourage cost containment, but result in under treatment, while FFS may result in over treatment. Both can be detrimental to patient care. In a review of 15,000 medical records it was found that the problem with the greatest waste of resources was performing unsuccessful (arguably unnecessary) back operations in the private sector (over-servicing), whereas the next most costly problem, in terms of extra days in hospital, was under-investigation and inadequate treatment of ischemic heart disease in the public sector (under-servicing).[47]

Payment methods that involve incentives to provide safe, high quality services are not widely used. However, a systematic review of the literature on the effects of financial incentives on medical practice concluded that financial incentives can be used to reduce the use of healthcare resources, improve compliance with practice guidelines and achieve certain health targets.[48] It seems a pity that, all too often, they are not.

Dispersion of Accountability and Responsibility

Medicine was once an individualistic, intuitive and personal enterprise, and in the private sector, this flavour is largely retained. However, public hospitals increasingly provide a complex, impersonal service.[31] Yet the system for admitting and treating patients in public hospitals has remained essentially unchanged for over a century. Patients are still admitted under an individual clinician who theoretically makes the crucial decisions about treatment and discharge. However, while clinicians may 'own' their patients, the day-to-day needs of patients are usually managed by a hierarchy of nursing and medical staff (see Box 3.8).[49] Admitting consultants may in fact have no face-to-face meeting with some of their patients. Indeed, there are hospitals in which even the trainee scheduled to operate on a patient may not actually see the patient until he or she arrives in the operating theatre. This is clearly conducive to poor care and to increasing the risk of operating on the wrong body part or patient (see Box 11.1).

Box 3.8 An outlying patient

Mrs. Checker was a 50 year old clerk working in the supply department of the hospital. She was overweight, and slipped whilst getting the newspaper in her garden and struck her leg on a garden tap. She suffered a fracture of her fibula and was admitted because it was swollen and painful and required reduction. The procedure was delayed because the operating theatre was busy and her injury was a relatively minor one. The orthopaedic ward was full and so she was placed in a medical ward. Two days later the fracture was reduced and her leg was put into plaster. When she got up to go home, she collapsed and died. At autopsy it was found that she had suffered a massive pulmonary embolus. At no stage was heparin prescribed for the prevention of deep vein thrombosis and nor was any other preventive measure taken. Her husband was told that she had died from a clot on the lung which had formed in her leg as a result of the swelling and trauma. The lack of preventive measures was not mentioned.

Poor Orientation and Evaluation

Scheduling time for a thorough orientation of new staff to a unit is the exception rather than the rule. In Britain it is still the case that a mass 'move-around' of junior doctors from one post to the next takes place on a given day every six months. Many moves involve changing from one town to another as well as one unit to another. Consumers 'in the know' understand the importance of staying out of hospital during the following week. Some units do have a proper orientation with information about what the unit does and what is expected of staff, with an opportunity to discuss guidelines, protocols, and timetables. However, most units expect new staff to pick up this information 'on the fly'. Likewise, when staff leave the unit, most simply work their last rostered shift and move on to the next job. A few units will evaluate the staff and give feedback and constructive advice about how they have performed, and what areas might need attention, but again, this tends to be the exception rather than the rule.

A 1995 survey of Norwegian pre-registration interns found that 50 per cent of the 'medical' and 65 per cent of the 'surgical' house officers reported they received no introductory information or supervision before starting their hospital duties. Two-thirds said they did not attend any educational programmes and 80 per cent did not receive systematic feedback on their work. Most house officers received no evaluation of their work at the end of the pre-vocational year.[50] In addition to inadequate feedback on performance,[51] pre-registration house officers also perceived a lack of support from senior staff. Such perceptions are widespread.[52,53,54]

Non-compliant Behaviour

Experience from incident reports, reinforced by direct communications from nurses, reveals that there is a small subset of doctors who quite consistently fail to attend when called, and pass tasks on to the next shift. Some also behave so unpleasantly when called to help, that this provides a powerful disincentive to junior, and occasionally senior, nurses to call them.

Poor role models

Internship was originally designed to facilitate the passage from student dependency to autonomous clinical practice,[55] with the senior medical staff acting as role models. That link is sometimes remote today, because interns interact more with fellow trainees than they do with consultants. There are problems with inadequate acquisition of skills that are related to poor supervision.[56] Many interns learn procedures while unsupervised,[57,58] and are subsequently judged by supervisors to have poor technique and inadequate mastery of procedures (see Box 3.7).[59] The role models provided and attitudes projected by some part-time senior staff may promote leaving the teaching hospital environment as soon as possible to work (at least part-time) in the private sector, thus perpetuating and aggravating this cycle.

What Next?

We have discussed over two dozen factors which adversely affect system design and function, and the behaviour and performance of healthcare professionals. A further important influence on this behaviour and performance, is the human predilection for 'naming, blaming and shaming' when things go wrong. This is the subject of the next chapter.

Notes

1 McGlynn, E.A. et al. (2003), 'The Quality of Health Care Delivered to Adults in the United States', *New England Journal of Medicine* 348:26, 2635–45.
2 Institute of Medicine Committee on Quality of Health Care in America (2001), *Crossing the Quality Chasm: A New Health System for the 21st Century* (Washington DC: National Academies Press).
3 Degeling, P., Kennedy, J. and Hill, M. (2002), 'Mediating the Cultural Boundaries Between Medicine, Nursing and Management – the Essential Challenge in Hospital Reform', *Health Services Management Research* 14:1, 36–48.

4   Braithwaite, J. and Westbrook, M. (2005), 'Rethinking Clinical Organisational Structures: An Attitude Survey of Doctors, Nurses and Allied Health Staff in Clinical Directorates', *Journal of Health Services Research and Policy* 10:1, 10–7.

5   Braithwaite, J., Westbrook, M.T. and Iedema, R.A. (2005), 'Giving Voice to Health Professionals' Attitudes About Their Clinical Service Structures in Theoretical Context', *Health Care Analysis* 13:4, 315–35.

6   Braithwaite, J. (2004), 'An Empirically-Based Model for Clinician-Managers' Behavioural Routines', *Journal of Health Organization and Management* 18:4, 240–61.

7   Walton, M. (2004), 'A Multifactorial Study of Medical Mistakes Involving Interns and Residents', Ph.D. Thesis, School of Public Health (Sydney: University of Sydney).

8   Thompson, R.C. (1924), *The Assyrian Herbal. A Monograph on the Assyrian Vegetable Drugs* (London: Luzac).

9   History of Medicine Division, National Library of Medicine, National Institutes of Health. 'Asclepius', *Greek Medicine* [web resource]. Available at: <www.nlm.nih.gov/hmd/greek/greek_asclepius.html> accessed 31 May 2006.

10 Florence Nightingale Museum (2003), *Florence Nightingale* (London: Florence Nightingale Museum Trust) [web page] <www.florence-nightingale.co.uk/flo2.htm> accessed 31 May 2006.

11 Wolfe, R.J. (2001), *Tarnished Idol: William Thomas Green Morton and the Introduction of Surgical Anesthesia: A Chronicle of the Ether Controversy* (San Anselmo, California: Norman Publishing).

12 Darwin, C. (1859), *On the Origin of Species by Means of Natural Selection or the Preservation of Favoured Races in the Struggle for Life* (London: John Murray).

13 Bernard, C. (1865), *Introduction à l'Etude de la Médecine Expérimentale* (Paris: Baillière).

14 Jarvis, W.R. (1994), 'Handwashing – the Semmelweiss Lesson Forgotten?', *Lancet* 344:8933, 1311–2.

15 Nelson, R.A. (1965), 'The Hospital and the Continuing Education of the Physician'. In J.H. Knowles, ed., *Hospitals, Doctors and the Public Interest* (Cambridge, Massachusetts: Harvard University Press) p. 238.

16 The 'British' System refers to the training and registration requirements which are common to most of the British Commonwealth countries ranging from the UK to countries like Malaysia, Australia and New Zealand.

17 Berwick, D.M. (1996), 'A Primer on Leading the Improvement of Systems', *British Medical Journal*, 312:7031, 619–22.

18 Wennberg, J.E., Barnes, B.A. and Zubkoff, M. (1982), 'Professional Uncertainty and the Problem of Supplier-Induced Demand', *Social Science & Medicine* 16:7, 811–24.

19 Wennberg, J.E. (1987), 'The Paradox of Appropriate Care', *Journal of the American Medical Association* 258:18, 2568–9.

20 Kohn, L.T., Corrigan, J.M. and Donaldson, M.S. (2000), *To Err is Human: Building a Safer Health System* (Washington: National Academies Press).

21 Chassin, M., Hannan, E.L. and DeBuono, B.A. (1996), 'Benefits and Hazards of Reporting Medical Outcomes Publicly', *New England Journal of Medicine* 334:6, 394–8.

22 Sirio, C.A. and Rotondi, A.J. (1999), 'The Value of Collaboration: Quality Improvement in Critical Care Units', *Critical Care Medicine* 27:9, 2034-5.

23 Chassin, M. (1998), 'Is Healthcare Ready for Six Sigma Quality?', *Milbank Quarterly* 76:4, 565–91.

24 Plsek, P.E. and Greenhalgh, T. (2001), 'Complexity Science: the Challenge of Complexity in Health Care', *British Medical Journal* 323:7313, 625–8.

25 Mant, A. (1997), *Intelligent Leadership* (Sydney: Allen and Unwin).

26 World Health Organization, Preamble to the Constitution of the World Health Organization as adopted by the International Health Conference, New York, 19–22 June, 1946, signed on 22 July 1946 by the representatives of 61 States (*Official Records of the World Health Organization* no. 2, p. 100) and entered into force on 7 April 1948.

27 National Heart Foundation, Australia, promotes healthy diet and exercise to prevent cardiovascular disease [web page] http://www.heartfoundation.com.au/index.cfm accessed 31 May 2006.

28 Menadue, J. (2003), *Better Choices, Better Health. Final Report of the Generational Health Review* (Adelaide: South Australian Government).

29 Porter, R. (1997), *The Greatest Benefit to Mankind: A Medical History of Humanity from Antiquity to the Present* (London: Harper Collins).

30 Committee of Inquiry into Medical Education and Medical Workforce (1988), *Australian Medical Education and Workforce into the 21st Century* (Canberra: Australian Government Publishing Service).

31 Knowles, J.H. (1965), *Hospitals, Doctors, and the Public Interest* (Cambridge Massachusetts: Harvard University Press).

32 Ludmerer, K.M. (1999), *Time to Heal: American Medical Education from the Turn of the Century to the Era of Managed Care* (New York: Oxford University Press).

33 Abelson, R. (2002), 'Limits on Residents' Hours Worry Teaching Hospitals', *The New York Times*, June 2, New York.

34 Kennedy, I. (2001), *Learning from Bristol: the Report of the Public Inquiry into Children's Heart Surgery at the Bristol Royal Infirmary 1984–1995*, CM 5207 (London: The Stationery Office). Available at: http://www.bristol-inquiry.org.uk/ accessed 31 May 2006.

35 Braithwaite, J. et al. (2006), 'Does Restructuring Hospitals Result in Greater Efficiency? – An Empirical Test', *Health Services Management Research* 19:1, 1–12.

36 Williams, J.G. (1991), 'Supervised Autonomy: Medical Specialties and Structured Conflict in an Australian General Hospital', Ph.D. Thesis (Adelaide: University of Adelaide).

37 Williamson, A.M. and Feyer, A.M. (2000), 'Moderate Sleep Deprivation Produces Impairments in Cognitive and Motor Performance Equivalent to Legally Prescribed Levels of Alcohol Intoxication', *Occupational and Environmental Medicine* 57:10, 649–55.

38 Dawson, D. and Reid, K. (1997), 'Fatigue, Alcohol and Performance Impairment', *Nature* 388:6639, 235.

39 Savill, R. (1995), 'Tired Doctor Cleared over Patient's Death', *Daily Telegraph* 20 May, p. 3.

40 Christie, R.A. (1980), 'The Pre-Registration House Appointment. A Survey in Manchester', *Medical Education* 14:3, 210–3.

41 Douglas, N., Robinson, J. and Fahy, K. (2001), *Inquiry into Obstetric and Gynaecological Services at King Edward Memorial Hospital 1990–2000, Final Report, Vol. 1* (Perth: Government of Western Australia).

42 Secondary analysis of the clinical file review of 372 high-risk complex cases showed that junior medical officers (levels 1–4 registrars) provided most of the care at the crucial times (clinical assessment, decision-making or intervention).

43 Flexner, A. (1910), *Medical Education in the United States and Canada: a Report to the Carnegie Foundation for the Advancement of Teaching* (New York: Science and Health Publications Inc.).

44 Haldane, L. et al. (1913), *University Education in London: Final Report of the Commissioners* (Haldane Report) (London: Her Majesty's Stationery Office).

45 Levin, R., Moy, E., and Griner, P. (2000), 'Trends in Specialized Surgical Procedures at Teaching and Nonteaching Hospitals', *Health Affairs* 19:1, 230–8.

46 Gosden, T. et al. (2000), 'Capitation, Salary, Fee for Service and Mixed Systems of Payment: Effects on the Behaviour of Primary Care Physicians' (Cochrane Review), *Cochrane Database of Systematic Reviews* 3, CD002215.

47 Runciman, W.B, Edmonds, M.J. and Pradhan, M. (2002), 'Setting Priorities For Patient Safety', *Quality and Safety in Health Care* 11:3, 224–9.

48 Chaix-Couturier, C. et al. (2000), 'Effects of Financial Incentives on Medical Practice: Results from a Systematic Review of the Literature and Methodological Issues', *International Journal for Quality in Health Care* 12:2, 133–42.

49 Hillman, K. (1999), 'The Changing Role of Acute-Care Hospitals', *Medical Journal of Australia* 170:7, 325–8.

50 Aarseth, O., Falck, G. and Brattebo, G. (1995), 'Do the Interns Receive the Supervision They are Supposed to Get?' *Tidsskrift for Den Norske Laegeforening* 115:17, 2087–90.

51 Wise, A., Rutledge, A. and Craig, M. (1990), *Preparing Proper Doctors: An Evaluation of the Intern Training in Queensland Hospitals* (Brisbane: University of Queensland).

52 Calman, K.C. and Donaldson, M. (1991). 'The Pre-Registration House Officer Year: a Critical Incident Study' *Medical Education* 25:1, 51–9.

53 Nerenz, D. et al. (1990), 'The On-Call Experience of Interns in Internal Medicine. Medical Education Task Force of Henry Ford Hospital', *Archives of Internal Medicine* 150:11, 2294–7.

54 Hume, F. and Wilhelm, K. (1994), 'Career Choice and Experience of Distress Amongst Interns: a Survey of New South Wales Internship 1987–1990', *Australian and New Zealand Journal of Psychiatry* 28:2, 319–27.

55 Fraser, J. (1973), 'The Pre-Registration Year and the Undergraduate Curriculum', *Proceedings of the Royal Society of Medicine* 66:1, 29–30.

56 Wigton, R.S. (1992), 'Training Internists in Procedural Skills', *Annals of Internal Medicine* 116:12 Part 2, 1091–3.

57 Falck, G., Brattebo, G. and Aarseth, O. (1995), 'Is the Training of Interns in Practical Clinical Skills Adequate?', *Tidsskrift for Den Norske Laegeforening* 115:17, 2091–5.

58 Reynard, K., Gosnold, J.K. and Grout, P. (1993), 'SHO Training. Assessment Initiative in Accident and Emergency', *British Medical Journal* 306:6887, 1273–4.

59 Poses, R.M. et al. (1990), 'Are Two (Inexperienced) Heads Better Than One (Experienced) Head? Averaging House Officers' Prognostic Judgements For Critically Ill Patients', *Archives of Internal Medicine* 150:9, 1874–8.

Chapter 4

Naming, Blaming and Shaming

The complexity and uncertainty of healthcare mean that things can, will and do go wrong. The nature of healthcare dictates that some of these incidents will end in tragic outcomes. In most countries those harmed have to seek redress via civil litigation (using the tort system). This often places people who were previously in a trusting relationship at loggerheads, and can be a life-changing experience for both the person harmed (the plaintiff) and the healthcare professional (the defendant) (see Box 4.1).

Box 4.1 When things go wrong[1]

'... the usual human response is to apportion blame, demand retribution and compensation and seek assurance that the error will not occur again. Such redress is usually done through the legal system. However, less than 1 per cent of people suffering preventable harm receive any compensation through the tort system and there is little relationship between successful litigation and the degree to which negligent practices contributed to harm. Theoretically tort should help promote high standards and provide compensation for injured patients. In practice it often does neither; is grossly wasteful of resources; and is time consuming, threatening, and unpleasant for both plaintiff and defendant.'

In tort, it is necessary to find fault before those harmed can be compensated. From the perspective of the plaintiff this involves a stressful, drawn out, uncertain process, whilst having to live with the consequences of the harm. From the defendant's perspective, a finding of negligence may ensue even when he or she was acting in good faith and there is no suggestion of moral culpability. Even when the finding is in favour of the defendant, he or she will often have been subjected to a relentless campaign of adverse publicity by the media. It has been said that the punishment is in the process; unfortunately this is true, and applies to both the patient (who in general has certainly done nothing wrong) and the defendant (who may also have done little or nothing wrong). Ironically, in cases where moral culpability does exist, the likelihood is that a settlement will be reached out of court, the elements of punishment and deterrence minimized, and no one, other than those directly involved, afforded the opportunity to learn from the experience (see page 89).

Why is the situation so unsatisfactory? In this chapter we will address the following questions:

- What is the origin of and basis for the existing system?
- What is wrong with the existing system?
- Why are we in crisis?
- What are the elements of an appropriate response to accidents in healthcare?
- What do examples of alternative systems look like?

Background

Hippocrates articulated the principle that health professionals should not harm their patients some 2400 years ago (see page 1).[2] The related concept that those who do should be held accountable is now accepted. In 1768, in *Commentaries on the Laws of England*, Sir William Blackstone coined the phrase 'mala praxis' which he defined as 'injuries ... by the neglect or unskilful management of (a person's) physician, surgeon, or apothecary ...'.[3] He pointed out that such an injury 'breaks the trust which the party has placed in the physician, and tends to the patient's destruction'.[3] Today, the term malpractice is in the common vocabulary of all English-speaking societies, and carries strong connotations of culpable behaviour.

Although widely accepted, the notion that a disastrous outcome 'must' have involved negligence or culpable behaviour on the part of a clinician is simply not grounded in fact (see Chapter 5). The idea that if someone was hurt then someone must be to blame is called 'outcome bias' and is firmly entrenched in human belief systems. In many cases, outcome bias has so distorted our processes for dealing with iatrogenic harm that neither those harmed nor the health professionals involved are justly or adequately dealt with.

In the case described in Box 4.2, both patient and doctor were subjected to a protracted legal process that was avoidable. Why should a woman, with young children, unwell with a distressing condition, have had to spend months preparing for an adversarial court case when the person being blamed accepted his role in the evolution of the problem and would have been happy for the matter not to be contested? Why should implications of carelessness and negligence be broadcast across an entire state, and to some extent across an entire nation, by both print and television media, when system failure played a major role in the genesis of the problem, and when there was no suggestion that anyone had acted other than in good faith? Surely a reasonable settlement could have been achieved in a more timely manner, with less expense and no need for an adversarial confrontation?

Punishment (direct or indirect) may well be appropriate when a doctor has acted negligently, and particularly if he or she subsequently behaves in a self-interested way and shows little concern over the consequences of that negligence. However, this was not the case here.

Later in this chapter we will argue that it is quite irrational at a societal level to persist with a system that is not only unfair to both plaintiff and defendant, but costly, inefficient and ineffective in achieving its purported objectives. It is also unethical to waste money that could be far better spent.

Box 4.2 *Kite vs Malycha*[4]

Jayne Kite saw Dr. Peter Malycha, a breast surgeon, in late 1994 for what appeared to be an inflamed blocked sweat gland in her armpit, early in her third pregnancy. There is a detailed account of the visit in her medical record, but no mention of a fine needle aspiration (FNA) biopsy which was done, apparently at Jayne Kite's request, at the end of the consultation. She did not phone for the result nor keep her one month follow-up appointment. She returned ten months later with a lump in her armpit which on open biopsy was shown to be breast cancer. The appropriate treatment was started.

Two years later she had an appointment with an oncologist who made a routine request from the pathology laboratory for copies of all the pathology reports, so he could review them. The laboratory sent the 1995 open biopsy result, but also sent a report on the 1994 FNA biopsy, which was highly suggestive of breast cancer. Although copies of the FNA report were recorded by the laboratory as having been sent to Dr. Malycha, to Jayne Kite's obstetrician, and to her general practitioner, there was no trace of any such report in the otherwise complete records of these three doctors. The pathology laboratory was not implicated, although in retrospect it seems that there was substantial circumstantial evidence that the reports may never have been sent, or were sent to the wrong place.

Legal proceedings were started immediately and the case was heard over three weeks in mid-1998. Dr. Malycha had felt that he should take responsibility for a systems error, that the case could or should not be defended, and that a reasonable settlement should be made. However, the medical defence organization decided to contest the case, as it considered that the delay in diagnosis would not have compromised the outcome. There was a daily media blitz which was highly critical of Dr. Malycha, by implication. He was found negligent in June 1998 and Jayne Kite received $516,000 in compensation.

The process was a life-altering event not only for Jayne Kite, but also for Dr. Malycha and his wife and children. The family were distressed by the implications of carelessness and moral culpability made by both the print and television media. They were uncomfortable about the trial itself; Dr. Malycha's opinion was that the case could not be defended, and he had never wanted the matter taken through the courts.

Judge Perry stated 'I accept that Dr. Malycha was a truthful witness, he was open and candid as to how he went about the task of examining Mrs. Kite on that day, and as to the events that unfolded thereafter, even when some of the matters he admitted to were against his interest. But as will be seen, an unusual combination of circumstances arose which has most unfortunate consequences both for him and particularly Mrs. Kite'.

Jayne Kite, tragically, died from breast cancer in 2003, leaving behind three children, ranging in age from five to ten years old, to grow up without their mother.

The Origin of and Basis for the Existing System – Tort Law

We will start with some definitions. A *tort* is a civil wrong or injury not covered by a contract, and tort law is the law used to address such wrongs or injuries. A fundamental requirement for obtaining compensation from the tort system is the finding of wrong doing or fault (which meets the legal definition of negligence). It follows that tort law is inherently linked to the apportioning of blame. *Negligence* is a tort (i.e. a civil wrong). In the medical context negligence is generally expressed in terms of a failure to exercise reasonable knowledge, skill and care (assuming, as is almost always the case, that there is a duty of care). Note that a defendant's state of mind is not central to a finding of negligence.

The first reported case of malpractice-related litigation in the USA occurred as early as 1794. It concerned Dr. Benjamin Rush, who was a signatory of the Declaration of Independence. He issued a libel suit in response to an allegation of malpractice concerning his treatment of yellow fever victims.[5] In the mid 1800s malpractice claims increased ten-fold in the US.[6] Editors of medical journals wrote strongly-worded editorials about this new problem.[7] Many orthopaedic cases were won by patients who would have accepted inferior treatment (often resulting in amputation) 20 years earlier, simply because the standards on which to judge care had not been established. Many surgeons responded to the increased claims by refusing to fix broken limbs.[8] The relationship between lawyers and doctors deteriorated, foreshadowing the gradual development of a deep-seated animosity between many members of these two professions.[9,10]

The number and size of malpractice awards began to accelerate again in the 1930s, particularly in certain regions of the US. California, only the sixth most populous state, suddenly became the state with the greatest number of malpractice suits. Similar increases in the rate of litigation soon became apparent in Ohio, Texas, Minnesota and the District of Columbia. Thereafter, the number of malpractice suits continued to grow until World War II, during which it declined. In the 1950s the frequency of litigation began to increase again. As in the previous century, this could be attributed, at least in part, to the rapid increase in the complexity and efficacy of medical practice. New diagnostic techniques, therapeutic procedures and powerful drugs were developed, all of which were accompanied by new risks to the patient and new challenges for the practitioner. The rise of the consumer movement in the 1960s added impetus to this trend. The size of monetary awards to patients began to increase dramatically, and the costs of medical litigation became unsustainable. By the early 1970s this had precipitated a 'medico-legal' crisis in California, which spread to several other states.[8]

This crisis led to changes to the insurance industry and the legal system in many states. Many proposals were debated, including limiting or capping awards, screening claims, using alternate methods of dispute resolution, payment schedules, better reporting systems, and many other aspects of reform. A method for detecting adverse events using medical record review was developed in response to this crisis, in order to cost a possible no-fault compensation scheme (see page 38). However, it is worth noting that no major systematic initiatives were undertaken to prevent iatrogenic harm from occurring in the first place.

The situation worsened steadily and the term 'crisis' was applied again in the 1980s. Limited reforms to tort law were implemented in various states, including 'caps' to damages, but the positive impact of these has not been substantial, and the cost of malpractice litigation in much of the USA (as reflected by doctors' insurance premiums) has continued to increase.[11,12,13,14] This is true of other countries as well.[15,16]

In England, patients began winning court cases against doctors in the 1940s, but actions for medical negligence in the UK remained the exception rather than the rule until the 1970s.[17,18] During the 1980s a dramatic increase occurred in the frequency of such actions. In part this appears to have been facilitated by an increase in the availability of experts prepared to provide opinions to back the claims of patients, and by the emergence of organizations prepared to assist and advise potential plaintiffs (see page 195).[19] Legal advisers to the medical defence organizations state that compensation payouts to patients in the UK increased more than 2000 fold in 50 years. In 1952 the annual indemnity bill of the Medical Defence Union was £34,472. In 2000 it was nearly £78 million.[16]

The situation has been similar in Australia. The number of claims against doctors started rising in the 1970s and increased markedly during the 1990s.[20] Doctors' insurers claimed that the likelihood of a general practitioner being sued increased from one in 160 in 1990 to one in 84 in 1994.[21] The cost of malpractice insurance rose rapidly (Table 4.1).

Table 4.1 Medical insurance premiums in Australia from 1960 to 2000[22]

Year	Premium
1960	$10
1970	$50
1980	$200
1990	$2,000
1995	$2,000–20,000
2000	$2,000–100,000

Apparently, this increase in premiums was not enough to keep up with the increased cost of litigation and the ensuing settlements to patients. In New South Wales, a major insurer went into receivership in 2002. This certainly did create a crisis. Many practitioners found themselves without cover in an environment in which that cover was essential, leaving the provision of healthcare seriously under threat. The government intervened and some degree of normality was restored, but the risks and costs of litigation still loom large in healthcare in Australia. Fundamental reform has not taken place, although the rights of plaintiffs have been curtailed.

Furthermore, the medical defence organizations have been very reluctant to provide access to researchers who wish the use the rich information in their possession to prevent iatrogenic harm. Several applications for access have failed in Australia and the UK, although some valuable publications have been produced on 'closed claims' in the USA.

What is Wrong with the Existing System?

The Tort System

There is overwhelming evidence that the tort system fails both plaintiffs and defendants. It is generally accepted that tort law is expensive, slow and inefficient.[23,24,25,26] The costs of the tort system are now similar in the US, UK and Australia, and amount to at least 1 per cent of total health expenditure. In extreme cases the costs of insuring against litigation are so high that they have led to the abandonment by some of certain fields of practice.[15,27]

Despite this substantial cost, the tort system serves only a small number (less than one in every hundred) of those deemed by experts to have been negligently harmed.[28] These are mainly the very rich and the very angry, because those seeking redress via tort find themselves up against formidable opposition in the medical defence organizations. In addition to having suffered iatrogenic harm, patients have to commit substantial resources to a major campaign to seek redress; legal aid is not available in these cases.

Perversely, although only a tiny fraction of those harmed receive compensation via tort, about half of those who do receive compensation are not considered to have suffered a negligent adverse event in the opinion of independent medical reviewers.[25] More often than not, they are reacting angrily to being 'fobbed off' by an unsympathetic and patronizing response to problems associated with their disease or injury. Moreover, more than half of the overall amounts expended do not go to those harmed but are consumed by legal costs.[26,27,28,29,30,31,32]

A fundamental weakness of both the civil and criminal courts as a mechanism for dealing with harm from healthcare is the emphasis on outcome.[33,34] Outcome is sometimes largely a matter of chance (see Chapter 5, pages 126–131). There is a strong argument for punishing unacceptable behaviour whatever its outcome, and for not punishing reasonable behaviour even if it results in unintended harm. We accept to some extent the 'moral look' argument that truly tragic outcome demands a proportionate response. One understands the imperative to take death seriously, but it is illogical for the same action (e.g. accidentally giving the wrong drug) to go completely unpunished if no harm ensues, but result in manslaughter charges if the patient dies.

There is a further difficulty in this excessive focus on outcome. An essential element for obtaining compensation for harm caused by healthcare (or for obtaining a criminal conviction) is that the poor outcome was in fact caused by the alleged negligence and not something else, such as the patient's primary condition. Because of the complexity of illness and treatment, causation may be difficult to prove. This is particularly true in the criminal courts where the proof needs to be beyond reasonable doubt; in the civil courts the balance of probabilities applies. It might be accepted that the doctor was negligent, but unless it can be established that his or her actions actually caused the harm, compensation will not be payable. This means that the defence may concentrate on any uncertainty in the causation of the alleged harm rather than on the standard of care. Most of those harmed find this difficult to understand and may, reasonably, feel ill-served by the system, particularly when having to bear the burden of the cost of the case.

The publicity associated with a civil action may be damaging to all parties, but particularly to the defendant, whatever the outcome of the case. Typically the critical or sensational aspects of the alleged wrong doings are covered extensively in the media during the early stages of a hearing, but a finding in favour of the defendant may get little, if any, attention. Conversely, many truly negligent cases are settled out of court, confidentially, to avoid this publicity, and the practitioner may escape with very little in the way of punishment. There is ongoing debate about the need to balance the interests of a possibly innocent person against the interests of society in having open and transparent legal processes.

Like the criminal law, tort law tends to treat cases in isolation, divorced from a practitioner's overall track record and the needs of society. It is difficult to obtain funding for the initiatives needed to improve safety and quality in healthcare, but few barriers exist to prevent the expenditure of huge sums of money on a law suit when something goes wrong that might have been prevented by that funding. The costs of malpractice litigation are part of the costs of healthcare within any society. Disproportionate expenditure on a law suit is associated with substantial opportunity cost. The argument is really about efficiency and balance. Money does need to be spent on resolving disputes over wrong-doing in healthcare, but this money should be spent efficiently and distributed in proportion to the importance of the particular cases. This is no different from saying that one should direct healthcare expenditure on treatment in such a way as to maximize benefit – the 'common good' argument put forward in on page 3. Although we have argued in this book that the healthcare system does not deal with these issues well, it seems that the tort system ignores them altogether. The emphasis in tort is primarily on the interests of the litigant, not on the wider needs of society.

A key element of accountability is explaining what went wrong. Patients often sue because they feel this is the only way for them to get an answer. Sadly, the adversarial processes of the law often fail to provide the sort of information that they require. Lessons from negligence cases are rarely used to improve care.[35] Tort law tends to provide a strong disincentive to open disclosure and may damage the doctor-patient relationship by promoting a lack of candor about mistakes.[36,37] A civil case does not achieve the same ends as a root cause analysis (see Chapter 9) and may leave many questions unanswered.

Possibly the worse indictment of the tort system is that in spite of the human suffering and massive sums of money involved, few systematic attempts have been made to analyze its merits scientifically. Although some work has been done in the USA, there is relatively little information on which to assess the cost-benefit ratio of tort (or indeed any other) approach to regulating the health system.[24]

The Criminal Law

Again we will start with some definitions. *Gross negligence* has been defined as a reckless indifference to an obvious or understood risk of injury to a patient. When a patient dies as a result of gross negligence, the criminal law can be applied in the form of a charge of manslaughter (Box 4.3).[38] *Recklessness* involves understanding an unreasonable degree of risk and nevertheless deciding to take that risk. A key element of recklessness is that it involves a deliberate decision. *Mens rea* translates literally as 'guilty mind' and is used to describe the state of mind that may lead to recklessness and warrant punishment.

Box 4.3 Two cases of manslaughter

Adomako[38] is an important case in English law, in which the House of Lords confirmed gross negligence as the test in cases of manslaughter by criminal negligence involving a breach of duty. Dr. Adomako took over the care of a patient half way through an anaesthetic. The circuit became disconnected and he was slow in diagnosing and responding to this event. It has been suggested that there were a number of systems factors that were not adequately addressed in this case. This was an overseas trained doctor working long hours in a small hospital as a peripatetic locum registrar without adequate supervision. The criminal law has not been effective in identifying those responsible for permitting these arrangements, and it is not clear that changes to improve the system were brought about by the conviction.

A consultant anaesthetist was sentenced to six months jail in Canada after leaving a patient unattended while making a phone call outside the operating room, and then lying about what had happened. The patient became disconnected from the anaesthetic machine, and died.[39]

Use of the criminal law is appropriate when genuinely culpable behaviour is involved. Those who commit serious crimes, involving fraud, child pornography, rape, or murder, must face charges and be punished if convicted. The mass murderer Harold Shipman is an obvious example of a doctor who deserved to be sent to jail (see Box 4.4).

Box 4.4 Harold Shipman – the audit and the inquiry[40]

In 1976, UK general practitioner Dr. Harold Shipman was fined for dishonestly obtaining and using controlled drugs. In 2000, he was convicted of murdering 15 patients and forging a will. An audit conducted on his clinical practice from 1974 to 1998 found a high death rate and made recommendations regarding review of general practice statistics to identify aberrant patterns in mortality rates, reform of the death certification process, and greater monitoring of restricted drugs. A formal inquiry was established. It was found that, over two decades, Shipman had murdered more than 200 patients.

It is clear that a charge of murder was appropriate in the Shipman case, and that a charge of manslaughter may be appropriate in cases such as those described in Box 4.3. However, in some countries, the police have laid charges of manslaughter in cases of unexpected death in which there does not seem to be any element of moral culpability (see Box 4.5).[41] In New Zealand, before 1997, simple negligence was enough to justify a conviction for manslaughter if a person died as a result of an accident. This applied to non-medical situations as much as to accidents in healthcare. It seems now to be generally accepted that the threshold of negligence for criminal prosecution needs to be reasonably high. An analysis of unexpected deaths should take into account the principle of *mens rea* and the context in which the action occurred. Medicine often creates situations in which there is really no option not to act. Dr. Gale, trying to save the life of a critically ill patient in a difficult emergency (Box 4.5), was in a very different situation from those outlined in Box 4.3.

In another New Zealand manslaughter trial, involving a drug error in an emergency, the judge, explaining the prosecution's case, said 'The Crown says Dr. 'Y' is a highly trained, experienced, responsible man whom the Crown says made a mistake, through carelessness, on this one occasion'.[42] In an English case involving two junior doctors who inadvertently administered the wrong drug (vincristine, see Box 11.1) into the spinal fluid of a patient, the judge said 'you are far from being bad men; you are good men who contrary to your normal behaviour on this one occasion were guilty of momentary recklessness'. These are not descriptions of the sort of morally culpable behaviour one would expect to find in the criminal courts. In both of these cases many factors increased the chance of an error being made. In the case involving vincristine, the patient arrived late, leading to changes in procedures, the doctors were unfamiliar with the protocols and procedures, the syringes were similar in appearance and design, and the pharmacy sent two pre-filled syringes in one bag, one for intravenous injection and one for injection into the cerebral spinal fluid.

Our view of these cases is well reflected by the comments of the Australian judge in *R v Callaghan* who said 'Defaults involving no moral blame at all are out of keeping with the conceptions of the purpose of the Criminal Code ...'.[43] The criminal law is a very heavy handed tool and should be retained for serious wrongdoing. We believe that there has been a tendency in some of these cases to mistake the seriousness of the consequences, which have been disastrous, with the culpability of the actions, which was minimal or non-existent (see again, Box 4.5). The requirement for gross negligence was affirmed in the UK in Adomako (see Box 4.3), and in New Zealand the Crimes Amendment Act 1997 established a 'major departure' test which has much the same effect; the events in New Zealand have been reviewed by Skegg.[41]

Why are We in Crisis?

The current medico-legal environment, with all its faults, has been perpetuated and reinforced by the coalescence of some powerful forces: uncertainty in medicine, attitudes to human error, a gap between patient expectations and reality and a strong human predilection for blame, fuelled, to some extent, by the media. It is, of course, also perpetuated by political inertia and perhaps in some countries by reluctance to challenge the powerful vested interests of the medical indemnity industry, which has a turnover of hundreds of millions of dollars.

Box 4.5 A tragic case, resulting in a charge and acquittal from manslaughter[44]

Richard Davis, a fit, active 13 year old boy, died after a minor out-of-hours procedure for an infected knee. The anaesthetic was administered by a senior consultant anaesthetist, Dr. Gale, and proceeded uneventfully until, at the end of the procedure, Richard was transferred from the operating table. At this point he regurgitated and aspirated at least some gastric contents. He developed difficulty with breathing. He sat up and removed the laryngeal mask which had been used to maintain his airway, and then proceeded to display the signs of acute laryngospasm and, shortly thereafter, of frothing negative pressure pulmonary oedema. He was returned to a supine position and his trachea was intubated by Dr. Gale. Dr. Gale found it almost impossible to ventilate Richard's lungs through the endotracheal tube. She took appropriate steps to determine that the tube was in the trachea and not blocked or kinked, and then removed and replaced it. She went on to perform other tasks one might expect in the management of a patient whose lungs and circulation were progressively deteriorating (the administration of 100 per cent oxygen and of adrenaline, for example). She called for help very early in the development of this crisis, but effective help took nearly 30 minutes to arrive. The contribution of junior doctors on the arrest team, who arrived earlier, was ineffectual. Richard's condition deteriorated rapidly.

When the second anaesthetist arrived, Dr. Gale handed him the reservoir bag of the anaesthetic circuit to hold while she suctioned the endotracheal tube again. The bag did not deflate through the disconnected circuit, alerting the second anaesthetist to the fact that the filter used to protect the anaesthetic breathing circuit had become blocked, presumably by the frothing pulmonary oedema. Removing the filter restored adequate ventilation, but Richard had unfortunately developed irreversible brain damage by this stage and life support was discontinued the following day.

At Dr. Gale's subsequent trial for manslaughter – for failing to recognize the filter blockage – evidence was presented to the effect that this blockage could not have occurred until quite late in the proceedings when the froth in the circuit started to dry and encrust the surface of the hydrophobic filter. All four expert witnesses called in the case said that the general conduct of the resuscitation was within the limits of acceptable practice. Dr. Gale was acquitted.

Blame

Blaming individuals is a common response to accidental harm in all sectors of society and its pervasiveness impedes the management of iatrogenic harm.[45,46,47,48,49,50] For example, a study of patients' complaints about medical practice in Australia found that only 16 per cent of respondents would have been satisfied with an apology, and that satisfaction was much more likely if strong action had been taken against the doctor (Table 4.2).[51] The investigators concluded that complainants' expectations were at odds with the regulators obligations – that is, complainants want punishment and restitution while the role of the regulators is to protect the public. Blame leads to punishment rather than to addressing any problems in the system that may have contributed to the accident. There is a place for blame, but in our view this is very limited in relation to unintentional accidents in healthcare.[52]

Today most managers in industry realize that a culture of blame will not bring safety issues to the forefront.[53] Blame leads to cover-ups. Safety depends on open communication to identify failures in the system. Safe organizations routinely examine equipment design, procedures, training and other organizational features.[54] In healthcare, considerable progress has been made recently towards a more widespread understanding of these issues, but the inappropriate attribution of blame still tends to dominate the philosophy of many managers and retard the progress of safety in medicine.[44]

Table 4.2 Why patients complain – results of a review of 290 complaints[51]

Patients' expected outcome from complaints	Percentage
Doctor reprimanded or disciplined	33%
Doctor deregistered	23%
Doctor counselled or advised	22%
Apology from doctor and acknowledgement of harm done	16%
Compensation	3%
Conciliation or a fairer outcome	2%

Attitudes to Human Error

Mistakes ought to be seen as opportunities for learning. However, this requires a willingness to admit errors and discuss them. There are many disincentives to doing this in healthcare, not the least of which is the implicit admission of fallibility on the part of the practitioner who has made the mistake.[55,56] There is also the fear of complaint or litigation, which may or may not be well founded.[57,58,59,60] Mistakes tend to be seen as serious threats to reputations, careers, and referrals.[61] That human error is, in fact, ubiquitous, normal and necessary for learning is discussed in detail in Chapter 5.[62]

The Uncertainty of Medical Knowledge

The belief, widespread in medicine, that scientific knowledge is certain, that it can be acquired and stored in a person's mind, and that this store can be steadily added to by the accumulation of more and more facts is without foundation. This belief is linked to the idea that properly trained and conscientious clinicians can diagnose and treat patients perfectly, without ever making a mistake. At the heart of the perfectibility model is the belief that if only doctors and nurses would try harder and were more knowledgeable and skilful then errors would not happen. That this is false is made clear in Chapters 5 and 6.[55,63,64]

The uncertainty of medical knowledge is an even more fundamental issue than the inevitability of human error. Fox identified two types of medical uncertainty: incomplete or imperfect mastery of available knowledge and the limitations of current medical knowledge.[63] No matter how brilliant a health professional, he or she simply cannot have access to all the information needed for day-to-day medical practice. Furthermore, facts believed to be correct often turn out to be wrong. When the authors of this book were trained the suggestion that one should administer a beta-adrenergic blocker to a patient in heart failure would have been considered seriously incorrect, but today this has been shown to be good, evidence-based practice in the correct circumstances.

In Chapter 6 we will examine the limitations and uncertainties of medical knowledge in more detail. Some doctors are reluctant to disclose these uncertainties to their patients. Perhaps they fear their patients will lose trust in them, or that their private patients will decline an offered procedure. Incomplete disclosure of this sort adds to the problem of unrealistic expectations on the part of patients, discussed in the next section. Medical uncertainty because of insufficient scientific evidence about a particular condition and its prognosis, or a particular treatment and its efficacy, is different from inadequate knowledge or skill on the part of the clinician. Patients need to be aware that medicine is not a perfect science and that the discovery of medical knowledge will always be a 'work in progress'. They also need to know that it is impossible for their doctors to have all the information at their fingertips. Insight into one's own limitations is a strength, not a weakness. The reality is that honest and clear communication leads to greater patient satisfaction, improved clinical outcomes, fewer complaints and less litigation.

The Gap between Patient Expectations and Reality

There are few data on the expectations of patients.[65] It may be argued that escalating litigation is evidence of unrealistic expectations, but, at least half the people who sue have been harmed by their treatment, and are disaffected over a failure to meet realistic expectations, not unrealistic ones.

Nevertheless some patients may expect more of healthcare than is reasonable, particularly in relation to risk. If expectations are unrealistic, where do these come from? Part of the problem may be that doctors have in the past tended to provide too little information about the risks and limitations of medical treatment. If doctors' emphasis is on achieving a good outcome, it is natural for patients to think that there are few risks. Advertising may be particularly problematic, especially in relation to cosmetic surgery and drugs. It is therefore unfortunate that the traditional prohibition from advertising by doctors has been eased in many countries. Health segments are now part of daily news programs, including reports of new technology and scientific breakthroughs which may offer unfounded hope to patients who face chronic or terminal illnesses.

Medical scientists will often be more positive about their research than their data really warrant because of the pressure to attract ongoing funding for their work. There is no branch of medicine or healthcare untouched by the technological revolution and its concomitant commercialism. In the past the costs of setting up a medical practice were relatively modest. Today, many doctors working in the private sector need expensive equipment. Investing in this equipment increases the already considerable incentives of private practice to place commercial interests above those of society in general, and individual patients in particular.

Laser refractive eye surgery provides a good illustration of some of these points. The initial development of this technology was newsworthy, and received much publicity. Applications of the advances soon manifested as a profitable and widely sought procedure for people in developed countries, and one which was adopted aggressively by the private sector as well as within public hospitals. For most patients this procedure is entirely discretionary. About 100,000 people choose laser eye surgery in preference to the perfectly viable alternative of wearing glasses every year in the UK, and over a million refractive procedures are performed annually, at a cost of over US$2 billion, in the intensely competitive USA market.[66] In 2003 the Medical Defence Union in the UK reported a 166 per cent increase in claims related to eye surgery. This probably reflected the simple fact that if you perform more procedures you get more complaints, but the National Institute for Clinical Excellence in the UK was sufficiently concerned about the lack of evidence in support of these procedures to publish guidelines for surgeons that emphasized the need for informed consent and an audit process. Both organizations identified overselling the benefits and understating the risks as a factor leading to the increase in dissatisfied patients. One might say that patient expectations were unrealistic, but there is little doubt that much of the responsibility for this lay with the health profession.

The Media

It is easy to blame the media for the bad press that healthcare often receives. The media also provides positive coverage of new developments and notable successes in surgery or medicine. However, this may also be undesirable, because it may fuel unrealistic expectations on the part of patients. The popular media are characterized by a tendency to superficial coverage of topics, a focus on the novel or sensational, and at times a lack of balance. For example, during the legal proceedings outlined in Boxes 4.2 and 4.5, the prosecution's allegations were reported in detail, but the defence evidence was given little attention. After the verdict in the case in Box 4.5, one newspaper carried the headline 'Child dies and doctor gets off'. This is hardly impartial reporting of a finding of not guilty.

The media are an integral part of modern life. The challenge for healthcare professionals is to interact responsibly with the media, and to develop relationships of trust with those journalists and editors who are interested in objective and accurate reporting. However, identifying these people and ensuring their copy is not subverted or misrepresented by their colleagues is a daunting problem.

Ethical Considerations

As discussed in Chapter 2, healthcare is inherently risky, and decisions must often be made between unattractive options. The risks and discomfort associated with a surgical procedure and the subsequent stay in hospital are only acceptable in relation to expected benefits. These risks include the risk of human error. Critical decisions may need to be made under extreme pressure of time (Box 4.5), and followed immediately with skilled actions. The problem of unavoidable errors, especially in crises, is discussed on page 121.

There may be no entirely objective ethical framework within which to analyze the optimal response to iatrogenic harm in healthcare (see Chapter 7). Many ethicists today would insist on considerable autonomy for patients in relation to the decision to undergo a healthcare procedure in the first place. It is essential that patients understand the risks they are taking and have some appreciation of the fact that there are factors within the healthcare system beyond the control of the clinicians involved. The time for articulating these limitations may not be immediately preceding a life-saving procedure in an emergency. To a large extent, individual practitioners, particularly if junior, and especially in an emergency, can only operate within the system as they find it. In the end, it is the public, through government, who decide what type of healthcare system to have. Those with influence (e.g. consultant clinicians and senior managers) have a social responsibility to ensure that the service provided is the best possible within the constraints of the available resources, and they also have a responsibility to articulate to the public any important deficiencies in safety or other elements of quality that may result from those constraints.

Accidental harm is always unfortunate, and often tragic, whether it occurs within healthcare or elsewhere. Anyone undertaking any dangerous activity has a duty to do so with reasonable knowledge, skill and care. The expectations articulated in this chapter in relation to health professionals apply to other people too. However, two features distinguish the ethical basis on which to evaluate the appropriate response to an accident in healthcare from that in other areas of activity. First, healthcare is provided with the express intent of helping patients. This creates an expectation and a relationship of trust between patients and healthcare professionals, in which the power is unequal. This is quite different from the situation in a road traffic accident, for example, in which the participants are usually strangers with an equal share in the duty of care. Second, health professionals often find themselves with little choice but to act in an emergency, sometimes when fatigued and in less than optimal circumstances.

Healthcare is accepted as an essential element of society. Healthcare professionals are part of society, and are patients themselves from time to time. Also, many lay people and patients find themselves in positions to influence the healthcare system. From any ethical perspective which emphasizes the collective good, there is an imperative for all concerned to work together to achieve the best overall outcome for society. It follows that there is a collective responsibility on behalf of all members of society to do the right thing in relation to accidents in healthcare. Self-serving profiteering from accidents in healthcare is unhelpful. Unreasonable claims by patients fall into this category. So does the approach taken by some lawyers of treating iatrogenic harm as a business opportunity warranting the investment of venture capital. These activities are to the detriment of society and can only be justified within an ideological framework that places the welfare of an individual above that of society as whole. We argue that basic healthcare is everyone's business, and that all sections of society, including healthcare professionals, patients and their families have a responsibility to behave reasonably when things have gone wrong.

What are the Elements of an Appropriate Response to Accidents in Healthcare?

The elements of an appropriate response to iatrogenic harm include *retribution* (or punishment), *accountability* (which includes the provision of an explanation, and an assurance that something will be done to prevent a recurrence) and *compensation* for any expenses or losses that result from the accident. Each of these elements is provided at present in various ways: through the criminal and civil law; registration or licensure; disciplinary procedures and in some countries no-fault approaches to compensation. Each of these provides one or more of the three elements in varying degree (Figure 4.1). The appropriateness of the response in any particular case lies largely in the degree to which the right balance between these three elements is achieved. It would be ideal if the perfect balance could be achieved by a single process, in a timely fashion, efficiently and affordably.

Retribution

Most people who have been harmed by others experience some desire for retribution. Simple revenge is not generally seen as acceptable in modern western societies, but punishment of wrongdoing remains an objective of the law. Punishment for wrong-doing in healthcare is achieved at present through the criminal courts or the use of exemplary damages (i.e. civil damages in which a stated objective is to punish the defendant rather than simply to provide compensation), and through disciplinary proceedings held by medical councils and other statutory or professional bodies. The process of civil litigation, through its reporting by the media, also punishes the defendant, but that is (arguably) not its primary objective (see Box 4.2).

It is essential that punishment, when appropriate, it is seen as fair to all concerned. Patients' interests must be safeguarded, but so must the reasonable interests of health professionals. It follows that punishment must be just. Punishing serious violations is usually just. Punishing simple error usually isn't. Getting justice wrong undermines the standing and therefore the long-term effectiveness of the law.

There is a utilitarian argument that can be made for the value of punishment in deterring undesirable behaviour, even if that punishment is not strictly warranted in a particular case. This argument, however, is predicated on the notion that deterrence is effective. As we will discuss in Chapter 5, it is not possible to prevent human error by direct deterrence. On the other hand, it might be possible to deter those running an organization from failing to ensure adequate standards in relation to infrastructure, procedures, staffing levels, training and so forth, and it is possible to deter deliberate risk taking. To be effective, deterrence must be aimed at those who can make decisions. Anyone can choose to be reckless, but usually only senior doctors and administrators can influence the way an organization is equipped, staffed and run. Junior doctors and nurses cannot usually do much to change the system, yet they often end up being blamed for things which go wrong, while those 'at the helm' do not.

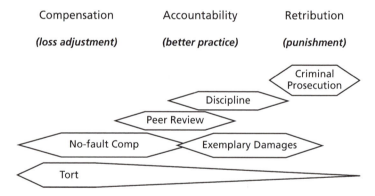

Figure 4.1   Dealing with accidental harm in healthcare: The elements of an appropriate response and some mechanisms by which these are usually achieved Some no-fault compensation systems have provisions for accountability as well

Accountability

Accountability implies being answerable to someone – in this case, to the patient as well as to those charged with running the healthcare system. It includes the provision of an explanation for what has happened and a commitment to ensure (as far as possible) that the same thing will not happen again. These things are often identified as important by patients who have been harmed – people want to know what went wrong, and what is going to be done to improve the system. Finding out what happened is the subject of Chapter 9. Accountability, in effect, is about responding to these findings and improving safety for patients, or addressing other important elements of the quality of healthcare.

Telling people what went wrong should be a timely, simple, accessible and unthreatening process. This is the concept of *open disclosure*. In practice, patients and their relatives often feel that they are being kept in the dark. They feel that things are 'covered up', and that they have been abandoned at the time of their greatest need. This leads to anger and frustration, and frequently motivates people to become aggressive litigants. It also erodes trust in the healthcare system and the medical profession.

Patients also appreciate an apology. If they have been wronged, they are owed this. The sooner it is given, the better. If it is unclear whether wrong has occurred or not, or even if it is clear that it hasn't, it is still reasonable and appropriate to provide an apology for the fact that harm has occurred. These matters are dealt with in Chapter 8. It is prudent to take advice from one's medical defence organization before admitting liability, but many medical defence lawyers today recognize that apologizing and admitting liability are not synonymous.

Compensation

If a patient suffers avoidable harm from healthcare, some form of compensation seems reasonable in the context of modern society and a caring profession. Compensation is largely provided through tort law in most countries. Indeed, the ostensible primary purpose of civil litigation is to adjust loss, rather than let it lie where it falls. In the context of healthcare, the adjustment is usually from the harmed patient to the insurer of the healthcare provider. There is much to commend this: if the provider has caused harm, he or she should share the consequences of that harm, and insurance is a practical way of doing this.

Compensation generally takes the form of money, which obviously cannot compensate for the loss of a loved one, or for serious permanent injury such as brain damage, paraplegia or a painful nerve lesion. On the other hand, money does compensate for loss of earnings, and the costs of treatment and rehabilitation required as the result of harm. Indeed, some of the most expensive settlements arise out of the need to cover the lifelong expenses of a permanently harmed baby. It follows that there is nothing unreasonable about large settlements per se. Much of the controversy over large settlements is about who should actually bear the costs of such compensation, and about the level of care and welfare which should reasonably be provided. Should a person be compensated to live in luxury or merely at the breadline? Should the previous financial status or prospects of the injured person make a difference? Are lifelong costs of babies injured at birth better laid at the feet of government than placed on the obstetrician (or his or her insurer), whose wrong doing may be very slight or non-existent, notwithstanding the enormity of the consequences? Controversy also arises in relation to the burden placed on injured patients to prove their entitlement to compensation, and over the time needed to bring a claim to fruition (see Box 4.1). In some jurisdictions, part of the compensation may be via creative solutions which meet the ongoing needs or particular desires of those harmed (see Box 8.6). On the other hand, in many jurisdictions, the entire settlement may be by way of a lump sum, and there have been unfortunate cases in which the entire amount has been lost, wasted or stolen within a few years.

The Ideal Response

We have devoted parts three and four of this book to analyzing and describing the ideal response to iatrogenic harm in healthcare. It is worth encapsulating the key points of this rather complex subject into one or two paragraphs.

The ideal response to a patient who has been harmed by healthcare should begin with the timely (i.e. immediate if necessary) and free provision of the healthcare needed to minimize that harm. Under the heading of accountability, the response should include an acknowledgement of the fact that something has gone wrong, an empathic apology, and an explanation. Compensation should be available as of right and without the need to prove fault (although it may be necessary to determine that the harm was avoidable, rather than an inevitable side effect of the treatment, and that it was caused by healthcare management). It should include the costs of any healthcare and rehabilitation needed as a result of the injury and provision for any loss of earning capacity that follows the harm. The response should include an appropriate analysis of why things went wrong and a concerted effort to correct any failings in the system and minimize the likelihood of a recurrence.

Finally, just and measured punishment may be appropriate in some cases, namely those in which a clear element of egregious behaviour can be identified. It is unjust, and entirely without value to punish simple error (see Chapter 5), either explicitly, or by sensational media coverage before the facts of the matter have been established.

What do Examples of Alternative Systems Look Like?

It is worth asking whether there are any examples of alternative approaches to litigation as a response to iatrogenic harm. A few countries around the world (for example, Finland, Sweden, Britain, the Netherlands, New Zealand and some states in the US) have adopted some aspects of no-fault compensation for at least some injuries caused by healthcare. This approach is very forward-thinking.

It seems that the collective expectations and cultural attitudes of society pervade the relationships of individuals with their healthcare professionals, and set the tone for dealing with accidental harm in healthcare. A readiness to turn to the civil courts for redress may have more to do with a certain view of the world, and of the place within that world of healthcare providers, than with the merits of any particular event. Very high incomes for doctors in some specialties may encourage law suits, for example. A universally accessible no-fault scheme is very unlikely to provide some of the very large settlements that have characterized tort-based systems. If many people insisted on their right to pursue large claims, it would be difficult to promote the more balanced and egalitarian approach implicit in a no-fault system. Part (but not all) of that world view will depend on the presence or absence of adequate and readily accessible alternatives to litigation. The ability of a country to provide such a system is closely related to its existing social infrastructure. Countries in which the permanently injured or chronically disabled are already cared for by the state have fewer barriers to implementing a no-fault compensation system for patients injured by healthcare than countries which do not. Two examples will be given.

The Experience in Finland

In Finland, the Patient Injury Act of 1986[67] created a duty for all health providers to insure against awards for medical injury. Because of Finland's large public health system, the majority of this cost is borne by the Government, but private providers are required to carry this insurance as well. Injured patients apply directly to the insurer, and receive compensation for avoidable harm caused by healthcare that falls within specified categories defined in the act (harm from treatment, infection, accidents and misdiagnosis). Cover is not entirely comprehensive, and the act does not exclude the use of alternative means of pursuing compensation. The public health system and the social welfare system underpin the insurance scheme. Those in need of treatment or support can generally obtain it as of right.

The right to sue is retained, but does not appear to be used very often. The system seems to work to the satisfaction of the Finnish people, and there appears to be little confrontation between doctors and patients. It is not clear why some of the tensions which have arisen in New Zealand (discussed below) in relation to the accountability of doctors have been less apparent in Finland.

The Accident Compensation Corporation in New Zealand

New Zealand has gone further than Finland, and in 1967 effectively replaced litigation with a fairly comprehensive system of no-fault compensation.[68] The system is known to most New Zealanders as the 'ACC', an abbreviation for Accident Compensation Corporation, although its actual title has been changed on several occasions.

The scheme currently seems to be operating satisfactorily, and the medico-legal environment in New Zealand seems to be relatively constructive at present. Nevertheless, the track record of the ACC has been variable, with some very difficult periods in relation to accountability. The scheme has been the subject of numerous reviews (five in the six years leading to 1991), often initiated by changing political ideology rather than any substantive deficiencies in its operation. Its financial fortunes have fluctuated, and the claim that the scheme is unaffordable has been made on a number of occasions (although not recently; in the early years of the twenty-first century it appears to be operating on a sustainable economic basis). There have been times when no lump sum compensation was available to injured people (including patients); given that the right to sue had been lost, this was clearly unsatisfactory, but lump sum compensation has now been reinstated. Currently, claims are settled in just over two weeks, on average, and compensation includes 80 percent of salary (capped at NZ$90,000), out of pocket expenses, and, where necessary, home help.

'Medical Manslaughter' in New Zealand

Probably the most troublesome consequence of the introduction of the ACC relates to a widespread perception that setting aside the right to sue in New Zealand left doctors unaccountable. It was perceived by many that there was no mechanism for providing an adequate response to malpractice. During the 1990s, New Zealand experienced an astonishing increase in cases of low level negligence prosecuted through the criminal courts. Ten health professionals were charged with manslaughter between 1982 and 2002 (in a country of under four million people). In most of these cases the charges arose out of errors made during normal clinical practice and included no element of egregious behaviour (see Box 4.5 for an example). It is likely that most, if not all, of these cases would have been handled through the civil courts in most other countries, and by inference, they might well have been in New Zealand, had the civil courts been an option.[52] Any reservations one might have about the appropriateness of civil litigation as a response to medical accidents pale into insignificance in contrast to those applicable to criminal prosecutions.

Fortunately, common sense prevailed. After several years of in depth advocacy from a small group of doctors and lawyers, a change was made to the law in New Zealand which limited manslaughter prosecutions for negligence to cases in which that negligence represented a major departure from a reasonable standard of care. This brought the law in New Zealand into line with that in comparable jurisdictions.

The Health and Disability Commissioner in New Zealand

Even in countries with recourse to the civil law, accountability must be facilitated by additional mechanisms. All states in Australian have independent commissions for managing health complaints, with both conciliation and investigative functions, and some have the power to co-regulate the health professions with the various professional registration boards.

In New Zealand, a Health and Disability Commissioner (HDC) has now been appointed, and provides a first port of call for any patient with a complaint.[69] The jurisdiction of the Commissioner extends to all healthcare providers, including those with administrative responsibilities. The Commissioner has produced a list of the rights of any consumer of health or disability service, and, after due process, can find a practitioner guilty of a breach of one of these rights (see Box 4.6).

The processes of the HDC may still end up oriented primarily on the identification of blame, although the approach is more inquisitorial than a civil

Box 4.6 The wrong drug – a smoking gun[70]

Mrs. Jones was admitted to a private hospital in February 2001 for an elective hysterectomy. Her specialist anaesthetist, Dr. Aders saw her for the first time in the holding area at the back of the hospital's recovery area, inserted an IV line and administered a drug. He intended to give Mrs. Jones the sedative, midazolam, but inadvertently administered a muscle relaxant instead, producing generalized (reversible) paralysis. Mrs. Jones described her experience as follows: 'It was a very few short seconds after that I first felt extremely odd. I started to try and say something. What I was feeling was far different from previous anaesthetic experiences. Dr. Aders then gave me a look as if I was being a difficult patient. By now I was struggling to try and fill my lungs with air on my own, I was also struggling to keep my eyes open or to move any part of my body. On trying to speak, I found it was impossible. I was able to try and mouth 'Can't breathe' and also to hit my chest a couple of times to try so desperately to get attention. I also remember my face frowning badly. I still had a level of awareness even though I could not breathe. I do not know at this stage what the medical staff were doing. At this stage I believed that I was dying.'

Dr. Aders responded promptly and appropriately. He checked his tray of drugs, diagnosed his mistake, administered oxygen immediately, and procured a rebreathing bag with which he assisted his patient's ventilation. He transferred her to the operating room and induced anesthesia. Surgery then proceeded as planned. However, the emotional trauma of this experience led to on-going anxiety, which Mrs. Jones reported as still present three years after the event.

She complained to the Health and Disability Commissioner (HDC) of New Zealand. He conducted an investigation, which began in August 2002. The final report was completed in March 2004 (three years after the event). He found that Dr. Aders was in breach of Mrs. Jones' right (under New Zealand law) to have services provided with reasonable care and skill. In effect this is a finding of negligence. In justifying his finding he made the following comments: 'A simple check of the label would have averted the error. Dr. Aders failed to check the label on the syringe. Checking the drug to be given is an elementary and mandatory part of anaesthetic practice. Dr. Aders accepts that, for whatever reason, he did not check what drug he was administering. I note that he has now adopted the practice of using different-sized syringes to differentiate between drug types. He no longer takes muscle relaxant drugs into the preoperative area, and reads the label out loud before giving the injection.'

The Commissioner recommended no further action in respect of this finding, other than 'follow-up actions' to disseminate his report to Mrs. Jones's surgeons, to the hospital and to the Australian and New Zealand College of Anaesthetists; he also placed the report on the HDC website for educational purposes.

action, and probably more satisfactory to all concerned. Patients do not need any financial resources to approach the Commissioner, and are provided with advocates to assist them with the process of laying a complaint. There is a strong emphasis on obtaining low level resolution to complaints if possible, and the option of referring the matter to the Medical or Nursing Council (or other relevant authority) for disciplinary procedures is used only when deemed appropriate.

As is evident from Box 4.6, the process is often quite slow and, as will be discussed in Chapter 9, often achieves disappointingly little in the promoting the better healthcare. Although the findings in the case in Box 4.6 were relatively favourable to the doctor, the process focused more on whether the doctor's actions were consistent with accepted standards of practice than on whether those standards are adequate. Nevertheless the approach taken seems very constructive in comparison to that of civil litigation.

Tort Reform?

It would seem that the New Zealand and Finnish systems would be reasonable starting points for reform in countries in which the tort system currently dominates. The ACC and HDC are highly valued by most New Zealanders. There is no agenda or identifiable energy for change. Even the majority of lawyers seem convinced that the ACC provides a better approach to accidents than the civil law; these alternatives to litigation seem to have become embedded in the culture of the country.

In fact, mediation and out-of-court settlements are already widely used to avoid adversarial, expensive court cases, even in countries with the tort system. It would seem highly desirable to formalize the premise that no-fault compensation should be the starting point for most negotiations, and to improve the machinery so that it is quick, efficient, and fully acceptable to those harmed.

The reforms introduced by the Woolf Report[23] in the UK are also worth considering, as they have substantially reduced delays in civil actions and have provided major incentives to both sides of any dispute to resort to mediation and to settle actions out of court. It would seem that the elements of a good scheme may be one based on no fault compensation for the majority of reasonable cases, with the right to sue being reserved for contentious or difficult cases.

Conclusions

In this chapter we have argued that many aspects of the medico-legal response to iatrogenic harm fall short of the ideal. A medico-legal environment based on conflict corrodes trust between patients and healthcare providers. Medicine is an imperfect science, and the pastoral care of the sick and disabled has always been a very important part of the role of healthcare professionals. Trust is critical to this role, and is an essential ingredient of the provision of optimal therapeutic care. In the absence of trust, how is the patient to evaluate the complex and highly technical issues associated with decisions about their healthcare?

Although it is clear that trust needs to be earned by healthcare professionals, it also needs to be respected by society. Trust is a manifestation of a relationship which operates to the satisfaction of all parties. If health professionals who are conscientiously practising to the best of their ability are subjected to unjust criticism and publicity, they are likely to indulge in at least some degree of defensive practice. A positive and trusting relationship with one's patients is one of the greatest rewards of working in healthcare, and is a major reason for keeping practitioners engaged, committed, and ready to go the 'extra mile'. The value of this to everyone should not be underestimated, and systems which actively impede this should be reformed.

In Chapter 1 we discussed the fact that society always pays for healthcare, whether through the private system, insurance, or the public system. The cost of the legal response to things which go wrong is part of the total cost of healthcare, as is the cost of the consequences of iatrogenic harm. Money wasted on unduly expensive litigation could be better spent supporting a patient who has become permanently incapacitated by a medical accident, or, even better, on preventing a similar accident in the future. It is of course necessary to ensure that those who suffer from medical negligence are provided appropriate compensation, and it is also essential to have legal checks and balances which safeguard the rights of both patients and healthcare professionals. However, this should be via an appropriate, timely legal response, not an adversarial, inefficient and very costly one.

In many countries, the costs of litigation are excessive. The process serves patients and healthcare professionals poorly and is more likely to increase defensive medicine than to promote safety. This represents a substantial opportunity cost: at least some of the money could be better spent. Furthermore, the pattern appears to be one of an escalating cycle of an approach to iatrogenic harm that is unnecessarily expensive. High quality, equitable, safe healthcare ought to be a possibility in most countries of the world. Getting the legal and regulatory side of healthcare right is part of achieving that end. We believe that fundamental reform is overdue in this area in many countries.

Notes

1   Runciman, W.B., Merry, A.F. and Tito, F. (2003), 'Error, Blame, and the Law in Health Care – an Antipodean Perspective', *Annals of Internal Medicine* 138:12, 974–9.

2   Hippocrates (400 BCE), *Of the Epidemics*, Book 1, Section II, part 5, translated by Adams, F. 'The physician must ... have two special objects in view with regard to disease, namely, to do good or to do no harm'. available at: <http://classics.mit.edu/ Hippocrates/epidemics.html> accessed 1 June 2006.

3   Blackstone, W. (1768), 'Of Wrongs and Their Remedies, Respecting the Rights of Persons', Book III, Chapter 8 of Blackstone's, *Commentaries on the Laws of England* p. 122. Available at: The Avalon Project at Yale Law School [web page] <http://www.yale.edu/lawweb/avalon/blackstone/bk3ch8.htm> accessed 1 June 2006.

4   *Jayne Carlene and Darren John Kite v Peter Malycha*; *Jayne Carlene and Darren John Kite v Peter Malycha and Peter Malycha Pty. Ltd.* Nos SCGRG-97-1621, SCGRG-98-141. Judgement No.6702, South Australian Supreme Court, 10 June 1998.

5   Sandor, A.A. (1957), 'The History of Professional Liability Suits in the United States', *Journal of the American Medical Association* 163:6, 459–66.

6   DeVille, K.A. (1990), *Medical Malpractice in Nineteenth Century America: Origins and Legacy* (New York: New York University Press).

7   Mohr, J.C. (1993), *Doctors and the Law: Medical Jurisprudence in Nineteenth Century America* (New York: Oxford University Press).

8   Mohr, J.C. (2000), 'American Medical Malpractice Litigation in Historical Perspective', *Journal of the American Medical Association* 283:13, 1731–7.

9   Elwell, J.J. (1860), *A Medico-Legal Treatise on Malpractice and Medical Evidence, Comprising the Elements of Medical Jurisprudence* (New York: JS Voorhies).

10 McClelland, M. (1873), *Civil Malpractice* (Chicago: WB Keen Cooke).

11 Marchev, M. (2002), *The Medical Malpractice Insurance Crisis: Opportunity for State Action* (Portland, Maine: National Academy for State Health Policy, USA).

12 Common Good (2002), 'The Effects of Law on Health Care', *Common Good Forum: Building a New System of Medical Justice* (Washington, DC: AEI-Brookings Joint Center for Regulatory Studies).

13 Brody, W.R. (2003), 'Is the Legal System Killing Healthcare?' (New York: Common Good at the Manhattan Institute).

14 Rosenblatt, R.A. et al. (1991), 'Tort Law Reform and the Obstetric Access Crisis. The Case of the WAMI States', *Western Journal of Medicine* 155:4, 428–9.

15 MacLennan, A.H. and Spencer, M.K. (2002), 'Projections of Australian Obstetricians Ceasing Practice and the Reasons', *Medical Journal of Australia* 176:9, 425–8.

16 Meikle, J. (2002), 'Huge Rise in Medical Negligence', *The Guardian*, June 3.

17 Forbes, R. (1948), *Sixty Years of Medical Defence* (London: Medical Defence Union).

18 Rosenthal, M.M. (1987), *Dealing With Medical Malpractice: The British and Swedish Experience* (London: Tavistock).

19 *Action against Medical Accidents* (AvMA) was established in 1982 and is a United Kingdom charity which promotes better patient safety and justice for people who have been affected by a medical accident [web page]: <http://www.avma.org.uk> accessed 11 June 2006.

20 Komesaroff, P.A. et al. (1996), 'Is there a Medical Litigation Crisis?', *Medical Journal of Australia* 164:3, 178–82.

21 Keaney, M.A (1996), 'Is Litigation Increasing?', *Medical Journal of Australia* 164:3, 178–9.

22 Medical Defence Organization insurance premium data from personal communication, Runciman, W.B.

23 Lord Woolf (1996), *Access to Justice: Final Report to the Lord Chancellor on the Civil Justice System in England and Wales* (London: Her Majesty's Stationery Office).

24 Ransom, S.B. et al. (1996), 'The Economic Cost of the Medical-Legal Tort System', *American Journal of Obstetrics and Gynecology* 174:6, 1903–9.

25 Studdert, D.M. et al. (2000), 'Negligent Care and Malpractice Claiming Behavior in Utah and Colorado', *Medical Care* 38:3, 250–60.

26 Localio, A.R. et al. (1991), 'Relation Between Malpractice Claims and Adverse Events Due to Negligence: Results of the Harvard Medical Practice Study III', *New England Journal of Medicine* 325:4, 245–51.

27 Manuel, B.M. (1990), 'Professional Liability – a No-Fault Solution', *New England Journal of Medicine* 322:9, 627–31.

28 Runciman, W.B. and Moller, J. (2001), *Iatrogenic Injury in Australia* (Adelaide: Australian Patient Safety Foundation).

29 National Audit Office, United Kingdom (2001), *Handling Clinical Negligence Claims in England*, Report by the Comptroller and Auditor General, HC 403 (London: National Audit Office). Available at: <http://www.nao.org.uk/publications/nao_reports/00-01/0001403es.pdf> accessed 1 June 2006.

30 Hiatt, H. and Weiler, P. (1999), 'No-Fault Medical Coverage Would Cure Many Ills', *The Boston Globe* 5 November, p. 5.

31 Mello, M.M. and Brennan, T.A. (2002), 'Deterrence of Medical Errors: Theory and Evidence for Malpractice Reform', *Texas Law Review* 80:7, 1595–637.

32 Drimmer, J. (1989), 'My Malpractice Ordeal is Over – After Only 26 Years', *Medical Economics* 2, 50–2.

33 Brennan, T.A., Sox, C.M. and Burstin, H.R. (1996), 'Relation Between Negligent Adverse Events and the Outcomes of Medical-Malpractice Litigation', *New England Journal of Medicine* 335:26, 1963–7.

34 Taragin, M.I. et al. (1992), 'The Influence of Standard of Care and Severity of Injury on the Resolution of Medical Malpractice Claims', *Annals of Internal Medicine* 117:9, 780–4.

35 Walton, M. (1998), *The Trouble with Medicine: Preserving Trust Between Patients and Doctors* (Sydney: Allen and Unwin).

36 Studdert, D.M. and Brennan, T.A. (2001), 'No-Fault Compensation for Medical Injuries: The Prospect for Error Prevention', *Journal of American Medical Association* 286:2, 217–23.

37 Kennedy, I. (2001), *Learning From Bristol: The Report of the Public Inquiry into Children's Heart Surgery at the Bristol Royal Infirmary 1984–1995* (London: The Stationery Office).

38 *R v Adomako* (1994) 3 WLR 288.

39 Williams, L.S. (1995), 'Anesthetist Receives Jail Sentence After Patient Left in Vegetative State', *Canadian Medical Association Journal* 153:5, 619–20.

40 Baker, R. (2001), *Harold Shipman's Clinical Practice 1974–1998* (London: Stationery Office).

41 Skegg, P.D.G. (1998), 'Criminal Prosecutions of Negligent Health Professionals: the New Zealand Experience', *Medical Law Review* 6:Summer, 220–46.

42 *R v Yogasakaran* (1990) 1 NZLR 399 (New Zealand).

43 *R v Callaghan* (1952) 87 CLR 115 (Australia).

44 The case is a genuine one, the names are pseudonyms. It is reproduced, with some changes, from Runciman, W.B. and Merry, A.F. (2005), 'Crises in Clinical Care: An Approach to Management', *Quality and Safety in Health Care* 14:3, 156–63.

45 Millenson, M.L. (2002), 'Breaking Bad News', *Quality and Safety in Health Care*, 11:3, 206–7.

46 Gault, W. (2002), 'Blame to Aim, Risk Management in the NHS', *Risk Management Bulletin* 7:1, 6–11.

47 Berwick, D.M. (2003), 'Improvement, Trust and the Healthcare Workforce', *Quality and Safety in Health Care* 12:Supplement 1, i2–i6.

48 Reason, J. (1997), *Managing the Risks of Organisational Accidents* (Aldershot: Ashgate).

49 Walton, M. (2004), 'Creating a "No Blame" Culture: Have We Got the Balance Right?', *Quality and Safety in Health Care* 13:3, 163–4.

50 Gault, W.G. (2004), *Experimental Exploration of Implicit Blame Attribution in the NHS* (Edinburgh: Grampian University Hospitals NHS Trust).

51 Daniel, A.E., Burn, R.J. and Horarik, S. (1999), 'Patients' Complaints About Medical Practice', *Medical Journal of Australia* 170:12, 598–602.
52 Merry, A.F. and McCall Smith, A. (2001), *Errors, Medicine and the Law* (Cambridge: Cambridge University Press).
53 Helmreich, R.L. and Merritt, A.C. (1998), *Culture at Work in Aviation and Medicine* (Aldershot: Ashgate).
54 Strauch, B. (2002), 'Normal Accidents – Yesterday and Today', in Johnson, C.W. ed., *Workshop on the Investigation and Reporting of Incidents and Accidents (IRIA 2002)*, GIST Technical Report G2002-2 (Glasgow: Department of Computing Science, University of Glasgow).
55 McIntyre, N. and Popper, K. (1983), 'The Critical Attitude in Medicine: the Need for a New Ethics', *British Medical Journal* 287:6409, 1919–23.
56 Leape, L.L. (1994), 'Error in Medicine', *Journal of the American Medical Association*, 272: 1851–1857.
57 Vincent, C., Stanhope, N. and Crowley-Murphy, M. (1999), 'Reasons for Not Reporting Adverse Incidents: an Empirical Study', *Journal of Evaluation in Clinical Practice* 5:1, 13–21.
58 Baylis, F. (1997), 'Errors in Medicine: Nurturing Truthfulness', *The Journal of Clinical Ethics* 8:4, 336–40.
59 Rosenthal, M.M. (1999), 'How Doctors Think about Medical Mishaps', in Rosenthal M.M., Mulcahy, L. and Lloyd-Bostock, S., eds, *Medical Mishaps: Pieces of the Puzzle* (Buckingham: Open University Press).
60 Kapp, M.B. (1997), 'Legal Anxieties and Medical Mistakes: Barriers and Pretexts', *Journal of General Internal Medicine* 12:12, 787–8.
61 Walton, M. (2001), 'Open Disclosure to Patients and Their Families After Medical Errors: a Literature Review' (Canberra: Australian Council on Quality and Safety in Health Care).
62 Allnutt, F. (1987), 'Human Factors in Accidents', *British Journal of Anaesthesia* 59:7, 856–64.
63 Fox, R.C. (1957), 'Training for Uncertainty', in Merton, R.K., Reader, G.G. and Kendall, P.L., eds, *The Student-Physician: Introductory Studies in the Sociology of Medical Education* (Cambridge, MA: Harvard University Press), 207–41.
64 Hilfiker, D. (1984), 'Facing Our Mistakes', *New England Journal of Medicine* 310:2, 118–22.
65 Bell, R.A. et al. (2002), 'Unmet Expectations for Care and the Patient-Physician Relationship', *Journal of General Internal Medicine* 17:11, 817–24.
66 Maller, B.S. (2000), 'Market Trends in Refractive Surgery', *International Ophthalmology Clinics* 40:3, 11–9.
67 Finland (1986), *Patient Injury Act 585/86.*
68 Accident Compensation Corporation of New Zealand [web page] <http://www.acc.co.nz> accessed 1 June 2006.
69 Health and Disability Commissioner, New Zealand [web page] <http://www.hdc.org.nz/> accessed 1 June 2006.
70 Health and Disability Commissioner (2004), 'Case 02HDC05291. Anaesthetist. Error in Administration of Anaesthetic' (Auckland: Health and Disability Commissioner of New Zealand).

Chapter 5

Human Error and Complex Systems

Humans Versus Systems

Human error underlies many of the things that go wrong in the delivery of healthcare, a quintessentially human endeavour. Errors may occur in deciding what to do, in the organization of healthcare, in the design or choice of equipment, in the imperfect execution of a procedure or in a simple slip or lapse.

This idea is reflected in the first part of the title of the seminal report by the Institute of Medicine, *To Err is Human: Building a Safer Health System.*[1] The second part of the title implies that the solution lies in the system. The challenge is to exploit the undeniable strengths of the human mind and spirit, but to deploy these attributes in a system designed to compensate for human fallibility.

The contributing factors and hazards that conspire together in never-ending combinations to cause incidents and adverse events in healthcare are shown in Figure 1.6. In this chapter we will address human contributing factors (errors and violations) and how they interact with failures in the system to breach its defences. We are equally interested in the extraordinary capacity of human beings to continuously intercept things that are going wrong and steer the trajectories of evolving events away from potential tragedy towards safe and successful outcomes. The importance of minimizing harm after things have gone wrong is discussed in Chapter 8.

Complex Systems

A system is any collection of two or more interacting parts. A system may be thought of as complex if the number of possible interactions is such that predicting its long term behaviour on the basis of knowledge of its component parts becomes difficult or impossible.[2] Charles Perrow argues that accidents are inevitable in complex systems.[3] Healthcare is a complex system (see Figures 1.5 and 1.6) comprising humans (patients and staff), infrastructure, technology and therapeutic agents; these components interact in highly complex, almost infinitely variable ways.

In his book *Normal Accidents*, Perrow characterizes processes on two dimensions.[3] The first dimension is *complexity*, on a continuum from linear to complex. Sorting mail in a post office is a linear process, and much manufacturing uses linear or production line processes. Managing patients in a hospital is a complex process, in which the possible variations of order in and inter-relationships between tasks are almost infinite. The second dimension is *coupling*.

Coupling is the relationship between an action and its consequences. Putting one's hand into a fire would be tightly coupled to getting burnt: a burn would result every time. Attending lectures at University is loosely coupled to attaining one's degree: one could miss several lectures and still do well in the end. Actions in healthcare vary from loosely coupled to tightly coupled.[4] The injection of concentrated potassium chloride intravenously instead of saline (for example) is tightly coupled to the immediate death of the patient. Forgetting to give an antibiotic before an operation is loosely coupled to the possible complication of a postoperative wound infection.

In evaluating the safety of complex systems, Perrow also takes into account the social utility of the system and the potential consequences of failure. For many systems, the benefits are such that it is reasonable to accept occasional disasters; aviation is an example, and so is healthcare. For certain activities, however, the catastrophic consequences of failure may be thought to outweigh any benefits. Perrow places the nuclear industry in this category.

The Differences between Healthcare and other Complex Systems

There is no doubt that healthcare is a complex system, and that it is one which shares many characteristics with other hazardous high-technology systems such as commercial aviation, nuclear power generation, railways, marine operations, chemical process plants and the like. Where there are functional and structural overlaps between healthcare and these other systems, it is possible to import valuable lessons regarding safety. However, it must also be appreciated that healthcare differs in several important ways from most other hazardous domains.[5]

Diversity Within healthcare there is an enormous diversity of tasks and of the means for carrying them out. By contrast, aviation, nuclear power generation and railways systems are relatively homogeneous. Transport systems move people and goods from A to B, mostly in a tightly scheduled fashion, and power generating systems push out megawatts in as stable a manner as possible. Each domain has a limited number of types of equipment. In modern commercial aviation two manufacturers – Boeing and Airbus – supply the vast majority of aircraft. Little or none of this standardization can be found in healthcare.[5] Indeed 'product differentiation' to promote marketing has had the opposite effect. For example, deliberately adding features to a ventilator, not because there is a need or demand for them, but simply to differentiate it from a competitor's product, increases complexity and the chance for errors for almost no added benefit.

Vulnerability Unlike passengers or consumers of electrical power, many patients are, by definition, vulnerable people. They are usually sick or injured, and often old or very young (see pages 34 and 35). This vulnerability increases their liability to serious damage by unsafe acts. There are few areas of human endeavour outside healthcare, including modern warfare, in which certain planned procedures routinely carry mortality rates well in excess of 1 per cent.

Activity patterns, uncertainty and lack of regulation Healthcare also differs from most other complex systems with respect to its activity patterns, which often have a great deal of immediate human involvement with high safety-criticality (see pages 119–121), with respect to its uncertainty (see Chapter 7), and with respect to its lack of regulation (see Chapters 7 and 11).

Error and Blame

Pioneers such as Perrow,[3] Reason[5] and Rasmussen[6] originally suggested that the operator, or human, is typically the component of a system that is the most difficult to change, and advanced the idea that the main response to an accident should be system-based, rather than person-based. According to this view, blame (inherent in the person-based approach) is particularly counter-productive. The emphasis on a system-based response to accidents has increased to the point where some commentators even suggest that the concept of error is itself unhelpful. Defining error, classifying it, or even identifying it is seen as very difficult, and it is argued that effort is better directed towards understanding and improving the function of the system as a whole without worrying about whether or not any particular event is an error. The research associated with this view is known as '*The New Look*'.[6,7]

These are the opinions of some experts in the fields of human cognition, human factors and safe system design, and they have much merit. However, the public seems often to take a different view. The media is full of stories of medical negligence, usually with calls for greater accountability for health professionals. In Great Britain and New Zealand there has been an increase in the use of the criminal law to prosecute doctors after the accidental death of patients. It seems clear that many people, including some judges, have great difficulty accepting a 'no blame' response to the harm caused by health care. Indeed, it can be argued that personal accountability is one of the fundamentals of a healthy moral society.

A number of authorities now argue that blame does have a legitimate place in improving healthcare.[8,9] Bagian[10] and Marx[11] in the USA and Reason[12] in the UK have developed processes for triage between blameless errors and acts of a more egregious nature (see pages 202–205). The former are subject to a systems-based process of root cause analysis while the latter are passed on to the appropriate authorities to be dealt with very much in a person-based fashion.[12]

Making a proper distinction between culpable acts and situations in which no culpability should apply is in the interests of natural justice and of prevention of harm in healthcare, and is the essence of a *just culture*.[11] Unlike the proponents of the 'New Look', we think a proper definition of the term 'error' is both possible and worthwhile. It is vital to distinguish between errors, the origins of which lie in human evolution and the defences to which lie in error proofing the system, and violations, the origins of which lie more in human behaviour and culture, and the defences to which lie in changing behaviour as well as better system design. We need to understand the types of error and violation, and how they come about, if we are to devise strategies to prevent them, or to intercept them before they cause harm. We will therefore consider errors, violations and deliberate harm, in turn, before addressing some human strengths and weaknesses and the troubled and troubling relationship between outcome and error.

Errors

In simple English, an *error* occurs 'when someone is trying to do the right thing, but actually does the wrong thing'. The key element is that there is a deviation from what is intended and that this deviation is not deliberate. A more formal definition of error is 'the unintentional use of a wrong plan to achieve an aim, or failure to carry out a planned action as intended'.[13] Outcome has no place in the definition of error, although in practice it often draws attention to the fact that something has gone wrong and influences our perception of an error.

There are many classifications of error. Phenomenological classifications can be useful in describing the types of error that occur in a particular context – inadvertent overdose or omission in drug administration, for example.[14] Traditionally, authorities such as Rasmussen and Reason have identified knowledge-based, rule-based, and skilled-based errors (slips and lapses); this classification is based on identifying the cognitive process involved in the generation of the error. Later, technical errors (flawed executions of correct actions) were added to this classification.[15] We propose an extension of these ideas that we think is useful for devising corrective strategies. For example, if the wrong dose of a drug was given it would be useful to know whether this was due to inadequate knowledge stored in the mind of the practitioner about the correct dose, or because of an error in the calculation of the dose. Each of these rather different types of error would be classified in the original Reason-Rasmussen model as a knowledge-based error.

The Basics

The knowledge base Humans inhabit the physical world. In order to function within this world, they need to assimilate information about their surroundings, interpret it, and respond to it. Information exists in the mind and in the world (Box 5.1). It is possible to demonstrate by a simple exercise (Box 5.2) that humans function not on the basis of the world as it actually is, but on the basis of an internal representation of the world, within their minds. Furthermore, this representation is based on a very limited, and often imperfect, subset of information. This is just as well. We are flooded with incoming information. Making sense of the world would be impossible if it were not for the fact that we sift the pertinent facts from the simply salient and integrate these into a coherent conceptualization of our surroundings. This conceptualization is called a mental model or schema: schemata may be literal, such as of the furniture in a typical dining room, or conceptual, such as of the properties of an exponential function.[16]

Box 5.1 Information available to the health professional

Information in the mind:
  - in his or her own mind (knowledge);
  - in other peoples minds, accessible by:
    consultation, or, for example,
    taking a history from a patient.
Information in the world:
  - physical – accessible by examining the surroundings or a patient;
  - written – accessible from patient records, books and journals; or
  - electronic – accessible by means of computers.

Bounded or keyhole rationality Consider a black-board full of information in a dark room. A small circular area of the board is illuminated by a spotlight, which reveals a small, randomly selected, portion of the information. Moving the light allows more of the information to be accessed, but it is not possible to see all the information at one time. Even after shining the light in many places, it is rather difficult to be sure that one has accessed all the information on the board.

In an analogous way, the set of information available for decision making at any particular time is usually incomplete and sometimes inaccurate. One can generally acquire more information, but it is hard to know what is missing and therefore difficult to be sure about when to stop chasing facts and get on with making a decision. This difficulty is referred to as *bounded*, or *keyhole*, rationality.

Box 5.2   An exercise to demonstrate the gap between information in the world and information in the mind

Close your eyes. Attempt to list, in detail, the objects in your immediate surroundings. Describe their features – the colours of the walls of the room, the clothes people are wearing, the types of trees in the garden, and so on. Then open your eyes. It should be apparent that there is much more information in the world about you than you can recall or have even noticed. Furthermore, in all likelihood, some of the information you recalled will be incorrect.

Minute by minute, we function on the basis of an internal representation of the world – *information in our mind*. This is a limited and often imperfect representation of the world as it actually is. However, for most purposes, it is adequate. If we need more information, it is usually present in our surroundings, as *information in the world*, and we can access it by simple inspection.

Rules or precompiled responses Humans have a strong predilection for pattern recognition and rule-based decision making. On the whole people prefer this to thinking from first principles, presumably because the latter requires more effort. This predilection for pattern recognition has been called '*reluctant rationality*'.

Positron Emission Tomography (PET scanning) of the brain has been used to demonstrate that the difference between these two types of thinking has a physiological basis. Novices presented with a complex task manifest a particular pattern of activity on their PET scans. Expertise, to a very large extent, represents the assimilation of large quantities of pre-stored schemata and associated rules. The expert can recognize complex situations and instantly respond with an appropriate set of actions. Little conscious thought is necessary. After training and the development of expertise in relation to the specified task, the areas of the brain which light up on scanning are different from those in the novice. Of course, there is a continuum rather than a dichotomy: at one end, actions are entirely automatic with no conscious thought at all; at the other, they are the result of a laborious and highly conscious process of thinking and reasoning (see Figure 5.1).

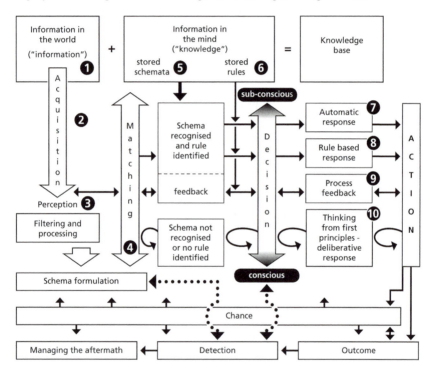

Figure 5.1 Schematic representation of the types of error that can be made (1–10, see Table 5.1 and accompanying text) **in making and carrying out a plan**

A Classification of Error

The processes involved in the generation of an action are depicted in Figure 5.1 and listed in Table 5.1. Information is acquired from the world, filtered and processed, and used to generate schemata representing a conceptual interpretation of the situation;[16] incoming information is compared with information in the mind (also stored as schemata). We propose to call the information stored in a person's mind *knowledge* to distinguish it from information in the world, which we will call *information* (other people's knowledge is treated as information). If a match is achieved between the interpretation of the present situation and a previously stored schema, a rule (also pre-stored) can be applied (if available), and an action generated. Sometimes, if the situation is familiar, an action can be generated automatically, with no conscious thought. On the other hand, if no match can be made, or no rule found, it becomes necessary to think from first principles – to deliberate. On the basis of this deliberation, a decision is made and an action generated. Actions generated (whatever the decision process) may or may not be the ones intended. Their execution may be flawed, sometimes because the cues necessary to guide them are under-specified or simply because the actions are poorly or wrongly carried out.[8] It is possible for things to go wrong with each of these processes (see Figure 5.1). Chance may play a role in influencing how and why things go wrong, and has an important influence on the outcome of any decision or action, erroneous or not.

Table 5.1 A classification of error

1.	Errors in information
2.	Errors in acquisition of knowledge
3.	Errors in perception
4.	Errors in matching (including fixation errors)
5.	Errors in knowledge stored as schemata
6.	Errors in knowledge stored as rules
7.	Skill-based errors – slips and lapses
8.	Errors in choice of rule
9.	Technical errors
10.	Deliberative errors

1. Errors in information   Many errors in healthcare arise because of faulty, incomplete or absent information. This information may relate to the patient's history or physical signs, facts recorded in the notes, results of blood tests recorded on computers, or information held in the minds of other health professionals. There is a real challenge in healthcare in providing all the information needed for proper decision making, in the right form, to the person who needs it, at the time it is needed. 'Handovers' at a change of shift are a rich source of problems in this area.[17] Electronic databases and record keeping may be helpful, but a fundamental aspect of bounded rationality remains – it is always difficult and sometimes impossible to know what one does not know (see Boxes 1.1, 5.6, 5.7).

2. Errors in acquisition of knowledge   Even if the required information is available, it is necessary to acquire it. This may go wrong in several ways. Firstly, there may be a simple failure to read the notes, to take a history or to examine the patient.

This is the fundamental problem underlying many adverse events. The information was readily available but it is quite clear that the decision-maker failed to access it. In its crudest manifestation a diagnosis of death by natural causes may be made and recorded before turning the dead patient over in bed and finding multiple stab wounds in the back. More realistically, finding the result of a laboratory investigation may be quite difficult, particularly if it is misfiled in a large set of notes; under these circumstances, a clinician may simply give up trying, and assume that all is well. Sometimes a clinician may not even be aware that the notes contain an unseen but important piece of information (see Box 5.7). There have been many cases of positive pathology results being filed in notes without being seen by doctors, with the result that a required action has not been taken (see Box 3.6).

3. Errors in perception The information may be inspected but misunderstood. One word may be mistaken for another, or instructions may be incorrectly heard. People do not read words letter by letter. They recognize the general shape and appearance of the word, as a whole. It is very easy to read what one expects to see, rather than what one actually sees. Unfortunately, it is the perceived information that will be acted upon, not the actual information. The presentation of different drugs in ampoules of similar appearance with hard-to-read labels is an excellent example of poor design which may predispose to errors in perception of crucial information. This is a common type of error in healthcare; it leads to the wrong conceptual schema being generated (see Box 5.3).

4. Errors in matching Cognition does not involve a direct response to perceived information. It is necessary for the overwhelming flood of facts to be filtered and matched before sense can be made of them. New information must be interpreted not only within the context of the instant but also in the light of what has gone before. Unfortunately this leads to a phenomenon that can be a powerful cause of failure in cognition. *Confirmation bias* or *fixation error* are terms describing the processes by which new information tends to be interpreted to fit a preformed ('strong but wrong') concept or schema.[16,18] This may have been formed moments before, as in an evolving crisis, or at some stage in the recent or distant past. Once one has decided on a diagnosis, new signs tend to be fitted into that diagnosis rather than being taken as evidence to the contrary. There is a tendency to interpret information to fit one's personal store of patterns. In a patient with back pain, an orthopaedic surgeon will perhaps see a problem in a joint where a neurologist might attribute it to a nerve and a psychiatrist to the brain. One criticism of the so-called medical model is that doctors diagnose conditions (schizophrenia, for example) which certain other people consider to be variations on the normal. What is at issue in these disputes is the need not just to *sense* the world around us, but to *make sense* of it. Making sense is influenced by personal experience – one person's understanding of a situation will not necessarily match another's. There is room for difference in this regard, but at a certain point a person's view of the world can be so fixated ('this and only this') that decision making will not produce a functional result (see Box 4.5).

5. Errors in knowledge stored as schemata Errors at this level are of two primary types: absent knowledge (knowledge that is not known because it has never been known or has been forgotten) and knowledge which is incorrect. This is the basis for many of the problems which lead to patient harm. A great deal of effort in healthcare is directed to improving knowledge, but part of the problem is the excessive emphasis placed on memory. In Chapter 7 we point out that it is not possible for individuals to know all the necessary information for making the best decisions in clinical medicine. Modern technology has, to some extent, overcome the limitations of knowledge and memory by providing access to accurate, up to date and relevant information at the time and place it is needed – by having access to computer systems at the point of care.

Box 5.3 Rescue from a fatal overdose

Mr. Clifford was a 48 year old man who, one year previously, had half of his large bowel removed for cancer. He was diagnosed a year later with a single metastatic secondary in the left lobe of his liver. It was thought to be worthwhile to remove the left half of his liver as the lesion might have been an isolated secondary. He underwent the procedure, and the surgeons had considerable difficulty in stopping the bleeding during the operation. After the operation, a nurse mistakenly gave him 50,000 units of heparin by subcutaneous injection when the order was for 5,000 units. Heparin in this lower dose is used to prevent deep vein thrombosis after operations of this kind. The ampoules are almost identical and both the nurse and the person who checked the ampoule failed to notice that the dose was ten times greater than intended. However, the nurse who gave the injection realized her mistake, and immediately reported this to the registrar on the ward. As there is an antidote to this anticoagulant, blood tests were done every hour and doses of antidote were given, appropriately. The patient did not suffer a major bleed and within 12 hours the situation had stabilized. The staff immediately explained what had happened to the patient. The nurse apologized and was tearful and extremely concerned for the welfare of the patient, as use of the antidote carries a significant risk of an adverse reaction. The patient ended up comforting the nurse, accepting the apology, and a few days later bought her a box of chocolates to thank her for promptly owning up to her mistake, which may well have saved his life.

---

6. Errors in knowledge stored as rules Experience in medicine involves building up identifiable patterns or schema of clinical situations and of responses to them. The ability to look at a clinical situation, make a diagnosis and know what to do has been called clinical acumen. Knowing what to do is encapsulated in a rule. Errors may arise because an important rule has never been stored or has been forgotten or because what has been stored is wrong. One example of this may be the incorrect injection of the entire contents of an ampoule because of an erroneous 'rule' that all ampoules contain the average dose for an adult.

7. Skill based errors – slips and lapses These manifest as forgetting to do something or enacting the wrong sequence of actions because of 'attentional capture' (see page 120). Complex sequences of actions can be involved because of what is known as 'chunking'. For example, entering one's house is not perceived as a vast sequence of unrelated facts (front door, carpet, wall colour, pictures, ceiling, lights etc.) but as a single conceptual whole – the experience of being 'home'. In a similar way, many actions are chunked and executed as integrated blocks of cognition and action. For example, tying shoelaces is typically a chunked activity. If interrupted, many people find it easier to start again from the beginning than to resume from where they left off, because the process has been learned as a whole, not as a sequence of linked parts. Chunking predisposes to the carrying out of complex, correctly executed but unintended and inappropriate sequences.

8. Errors in choice of rule Here rules which are not intrinsically wrong are wrongly chosen and applied. For example, a particular drug may be used to treat an abnormal rhythm of the heart. A doctor might diagnose a dysrhythmia correctly, but choose a rule for treating another dysrhythmia to treat it. Thus, a perfectly good rule might be applied in the wrong context. This type of error is midway on the continuum between subconsciously capturing a completely inappropriate set of actions and having to think from first principles. It can be thought of as the cognitive analogue of a slip.

9. Technical errors Technical errors involve the imperfect execution of correct actions because of under specification of the situation or a mismatch between the demands of the task and the skill of the operator. Thus a person attempting to place the tip of a needle in the epidural space during labour may fail in this endeavour because he or she cannot actually visualize the precise location of the tip of the needle. Some practitioners are highly skilled and others are less so. Training and practice improve skill. In effect, technical errors represent mismatches between the skill and ability of the practitioner and the challenge posed by the task in the prevailing circumstances.

10. Deliberative errors Deliberative error occurs when rules run out and people have to work things out from first principles, either because the situation is new or because they recognize that they have never developed or stored a rule for it before (see page 121). An important practical difference between rule-based and deliberative decisions is that the former can usually be made almost instantaneously, whereas as the latter typically take longer. The situation described in Box 4.5 was one in which the rules failed, and the need was for a response which had to be worked out from first principles. This example provides a good illustration of the very real difficulties faced when deliberative decisions have to be made rapidly.

Chance

All types of error may be influenced by chance, as cognitive function can be degraded by extraneous factors which may just happen to intrude at a crucial moment (a distraction or a sudden change in ambient light or sound). The *detection* and *outcome* of an error may also be heavily influenced by chance. The outcome will also depend on whether the problem is detected before harm has occurred and on how the *aftermath* is handled (see Chapter 8). For example, a breathing circuit disconnection under anaesthesia in a paralyzed patient is of no consequence if detected and corrected immediately, but will result in brain damage or death if detected late and/or not corrected in a timely manner.

Combinations of errors   The lines between these different types of error are not clearly drawn. Many errors are made up of combinations of these different failures in cognitive processing. For example the error in Box 5.3 may have had elements of errors of Type 2 (in the acquisition of knowledge), Type 3 (in the formation of a schema of 5,000 Units instead of 50,000 Units because of matching of the actual ampoule with a strong frequently reinforced (very similar) image of commonly used 5,000 Unit ampoules), and Type 5 (in the lack of knowledge that a near identical 50,000 Unit ampoule even exists). More than one error may be made in some instances – this may compound the problem, but occasionally saves the day (see Box 5.4). The model proposed here may seem complex, but in fact leaves many aspects of human cognition unaccounted for. For example, it has not factored in the concept of ironic processes of mental control.[19] These are well illustrated in the context of sport: for example, concentrating on avoiding a water hazard in golf may prove not only useless but in fact positively counterproductive. Similarly, trying to go to sleep tends to result in one's staying awake. There is much about the working of the human mind that we have still to understand.

Errors and Categories of Human Activity

Human activities fall into four categories; this classification applies to workplace activities, but also, more generally, to all aspects of daily life. These categories are:

- Routine operations.
- Maintenance activities.
- Dealing with abnormal conditions (sometimes in emergencies).
- Creative activities (sometimes in emergencies).

The amount of time that people spend on each category of activity depends very much on the *type of work* in question and on their *role* in that work. Bus drivers, laboratory workers, commercial airline pilots or surgeons specializing in cataract procedures may spend the majority of their time on routine operations, and a fair amount on what might be described as maintenance activities. However, racing

---

Box 5.4 Saved by a double error

Cardiac output may be measured by injecting 10ml of cold fluid into a special catheter placed into the heart, and then measuring the profile of the change in temperature after blood leaves the right-side of the heart with a thermistor in the main artery going to the lungs. Triplicate measurements are usually made, by means of three injections of 10ml of 5 per cent dextrose. On a particular occasion, when the first of the set of three rapid injections was made, the fluid squirted from the tap at the end of the catheter into which the injection was being made into the eye of the person making the injection. This was because the tap had inadvertently been turned to the 'off' position. As this stung badly, the operator checked the ampoules from which the cold '5 per cent dextrose' had been drawn. These turned out to contain 10 per cent potassium chloride. If the tap had been turned on correctly so that the fluid had gone as intended into the right-side of the heart, the patient would have died within seconds of the injection. As it was, the fluid squirted harmlessly away, except for a few drops which stung the eye of the injector and saved the day.

---

drivers, interventional radiologists, fighter pilots or trauma surgeons might spend much more time dealing with highly variable or abnormal conditions which may sometimes require creative approaches. To some extent, spending too much time in one or two of these modes of operation can compromise ones performance in the other areas. People are more prone to certain types of errors with certain types of activity.

Slips and lapses are typically a problem in routine or repetitive activities. They generally occur because of inattention, distraction and multi-tasking. Many drug administration errors are of this type. For example, during an anaesthetic a drug may be omitted simply because the practitioner was distracted at the time it ought to have been given. Alternatively a wrong drug may be given, automatically, and without conscious thought, because the practitioner's mind is elsewhere, because of distraction (attentional capture).

Rule-based errors are also associated with routine activities. Humans are attracted to particular rule-based solutions on the basis of a number of factors. The first relates to the *recency* with which a situation has been seen before – one is more likely to choose a solution that has worked recently than one buried in the distant past. The second relates to the *strength* with which a particular experience has embedded itself in the mind. For example, the fact that a particular situation resulted in a catastrophic outcome on one previous occasion is likely to colour a practitioner's view of matters strongly, even though a logical view of events might be that the catastrophe represented a vary rare complication (anaphylaxis for example) and is most unlikely to happen again. Doctors are taught not to base their practices on anecdote, and one aim of medical training is to build up a sizable store of appropriate rules based on evidence and logic, but in fact personal experience is often the primary driver in their decision making. It is thus possible to have a *strong* match between a pre-stored solution and a particular set of circumstances, which is in fact *wrong*.[16,18] Without doubt, experience is more influential than information in colouring practice.

Deliberative errors   People resort to deliberation only when rules run out. Deliberation is therefore typical of abnormal or unfamiliar situations. In a situation which has not been seen before, there is no choice but to think from first principles. Certain forms of creative activity involve deliberation – writing a book for example. The need to deliberate does not in itself create any particular difficulty, provided enough time is available. Some professions focus on deliberative activities – engineers working on novel problems, for example. Training and experience equip the professional to develop rules to solve problems for which the solution has not previously been worked out. Most of healthcare involves applying established approaches to the treatment of medical conditions, rather than working from first principles. Most decisions are rule based – if the patient has a stiff neck and pyrexia, meningitis must be ruled out. The pattern must be recognized, and the appropriate response known.

Crises   In healthcare, there are occasions when time is strictly limited. In an anaesthetic crisis, a problem in oxygenating the patient may need to be resolved within three or four minutes if irreversible brain damage is to be avoided. So long as rule-based decision making works, limitations of time do not pose an insuperable problem. A *crisis* may be defined as a situation in which the rules have run out and time is limited.[20] Imagine trying to work out from first principles the cause of a failure in the mechanism for opening a parachute. This problem would provide nothing to worry about if it were presented to a person working at a bench in a laboratory. For the parachutist who has begun his or her (rather too rapid) descent towards the earth, thinking from first principles is not appropriate. The rule is: pull the cord for the reserve chute. If this rule works, the crisis is brought to an abrupt end. If it fails, a catastrophic outcome is likely. It is surprisingly easy to overlook the importance of limited time when retrospectively judging the performance of health care professionals in emergencies (see Box 4.5).

Errors of judgement   The term 'error of judgement' is in common use, but we do not find this concept particularly helpful. In effect, judgement is a form of deliberation and it is difficult to distinguish errors of judgement from errors of deliberation. In practice, the tendency is to call a decision an error of judgement if it works out badly, and to praise an individual's judgement if it works out well. This is inconsistent with our view that decisions should be judged on the merits of the argument rather than on their outcome. The term error of judgement implies that the decision was not flawed on solely objective grounds. It is therefore a *normative* description of the error. It suggests that in the judgement of the person making the assessment, the decision was not a good one. There is circularity in this view. It leads to the conclusion that the evaluation of judgement in any single event is probably a matter of opinion. Over a series of events one might be able to obtain statistical data to support or refute such opinion. This would elevate the decision to one based on evidence rather than opinion, so judgement would no longer be at stake.

Violations

Violations differ from errors in that they involve an element of choice and usually involve a 'trade-off'. A simple-English definition of violation is '*an act which knowingly incurs a risk*'. A more formal definition can be put together from elements of two different definitions proposed by James Reason:[8,16] '*A violation is a deliberate – but not necessarily reprehensible – deviation from safe operating procedures, standards or rules.*' Violations range from routine acts which may be virtually subconscious or even well intended to the deliberate compromise of other people's safety for personal benefit or gratification. Reason makes the point that 'the boundaries between errors and violations are by no means hard and fast, either conceptually or within a particular accident sequence'.

A Classification of Violation

Routine violations These can be seen daily in most workplaces, and typically involve the cutting of corners in everyday tasks. Violations often involve a trade-off between safety and (perceived) efficiency. A classic example is the failure of health professionals to wash their hands between contact with successive patients. There is a wealth of literature to show that this simple measure substantially reduces the risk of nosocomial infection.[21] Failure to follow this rule may initially reflect pressures of everyday work, a lack of adequate facilities for hand-washing or failure on the part of senior members of staff to provide appropriate role models in this regard. After a while, violations may become subconscious. It could then be asked whether they constitute an error, rather than a violation. The fact that they are daily occurrences helps to distinguish them from errors. Errors are nearly always exceptional events. The element of choice in a routine violation may only relate to the first few times the violation is committed. Nevertheless it is usually possible to change one's behaviour in respect of a violation by deciding to stop violating. In the case of error, decision alone cannot prevent recurrences.

Corporate violations Many violations are 'corporate violations' rather than individual violations (see Box 5.6). Doctors, especially junior doctors, often work very long hours. The evidence on fatigue indicates that this is unsafe (see page 236).[22] However, the necessity for working long hours is forced upon individuals by the system. This has been called a *systems double-bind*.[16] This for example, was the case when a young doctor injected penicillin into the wrong line in a patient after working for 110 hours in one week (see Box 3.5).[23] These excessive hours of work may well have contributed to her mistake, but the decision to keep going reflected commitment to the job rather than any morally reprehensible lack of concern for the safety of her patients.

Exceptional violations occur under conditions in which some rule which is normally accepted as appropriate cannot easily be followed. Under exceptional circumstances it may even be preferable or unavoidable to violate a rule. These violations are called *appropriate* or *necessary*. For example, in a life-threatening emergency, those involved may deliberately chose to dispense with record keeping, even though it is a clear rule that adequate, timely records should be kept.

Optimizing violations by contrast, are violations for self-gratification or personal benefit. Driving too fast, in the pursuit of excitement rather than because of an emergency, would be an optimizing violation. Although those committing violations have no intention of harming anyone, they are behaving unethically as the decision involves a deliberate choice to gain personal satisfaction or benefit at the cost of increasing the risk to someone else (see Box 5.5). Unnecessarily rude, aggressive or overbearing behaviour may be regarded as a variant of such a violation and may unsettle other people and impair their performance.

Violations as antecedents to errors and adverse events Violations are highly undesirable primarily because they increase both the likelihood of error and the propensity for harm if an error is made. For example, speed itself may not cause motor accidents, but it reduces the time available for the driver to react to unexpected situations and increases the chance of error. If an error occurs, and an accident follows, the energy associated with the crash is increased and so is the risk and severity of harm.

Box 5.5 A dangerous optimizing violation – a case of hit and run

One of the authors was a member of the team called to the post-operative recovery ward of a large private hospital to resuscitate and retrieve a patient who had collapsed after an operation for perforation of the large bowel.[24] On arrival, the patient was grey and pulseless and was being artificially ventilated by mask by a senior recovery nurse. The surgeon had left immediately after the case, and the anaesthetist had been on his way out of the hospital when the patient had collapsed. The anaesthetist had glanced at the patient, ordered an increase in the rate of fluid infusion, suggested that the nurse assist ventilation if necessary, instructed the staff to call for a retrieval team, and walked out. Fortunately, the patient responded to resuscitation when this was started by the retrieval team and after several weeks in Intensive Care at a teaching hospital was discharged to a general ward. When questioned, the anaesthetist, who had recently qualified as a specialist, simply stated that the realities of competitive private practice were such that if he had kept the surgeon waiting for the next case at another hospital, he may have lost that surgeon's patronage. He stated that retrieval teams were there to take care of the sort of problem that he had encountered.

Deliberate Harm

Harold Shipman, the English general practitioner who murdered over 200 of his patients, provides an illustration of a practitioner who deliberately harmed people (see Box 4.4).[25] Despite the extraordinarily high profile of his case, deliberate harm is rare in healthcare; accidental, unintended harm exceeds deliberate harm by several orders of magnitude. Obviously, deliberate harm constitutes a violation but in general the term violation applies to situations in which harm is not intended (although the operator may know that the safety margin has been reduced).

There is a continuum from violations in which harm is very unlikely to those in which it is almost inevitable. Lawyers would use the term recklessness to describe violations in which harm is likely and may be severe; if death ensues, such a violation may attract a charge of manslaughter. The difference between recklessness and deliberate harm may be slight (see Boxes 4.3 and 5.5),[9] and the legal sequelae often depend on the outcome of an action rather than of the degree of culpability associated with it.

Human Strengths and Weaknesses

Man, Machines, Error and Effort

On man and machines One of the most distinctive features of mankind's success in the last 10,000 years, has been the development of machinery. The increase in the quantity, complexity and capability of machinery has been exponential. Since the industrial revolution, society has been redefined by machinery. Machinery is integral to human existence today, and our experience of machinery has almost certainly coloured our perception of human cognition, or at least of what we think human cognition might be like.

Machines are, on the whole, predictable and reliable. These are highly valued attributes in machinery, but it is a mistake to think that failure to exhibit these attributes to the same degree is a weakness on the part of humans. Humans are not machines and are not even like machines. The reality is that humans create machines to do some things better than we can ourselves, or to do things we don't want to do or cannot do. In comparison with machines, humans are relatively unpredictable and unreliable, but are also creative, imaginative, empathic, self-aware and distractible. Distractibility, in particular, predisposes human beings to error. However, distractibility is also a survival advantage. A machine will continue its repetitive task, without stopping, even if its surroundings catch on fire and threaten its very existence, while a person will notice that something is amiss and respond appropriately. Like the other characteristics listed, distractibility has contributed to mankind's success. Failure to behave like machines should not be seen as a human frailty, but rather celebrated as a human strength. The human propensity for error is associated with this strength – put simply, error is the downside of having a brain.

Hard and soft engineering Machines do some things well and other things poorly. Humans, similarly, are very good at some things and bad at others. Norman has drawn attention to an approach to design which he calls 'soft engineering'.[26] This approach is based on assigning to machines the things that machines do well and to humans the things that humans do well (see page 258). 'Hard engineering', by contrast, is predicated on the concept that the engineered solution ought to solve the entire problem. In some circumstances this might work well, but in others a better solution will be obtained by leaving to humans those activities at which humans are better than machines. Improving safety is as much about appropriately assigning tasks between machines and humans as it is about automating tasks or creating new technology. Reason has emphasized that human attributes are essential for efficiently navigating the complexity of healthcare. He has made the point that the capacity for humans to retrieve apparently hopeless situations by the use of imagination and lateral thinking is at times extraordinary, but often fails to attract the same amount of attention as the errors which set up the difficult situation in the first place.

The 'catch-22' of human supervisory control This phrase was coined by Reason to describe a common paradox in healthcare and other industries.[16] In certain activities, notably anaesthesia and nuclear power generation, humans are used to monitor essentially stable situations over long periods of time. One of the main reasons for using a human in this situation is because of the human capacity to respond appropriately to unexpected situations when they do arise. The irony, however, is that the capacity to respond in this way depends to a large extent on regular training and practice. The process of routine monitoring does not enhance the skills required to manage a crisis when it develops. Taking the anaesthetic example, the better an anaesthetist does the job of routine monitoring the less often she or he will have the opportunity to practise crisis management. Ultimately, the hours, days and years spent on supervisory control do not equip the anaesthetist for the task that really does require a human, and a human with up to date expertise and regularly practised skills at that.

Forced and unforced errors In the context of sport, the concept of a forced error is well understood. A tennis player who hits a ball out of court has presumably made an error if his or her intention was to hit it in court. Observers clearly distinguish between a situation in which a shot ought to have been within the capability of the player and a shot which has been set up by the opponent in such a way that it was beyond the player's capability to return the ball, and perhaps beyond the capability of any reasonable player. The latter situation is described as a forced error. This analogy applies to healthcare. Because of the necessity to proceed, particularly in an emergency, surgeons, anaesthetists and other doctors sometimes find themselves stretched to the limit of their abilities. Under these circumstances most types of error will occur more frequently than in situations of a more routine nature. Not surprisingly, recent research in a human patient simulator has demonstrated that placing anaesthetists under stress in difficult circumstances reliably results in both forced and unforced errors.[27]

Effort, management and errors   Because error is unintentional, it is clearly not possible to avoid errors altogether simply by deciding to try harder. However, Gawande has made the point that effort does matter, although effort is more effective in the avoidance of violation than in the avoidance of error.[28] Effort does contribute to error reduction, because distraction can contribute to error, and extra effort can increase the degree to which an individual concentrates on a difficult activity. Maintaining maximal effort at all times is, however, almost impossible. The relationship between management and front-line staff is important in this regard. The intangible benefits of engaging the workers fully in promoting safe and efficient healthcare are substantial, but difficult to quantify in a way that can be demonstrated on a balance sheet. Management that is predicated on simplistic, financial principles is often de-motivating. Creating an environment in which safety is paramount is in part dependent on creating an environment in which morale is high and people feel motivated to do their best for patients (see pages 267 and 268). However, continuous sustained concentration and vigilance are tasks for which humans are ill-equipped, and the use of machines to help in these circumstances should be considered where possible.

Outcome, Error, Blame and Chance

Error is often defined in relation to outcome, erroneously in our view. Outcome is not a good way of deciding whether a particular decision is a mistake or a particular action constitutes an error. There are many examples of 'fortunate errors' which result in unexpected but welcome outcomes (see Box 5.4). Conversely, it is quite possible to have a bad outcome without any error at all. Every year, many people attempt ascents of Mount Everest. The challenge associated with this is enormous. Failure to reach the summit does not necessarily imply error in the attempt (unless one takes the view that such attempts are misguided by definition). Similarly, doctors occasionally undertake cases that are very difficult indeed. Failure to save a life in a complicated emergency operation – a ruptured aortic aneurysm for example – may simply reflect the fact that the challenge was overwhelming. On the other hand, things can go spectacularly wrong on the basis of quite small failures, particularly when complex systems and sophisticated technology are involved. The stories in Boxes 5.6 and 5.7 illustrate a number of key points about the often contentious relationships between error, outcome, blame and culpability.

Errors are unintentional   In the Erebus disaster, if the pilot intended to fly into Mt Erebus, this would have been suicide and mass-murder, not an error. On the other hand, choosing to fly below the regulation limit was intentional, although the pilot's decision did not involve intent to harm either himself or anyone else. Furthermore, it was dictated by company policy – a corporate violation.

Deterrence does not reliably prevent error, but may deter violations There could be few deterrents greater than the prospect of flying an aeroplane into the ground, yet this has been done many times by pilots who understand the consequences. If the thought of instant death cannot prevent errors, it is unlikely that draconian punishment will do so. This assertion is probably not completely true; to some extent a real and present danger will tend to focus the mind and reduce the chance of succumbing to distraction. However, it is clear that a decision to avoid violations is more likely to be effective than one to avoid error. For example, the airline was quite able to decide to discontinue the service to Antarctica, after this disaster, and thereby (somewhat indirectly) gave effect to a decision not to continue violating the rule against low flying.

Box 5.6 Minor errors leading to a major outcome[29]

The Erebus Disaster. On the 28th of November 1979, flight TE901 departed from Auckland on a scenic trip to the Antarctic. Neither the captain nor the first officer had been to the Antarctic before. No physical chart showing the planned route was used. The area which had been approved for descent was obscured by cloud, so the crew of the aeroplane decided on an alternative area to the North of Ross Island which was clear of cloud. They obtained clearance for this plan from the McMurdo control station. As they descended, the altitude warning device sounded. The pilot applied full power, but it was too late to avert disaster, and the aircraft struck the slope of Mt Erebus, resulting in the loss of 207 lives. It turned out that the plane's flight path was not over the flat ground of McMurdo Sound as the crew had believed, but over Lewis Sound instead. The crew failed to see Mt Erebus, an active volcano 3,794 metres in height, because of the effect of the flat white light at the time.

After a prolonged and controversial enquiry it ensued that on the day of the accident the coordinates in a computer involved in the guidance of the plane were altered. Ironically, this was done to correct a previous error, but the crew was not told. The result was a small but critical change in the flight path. A contributory factor related to the descent of the aeroplane. Pilots are expected to remain above a defined minimum height, and usually stay well above this minimum. Had this rule been followed the aeroplane would simply have passed above Mt Erebus. However, on sightseeing flights to the Antarctic, it was routine to descend below 1800 metres. This (corporate) violation was integral to the commercial purpose of these journeys – the provision of a good view of Antarctica to the passengers.

This is a classic example of an error originating from incorrect information which led to a faulty perception of reality in the context of a routine violation. The captain was making decisions on the basis of information that was flawed. His mental perception of the world did not match reality and in this particular case the mismatch proved fatal, because of the additional contribution of the flat light and altered flight coordinates.

The consequences of an error may be quite out of proportion to its nature and extent In Mt Erebus' case, an apparently trivial failure in communication over the change of coordinates in a computer (in combination with other errors and violations) resulted in 207 deaths.

Chance often plays a major role in determining outcome It was the combination of errors (Type I – wrong coordinates and Type III – flat white light; see Figure 5.1 and Table 5.1), a corporate violation (low flying: see page 122) *and* bad luck which resulted in a flight path directly over (or into) Mt Erebus. Better luck might have created a situation which was still erroneous, but safe.

Blame is often a response to outcome rather than culpability The investigators made an initial finding of 'pilot error'. If similar errors had been made, but a disastrous crash not occurred, it is likely that any punitive action would have been minor. In fact, there is a reasonable chance that the error would never have been identified at all. The moral wrong associated with the actions and decisions would not, however, have been any different. In legal terms, there was a *duty* of care and the potential for disaster implied that a very high *standard* of care was warranted; however, the fact that a disaster occurred says very little about the standard of care actually observed. In the language of safety and quality, risk places a huge onus on all concerned to do everything possible to improve safety, but the outcome of an individual case is not a reliable guide to standard of practice (see page 202–205).

Experts make errors In the Erebus story, the people responsible for making the change in the computer track, and the flight crew, were expert. It is often argued that experts are highly trained and should not make errors. This is of course fallacious. Experts do make errors, although some of the errors they make are distinct from those made by novices. Expertise underpins the ability of experts to undertake complex tasks which would be totally beyond the novice, but it also predisposes experts to certain types of error, notably slips and lapses when multitasking. In this case, although expert they were inexperienced in Antarctic conditions and hence might be said to have lacked expertise in this particular context.

The same points may be made about errors in healthcare (see Box 5.7) In the case of Mr. Davidson, the errors of misfiling the drug order, of the (unfamiliar) anaesthetist not noticing that the need for an order documented in the medical record was not on the drug ordering sheet, and of the ward staff assuming the post-operative orders were correct, were all quite trivial on their own. It was bad luck that an emergency case led to a change of anaesthetist. The outcome was quite disproportionate to the nature and severity of the errors. The family of the patient was incredulous that the staff at the hospital had failed to take care of the very thing the patient had insisted on telling them at admission, and for which the patient continuously wore an alert bracelet. All the staff were experts. It was bad luck that a different anaesthetist had to do the case. It was unfortunate that the patient was selected for a protocol for alcohol withdrawal which left him sedated and unable to check his own medication. In retrospect, he may have been better managed as a day patient. In both the Mt Erebus case and in this case, relatives of those harmed could easily focus on one of the errors and say 'this simply is not good enough'. The reality is that, in the circumstances, these problems were easy to miss, even by conscientious professionals. These cases lend weight to the argument for 'no fault' compensation promoted in Chapter 4. There is no question that it would be perfectly reasonable to provide compensation to those adversely affected by these events, but there is also no question that it would be unreasonable to blame any particular individual.

Box 5.7 A (preventable) massive stroke after a minor procedure

Mr. Davidson decided to have surgery to release a fibrous contraction of the palm of his right hand (a Dupuytren's contracture). He had previously had two operations for major bleeds from the lining of his stomach, and wore a 'Medic-Alert' bracelet stating that it was vital that he always be given medication to inhibit the secretion of gastric acid. Because he was a fairly heavy drinker, he was not selected for day-stay surgery, but was admitted to hospital so that he could be entered into a sedation protocol around the time of the procedure, to prevent alcohol withdrawal symptoms.

The intern who admitted Mr. Davidson documented his problems clearly in the medical record and listed the drugs he should be given. He also filled in a drug-ordering chart which included an order for omeprazole, the acid-inhibiting drug the patient was normally on to preserve his stomach lining. The anaesthetist saw Mr. Davidson whilst he was being admitted and checked and noted the orders on the drug chart.

In fact Mr. Davidson ended up being anaesthetised by another anaesthetist, because the person who saw him pre-operatively and who was scheduled to do the list ended up working all night with a difficult case, and being sent home by the duty anaesthetist to get some sleep. The drug order sheet was mistakenly filed in a previous volume of the patient's medical records by the ward clerk, not the volume in use at the time. The post-operative orders were written up by the second anaesthetist, not a usual member of that team, and did not include omeprazole.

As the patient was sedated post-operatively, as part of the protocol for heavy drinkers, he did not demand his medications. Two days after the procedure he suffered a massive bleed from his stomach, requiring admission to the intensive care unit. He required 30 units of blood and extensive resuscitation, including intubation and ventilation. Most of his stomach had to be removed during an emergency operation to stop the bleeding.

After the operation, it was noted then that he had suffered a massive stroke involving the dominant side of his brain and was paralyzed on one side of his body and unable to speak. This meant that he could not care for himself or make himself understood. Mr. Davidson ended up permanently institutionalized and depressed, with a very poor quality of life.

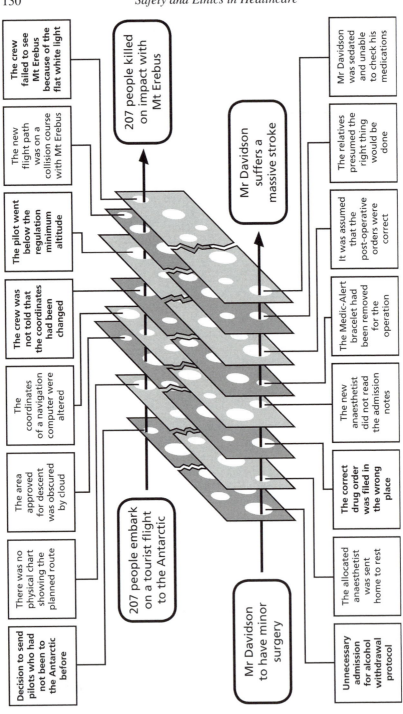

Figure 5.2 'Swiss cheese' diagram. The latent and *active* errors which caused the events in Boxes 5.6 and 5.7

The 'Swiss Cheese' model James Reason has provided a graphic conceptualization of accident causation.[5] He depicts complex systems as containing multiple defences against error. These defences are represented as slices of Swiss cheese (see Figure 5.2). In each slice latent factors (weaknesses in the system) and active errors are represented by holes. An error trajectory may pass through these holes, but having traversed a hole in one barrier will usually be stopped by the next. Accidents occur when the latent factors or errors (depicted by the holes) line up and an accident trajectory passes through all the available defences (or slices of cheese). Figure 5.2 shows the actual sequence of some of the particular factors which led to the outcomes in the two cases described in Boxes 5.6 and 5.7. Such sequences are similar to those teased out by the flowchart exercise in root cause analysis (see Chapter 9).

Foresight versus Hindsight In retrospect it might be quite clear that a particular chain of events led to a disaster, and quite easy for each link in the chain to be identified and characterized. However, before any event, one does not know which one of many possibilities might actually go wrong; to the operators of a complex system there are so many potential branching pathways, each of which can be subject to a variety of vagaries, that it is quite artificial and inappropriate to pass judgement through the clarity of the retrospectroscope (see Figure 5.3).[30] The value of identifying the latent errors in the system is that it may be possible to correct or remove them, thus avoiding the trap being reset for future operations (see Chapter 9).

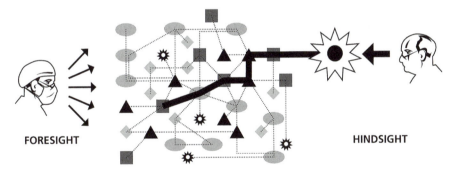

FORESIGHT   **HINDSIGHT**

Figure 5.3 Foresight versus hindsight[30]

Conclusion

As we pointed out in Chapters 1–3, a patient may be placed at risk either because of an error (a wrong plan or a reasonable plan poorly executed) or a violation (usually a shortcut taken out of habit or convenience). The significance for the complex system of healthcare is that to defend against errors, the system has to be error proofed, whereas violations are amenable to changes in individual or corporate behaviour. Both are best addressed by *forcing functions* involving redesign of the system (see page 258). Also, errors are generally not blameworthy, whereas violations may be. The temptation to automatically apportion blame when there has been a bad outcome should be resisted if a 'just culture' is to be developed.

When considering errors and violations it may be thought that decisions (and therefore the actions arising from decisions) can be judged on the basis of knowing the correct thing to do. This assumption may not always be true. Knowing what to do will be the subject of the next chapter.

Notes

1   Kohn, L.T., Corrigan, J.M. and Donaldson, M.S. (2000), *To Err is Human: Building a Safer Health System* (Washington DC: National Academies Press).

2   Webster, C.S. (2004), 'Implementation and Assessment of a New Integrated Drug Administration System (IDAS) as an Example of a Safety Intervention in a Complex Socio-Technological Workplace', Ph.D. Thesis (Auckland: University of Auckland).

3   Perrow, C. (1984), *Normal Accidents – Living With High Risk Technologies* (New York: Basic Books).

4   Simon, H.A. (1964), 'On the Concept of Organization Goal', *Administrative Science Quarterly* 9:1, 1–22.

5   Reason, J. (2000), 'Human Error: Models and Management', *British Medical Journal* 320:7237, 768–70.

6   Rasmussen, J. (1986), *Information Processing and Human-Machine Interaction: An Approach to Cognitive Engineering* (New York: North-Holland).

7   Woods, D.D. et al. (1994), *Behind Human Error: Cognitive Systems, Computers and Hindsight* (Dayton, Ohio: Crew Systems Ergonomic Information and Analysis Center, Wright Patterson Air Force Base).

8   Reason, J. (1997), *Managing the Risks of Organizational Accidents* (Aldershot: Ashgate).

9   Merry, A.F. and McCall Smith, A. (2001), *Errors, Medicine and the Law* (Cambridge: Cambridge University Press).

10 Department of Veterans Affairs, United States (2002), *VHA National Patient Safety Improvement Handbook* (Washington, D.C.: Department of Veterans Affairs, Veterans Health Administration).

11 Marx, D. (2001), *Patient Safety and the "Just Culture": a Primer for Health Care Executives* (New York: Columbia University). Available at: <http://www.mers-tm.net/index.html> accessed 5 Jun 2006.

12 National Patient Safety Agency (2005), *Incident Decision Tree* [website], National Patient Safety Agency, United Kingdom. Available at: <www.npsa.nhs.uk/health/resources/incident_decision_tree?contentId=3020> accessed 5 Jun 2006. Based on James Reason's culpability decision tree in Reason, J. (1997) cited above.

13 Runciman, W.B., Merry, A.F. and Tito, F. (2003), 'Error, Blame and the Law in Health Care – an Antipodean Perspective', *Annals of Internal Medicine* 138:12, 974–9.

14 Webster, C.S. et al. (2001), 'The Frequency and Nature of Drug Administration Error During Anaesthesia', *Anaesthesia and Intensive Care* 29:5, 494–500.

15 Runciman W.B. et al. (1993), 'Errors, Incidents and Accidents in Anaesthetic Practice', *Anaesthesia and Intensive Care* 21:5, 506–19.

16 Reason, J. (1990), *Human Error* (New York: Cambridge University Press).

17 Philibert, I. and Leach, D.C. (2005), 'Re-framing Continuity of Care for This Century', *Quality and Safety in Health Care* 14:6, 394–6.

18 Gaba, D., Fish, K. and Howard, S. (1994), *Crisis Management in Anaesthesiology* (New York: Churchill Livingstone).

19 Wegner, D.M. (1994), 'Ironic Processes of Mental Control', *Psychological Review* 101:1, 34–52.

20 Runciman, W.B. and Merry, A.F. (2005), 'Crises in Clinical Care: an Approach to Management', *Quality and Safety in Health Care* 14:3, 156–163.

21 Centers for Disease Control and Prevention (2002), 'Guideline for Hand Hygiene in Health-Care Settings. Recommendations of the Healthcare Infection Control Practices Advisory Committee and the HICPAC/SHEA/APIC/IDSA Hand Hygiene Task Force', *Morbidity and Mortality Weekly Report* 51:RR16.

22 Dawson, D. and Reid, K. (1997), 'Fatigue, Alcohol and Performance Impairment', *Nature* 388:6639, 235.

23 Savill, R. (1995), 'Tired Doctor Cleared Over Patient's Death', *The Daily Telegraph*, 20 May, p. 3.

24 Retrievals involve the collection and transport of critically ill patients with intensive medical care being provided by specially trained medical and nursing personnel during the journey to an inpatient facility.

25 The Shipman Inquiry (2002), *First Report: Death Disguised* (London: The Stationery Office).

26 Norman, D.A. (1988), *The Psychology of Everyday Things* (New York: Basic Books).

27 Merry, A.F. et al. (2006), 'A Simulation Model for Reduction in Error', *Anaesthesia and Intensive Care*, forthcoming.

28 Gawande, A.A., et al. (2003), 'Analysis of Errors Reported by Surgeons at Three Teaching Hospitals', *Surgery*, 133:6, 614–21.

29 Cairns, F.J. et al. (1981), 'Air crash on Mount Erebus', *Medicine, Scinece and the Law*, 21:3, 184–188.

30 Adapted from Cook, R.I., Woods, D.D. and Miller, C. (1998), *A Tale of Two Stories: Contrasting Views of Patient Safety* (Chicago: National Patient Safety Foundation).

Chapter 6

Knowing What to Do

We have seen that patients may be put at risk by wrong decisions (either by failing to get appropriate care or by getting inappropriate care) and by things going wrong even when a correct decision has been made. The question arises, how do we know the difference between a correct decision and an incorrect one? How do we know what we should be doing in healthcare?

In a patient-centred healthcare system, it might be thought that patients should make all the decisions related to their own care. Certainly, decisions should take account of patients' wishes, but they should also be soundly based in relation to the needs of the individual (which may not be the same as his or her wishes) and of the community (which may imply something else; see page 3). Total autonomy for individual patients may not always be appropriate, and is not generally practicable. Patients are dependent on healthcare professionals for information about their health and for guidance in interpreting that information. Ideally, decisions in healthcare should reflect consensus, with the patient at the centre of a notional collective which includes clinicians, administrators, funders and those responsible for setting policy (see Figure 1.1). All of these people need unbiased, reliable, up-to-date information on which to base decisions.

Many doctors believe that their practice has always been based on scientific evidence. To an extent, this has been true since Hippocrates first set aside superstition as a foundation for medicine, and embraced objectivity and observation. During most of the twentieth century, medical practice was grounded in the belief that knowledge, training and experience qualified doctors to make decisions on behalf of their patients. Emphasis was placed on the scientific foundations of medicine. The lessons of the laboratory were expected to translate into clinical practice. By today's standards doctors tended to be paternalistic towards their patients, but they also tended to accept the heightened responsibility that goes with paternalism.

Gradually it has become clear that scientific principles derived from laboratory and animal experiments do not always translate into clinical practice in the way one might expect. Healthcare professionals have realized that assumptions, however apparently logical, do need to be tested in clinical practice, and the *randomized controlled trial* (RCT) has emerged as the (perceived) gold standard for such testing. This development has not displaced the scientific foundations of clinical practice, but instead has supplemented them. It has added to the information that needs to be taken into account when considering the *evidence* for or against any particular treatment, and has given rise to a new understanding of the concept now called *evidence based medicine* (EBM). At first, there were only a few RCTs, and the results of these were published in a limited number of journals, so keeping up to date with the evidence was not unduly onerous. More recently, there has been an explosive increase in both trials and journals, and it has become impossible even to read everything published in any particular medical field, let alone critically evaluate and synthesize the new findings that emerge every day. There is a real risk that important new findings will be allowed to languish in libraries for years before being adopted into practice. Lags of 20 years are commonplace. Even worse, there is a risk that instead of these findings being accepted and applied to clinical practice, new trials investigating the same, already answered question will be carried out at great expense, with inconvenience and risk to patients. Not only is this needless, it is unethical. EBM is, as much as anything, a response to this problem (see Boxes 6.1 and 6.4).

Box 6.1 Delays in recognizing evidence

Antman et al. showed that recommendations for the routine use of thrombolytic therapy after acute myocardial infarction first appeared 14 years after evidence for benefit became available.[1] Conversely, the prophylactic use of lignocaine in this context continued long after evidence for lack of efficacy was published. Beta-adrenergic blockade after acute myocardial infarction reduces subsequent premature mortality by 20 per cent. This was evident on the basis of published trials at a statistically significant level ($P < 0.05$) by 1981. By 1997 some 20 further trials involving 15,000 patients had been undertaken to re-investigate this point.

The reader is directed to Chapter 1 of *Systematic Reviews in Healthcare*[2] for a full discussion of these important issues, numerous relevant references, and an explanation of the technique of cumulative meta-analysis, by which it is possible to identify the point at which it would have been possible to identify a significant treatment effect on the basis of repeated trials.

The philosophical origins of EBM as we think of it today lie in mid-nineteenth century practice,[3] but the concept did not gain traction until the later part of the twentieth century. Since then, there has been a dramatic growth of interest in EBM, to the extent that The Institute of Medicine has identified evidence-based decision-making as one of the core components of delivering safe, effective, efficient and patient-centred care.[4] A number of organizations have emerged whose sole purpose is to facilitate the synthesis of current evidence on important topics, with a view to guiding clinical practice and public health policy (see Appendix IV).

There has also been a growing body of criticism of the concept of EBM and of its tools, notably meta-analysis. This criticism has often been directed at an over reliance on the results of RCTs (and meta-analyses of these RCTs) in guiding clinical practice. Some of this criticism, however, represents a misunderstanding of what EBM actually is.

Sackett has defined EBM as 'the conscientious, explicit and judicious use of current best evidence in making decisions about the care of individual patients. The practice of EBM means integrating individual clinical expertise with the best available external clinical evidence from systematic research'.[3] Research includes clinical research (of which RCTs are only a part), research from basic science, and research which synthesize expert opinion. By this definition, EBM involves practising in accordance with an appropriate synthesis of evidence from sources as diverse as personal experience and RCTs, stored in repositories ranging from the minds of patients to the internet (Box 6.2).

Box 6.2 Sources of information related to medical decision making

- Research.
- The clinician's mind.
- Other peoples minds (including the patient's).
- Text books.
- Medical journals.
- Electronic repositories of information.
- The internet:
  - formal, moderated sources (e.g. Medline, Pubmed),
  - informal, unmoderated sources.

An Outline of this Chapter

Because there is a finite amount of money available for healthcare, it should be spent in the best possible way. If precious resources are to be invested in research and in the laborious process of synthesizing and critically appraising its findings with a view to guiding practice, it is worth ensuring that the research is ethical and of high quality, and that it is directed towards answering questions to which we need answers. After considering the quality and appropriateness of research, we will discuss problems with interpreting the literature, and then go on to consider the tools of evidence-based medicine and the question of ensuring that patients are properly informed.

The Quality of Research and its Interpretation

The Quality of Research

Ethics Research should be conducted in accordance with appropriate ethical guidelines. In most countries, medical research must comply with guidelines issued by the relevant National Research Council.[5] These Councils usually have statutory backing in that institutional human research ethics committees are bound to consider research proposals in accordance with recommended processes and guidelines. Many research projects have special problems that need addressing. In critically ill patients, for example, the issue of consent may be difficult to deal with, but is, if anything, even more important than in healthier subjects.[6] There is risk associated with any human endeavour, and when research is undertaken a responsible judgement must be made by the investigators that the risk is worth the potential benefit (see Box 6.3).

Box 6.3 Dying for (yet more) evidence[7]

It is now widely accepted that one or more RCTs constitute level one evidence (see page 145). These trials are expensive to do and logistically difficult to manage. Increasingly, the only people who can afford to fund them are pharmaceutical and medical device companies. The problem is that such companies have a vested interest in the outcome, which may influence their approach. For example, they may want to prove that a new drug performs in a similar manner to an existing drug of proven efficacy. Because the difference between the new drug and the existing drug is likely to be marginal, they may be motivated to compare their drug against controls who receive no drug at all.

It has been reported that tens of thousands of patients have been allocated to the control arm of RCTs which were unnecessary, in that an effective drug already existed. The example was given of aprotinin, used to reduce blood loss during surgery, which had been tested on more than 2,000 patients in a dozen RCTs by June 1992, with unequivocal results for efficacy. However, since then 50 subsequent trials involving more than 5,000 patients have been conducted gathering superfluous additional data. The desire to get publications has been cited as a possible reason for these unnecessary studies; failing to bother to conduct proper literature searches is another. This, of course, calls into question the rigor of ethics committees in their appraisal of research protocols. However, the task faced by ethics committees is an onerous one and the incumbents are nearly always unpaid volunteers who lead busy professional lives.[7]

Interestingly, a very recent safety study, which was not randomized, has raised the possibility that aprotinin might cause harm in certain groups of patients. The need in relation to new drugs is not for repeated studies of efficacy, but for effective phase 4 (i.e. post-marketing) studies with the power to identify uncommon or unsuspected side effects (or benefits) that are unlikely to manifest in a study the size of a typical RCT.

Research is about *adding* to the existing body of knowledge. It is a waste of time and resources, and unethical, to expose patients to the risks and inconvenience of research on a question that has already been answered. A systematic and comprehensive review of the literature is the starting point for any research; this should include a summary of what is and is not known on the subject to justify the proposed investigation.

Research projects need to be properly designed It is beyond the scope of this chapter to address research design comprehensively, but every effort should be made to 'get it right' to do credit to the effort and resources that will be expended. Some repeatedly identified deficiencies in clinical trials are listed in Box 6.4.

Box 6.4 Some repeatedly identified deficiencies in clinical trials

- Inadequate review of the literature in relation to the study.
- Inadequate formulation of hypotheses.
- Inadequate blinding.
- Incorrect statistical analyses.
- Inadequate discussion of limitations.
- Ghost or guest authorship.
- Publication bias (positive results are more likely to be published than negative).
- Fraud (e.g. data that has simply been fabricated or misrepresented).

The Interpretation of Research

Problems with the interpretation of research include the variable quality of research publications, publication bias and the use of inappropriate statistics.

The variable quality of research publications A persistent problem with the interpretation of the results of research relates not only to the quality of the research, but to the quality of its publication. At first blush, this is surprising, at least in respect of peer reviewed journals. However, the assumption that the process of editorial peer review ensures adequate quality in either the conduct or the reporting of research seems to be unfounded. In 1983, Bailar and Patterson identified that part of the problem of poor quality in published research was a lack of empirical research into the peer review and editorial processes at the heart of medical literature, and called for studies to be done on these processes.[8] Editors at JAMA responded by convening a conference at which the results of such research could be presented. By 2002 nearly 200 papers per year dealt with this subject. However, in an editorial on the fourth such conference, Rennie quoted the following comment he made after the third conference, and indicated that it still applied:[9]

> ... there are scarcely any bars to eventual publication. There seems to be no study too fragmented, no hypothesis too trivial, no literature citation too biased or too egotistical, no design too warped, no methodology too bungled, no presentation of results too inaccurate, too obscure, and too contradictory, no analysis too self-serving, no argument too circular, no conclusions too trifling or too unjustified, and no grammar and syntax too offensive for a paper to end up in print.

A problem in synthesizing evidence lies in the quality of the original publications (Table 6.1). For example, in a review of pain relief after thoracotomy, only 16 studies were considered interpretable out of over 100 identified in a search of the literature.[10] In a recent study of 60 placebo-controlled trials, the quality of reporting was considered high in only 18. The quality of the reporting was generally related to the quality of the studies, although in some cases poor reporting concealed somewhat better quality in the actual design and conduct of the research.[11] There are certainly examples of systematic review reaching one conclusion,[12] only to be superseded by a large randomized trial which reaches a different one.[13]

Publishing poor quality research is increasingly unacceptable. Given the challenges of keeping up with the evidence, adding to the existing cacophony will simply make the signal even more difficult to detect. Editors are increasingly committed to the elimination of flawed clinical trials from their journals, and many now require evidence of conformity with the proper principles of research before they will even send a paper for peer review. Check lists have been developed to assist with the critical evaluation of the quality of clinical trials (see Table 6.1).

Publication bias Publication bias is particularly troublesome to those seeking the truth. Whittington and co-authors conducted a systematic review of published data on the use of selective serotonin reuptake inhibitors (SSRIs) in children and then evaluated the effect of repeating this analysis after including unpublished data.[14] The former analysis suggested a favourable risk-benefit profile for some SSRIs. However, addition of unpublished data led to the conclusion that the risks could outweigh the benefits of these drugs (except for fluoxetine). This was a very worrying finding. Further analysis has cast serious doubt on the value of SSRIs in anyone, with suggestions that tiny statistical differences may have been inflated into apparently large effects.[15,16]

Why do data not get published? The most obvious reason is that negative results tend to be less exciting than positive ones. The finding that a new drug or technique saves lives is headline grabbing news which sometimes has substantial commercial value. The finding that a new drug has no benefit tends to raise questions as to why it was studied at all. Research into established treatments that demonstrates their lack of efficacy may be even less welcome. The people charged with the peer review process may well have reputations based on practising and supporting the discredited treatment.[1] This does not mean that they will be biased in their reviewing of the research, only that they might be. The so called 'grey' literature is therefore important. This includes PhD and Masters theses and proceedings of conferences. Organizations such as the Cochrane Collaboration make a point of seeking out data from these relatively inaccessible sources.

There is an even more insidious problem. A great deal of clinical research is funded by pharmaceutical companies or manufacturers of devices. The commercial imperative to publish is high for positive results, and low for negative. The support provided to authors to facilitate timely publication of data in the

Table 6.1   Check list for evaluating the quality of a clinical trial (developed by Huwiler-Muntener[11] following the CONSORT Statement)[17]

1. Does the title identify the study as a randomized controlled trial?
2. Is the abstract presented in a structured format?
3. Are the objectives stated?
4. Is the hypothesis stated?
5. Is the study population described?
6. Are inclusion and exclusion criteria described?
7. Are the interventions described?
8. Are the outcome measures described?
9. Is the primary outcome specified?
10. Is a minimum important difference for the primary outcome reported?
11. Are power calculations described?
12. Is the rationale for the statistical analyses explained?
13. Are the methods for statistical analyses described?
14. Are stopping rules described?
15. Is the unit of randomization described?
16. Is the method used to generate the allocation schedule described?
17. Is the method of allocation concealment described?
18. Is the timing of assignment described?
19. Is the method to separate those generating the allocation sequence from those assigning participants to groups described?
20. Are the mechanisms of blinding described?
21. Is the number of eligible patients reported?
22. Is the number of randomized patients reported for each comparison group?
23. Are prognostic variables by treatment and control group described?
24. Is the number of patients receiving intervention as allocated reported for each comparison group?
25. Is the number of patients analyzed reported for each comparison group?
26. Are withdrawals and dropouts described for each comparison group?
27. Are protocol deviations described for each comparison group?
28. Is the estimated effect of the intervention on primary and secondary outcomes stated, including a point estimate and measure of precision (confidence interval)?
29. Are the results stated in absolute numbers?
30. Are summary data and inferential statistics presented in sufficient detail to permit alternative analyses and replication?

former case is often substantial; in the latter this support may be less than enthusiastic.

Not all companies were willing to provide their unpublished data to the authors of the Whittington study cited above – although it should not be forgotten that some were. The reality is that bias begins even before the outcome of the research is known. Companies decide what to fund and what not to fund, and it is a reasonable assumption that the majority of these decisions are driven by considerations of profit rather than those of public good. It could be said that the major current problem with EBM is that commercial interests create the evidence.

Steps have been taken to try to improve this situation. Registering a clinical trial at its outset (before the data have been collected and the results are known) is one way of improving this situation. The International Committee of Medical Journal Editors (ICMJE) now requires clinical trails to be registered and has endorsed the World Health Organization's minimal registration set of twenty fields.[18] The ICMJE does not advocate any particular registry, but has listed criteria for acceptability of a registry. The WHO is developing an approval process to assist compliance with trial registers and many governments now have national registries.

The use of inappropriate statistics in medical research It has been demonstrated repeatedly that the standard of statistics in medical research is often poor. It seems that many clinicians find statistics arcane, frequently treat the statistical analysis of their data as a 'black box' into which they feed results and from which P values emerge, and often fail to grapple with the fundamental statistical principles which underlie their conclusions. In part this reflects a lack of emphasis on statistics in medical training, at both undergraduate and postgraduate levels. For example, a P value of 0.05 is usually used to denote 'significance'. It would often be more appropriate to use the actual P value than this arbitrary convention, and to evaluate the result in the context of all the circumstances, including the details of the trial and the presumed risks and benefits of the intervention.

There are numerous types of statistical deficiencies in medical research. One of the most common involves the failure to calculate the number of participants needed to have a reasonable chance of showing a difference between groups if one actually exists. Having too few participants in trials leads to *type two errors*, by which it is concluded that no difference exists when in fact there is a difference. This is particularly relevant to the discussion of EBM, because trials of this type are often taken to indicate that there is no effect, when in fact all they have done is fail to show an effect. Interventions to improve safety typically require very large trials if efficacy is to be demonstrated (see the discussion of pulse oximetry below). Another common mistake is to assume that association implies causation (Box 6.5).

Does this mean that the situation is hopeless? Not at all. An awareness of the issues facilitates a skeptical approach to analyzing the evidence. Skepticism is always warranted in interpreting the results of research, especially in relation to small effect sizes at marginal levels of significance and data from small numbers of patients or single studies. History is littered with discarded drugs which were heavily promoted and widely used after being subjected to hundreds of inadequately designed studies (high dose dexamethazone in septic shock,[19] dopamine to 'prevent' renal failure,[20] albumin for intravascular volume).[21] Nevertheless, as demonstrated in Antman's study (see Box 6.1), and in other large, well designed studies, there are clear answers to some questions, and it is important that this information is understood and applied reasonably soon after it has been obtained. The techniques of EBM are designed to help healthcare professionals to do this, and to distinguish situations where the answers are available from those in which they are not.

Box 6.5 The difference between association and causation

Epidemiological studies often demonstrate an association between two factors. For example, an association has been shown between moderate alcohol consumption and a reduced risk of coronary artery disease.[22] This is not, in itself, conclusive evidence that alcohol reduces coronary artery disease. For example, grey hair is probably associated with an increased risk of osteoporosis, because both are associated with aging. There may be other confounding factors that need to be taken into account when interpreting the meaning of an association. Criteria have been described for attributing causality to associations.[23] These include:

- A consistent relationship across multiple studies.
- A strong association.
- A dose response relationship.
- Evidence from temporal sequencing of events (i.e. how patterns change after specific alterations in the behaviour of a group of individuals).
- A biologically plausible mechanism.

Some Tools of Evidence Based Medicine

There are a number of techniques for evaluating and synthesizing data. We will deal here with just two of these: systematic review and meta-analysis. They are often confused, but they are in fact quite distinct. A systematic review is one that has been prepared using a systematic approach to minimizing bias and random errors in selecting the literature to be reviewed, whereas a meta-analysis amalgamates data from a number of studies in order to reach a more reliable conclusion.[2]

Systematic Review

Systematic reviews of the literature are the cornerstone of EBM. The difference between a systematic review and a traditional narrative review is that the method of identifying references for inclusion in the review is explicit in the former, but not in the latter.

Oxman assessed 50 traditional reviews published between June 1985 and June 1986 in four major medical journals against six criteria of quality and found only one that satisfied all six.[24] Study selection is only one source of potential bias in the construction of a review. The weighting given to findings from different studies and to the extraction of data and amalgamation of results are also open to bias. The degree to which subjectivity can influence the outcome of a traditional review was illustrated by two reviews of the use of spinal injections of steroids in the treatment of chronic pain published less than a year apart,[25,26] with quite different conclusions.

Systematic reviews are an attempt to produce *reproducible* summaries of defined topics.[24,27] The possibility of bias may not be completely eliminated, but because the process by which the review has been constructed must be described, a second reviewer should be able to repeat the same process and come to the same conclusions. As a minimum, this makes any source of bias explicit. This is not true for a narrative review. The Cochrane collaboration has developed a standardized and structured approach to the conduct of systematic reviews (called Cochrane reviews), in which the objective is to provide demonstrably balanced and comprehensive answers to clearly defined questions. When updated on a regular basis, they provide a definitive statement of current knowledge.

Is it therefore the case that the conclusions of Cochrane reviews are always correct and widely accepted? We think not. In the end, the critical interpretation of the results of such a review depends on the wisdom of individuals or small groups of people, and the Cochrane process is heavily weighted to RCTs. However, many questions are difficult to answer by means of RCTs. A classic example of a controversial finding by a Cochrane review relates to the use of pulse oximetry in anaesthesia:[28]

'The studies confirmed that pulse oximetry can detect hypoxaemia and related events. However, we have found no evidence that pulse oximetry affects the outcome of anaesthesia. The conflicting subjective and objective results of the studies, despite an intense, methodical collection of data from a relatively large population, indicate that the value of perioperative monitoring with pulse oximetry is questionable in relation to improved reliable outcomes, effectiveness and efficiency.'

It would be difficult to find a specialist anaesthetist who would give up using pulse oximetry on the basis of this conclusion. Many anaesthetists believe that pulse oximetry has dramatically improved safety in their specialty. We think that the conclusion in this particular Cochrane review was reached without taking account of all relevant evidence. Specifically, we think the process failed to adequately incorporate a very substantial body of expert opinion, and important evidence from sources other than RCTs.[29] Qualitative analysis of 2,000 incidents pointed to a reduction in cardiac arrest when pulse oximetry was used over a decade ago.[30] A recent review of 4,000 incidents and over 1,200 medico-legal notifications reported by anaesthetists revealed no cases of hypoxic brain damage or death from inadequate ventilation or misplaced tubes since the introduction of oximetry and capnography, whereas these were recurring problems up to 15 years ago.[31]

Hierarchies of Evidence At the heart of the dispute about the value of EBM lies the concept of a hierarchy of evidence (Table 6.2). According to common versions of this hierarchy, meta-analyses of data synthesized in a systematic review are the most reliable source of evidence, with individual RCTs second. Expert opinion rates well below this.

Table 6.2 Hierarchical categories of evidence defined by Eccles et al.[2]

Ia:	evidence from meta-analysis of randomized controlled trials
Ib:	evidence from at least one randomized controlled trial
IIa:	evidence from at least one controlled study without randomization
III:	evidence from non-experimental descriptive studies, such as comparative studies, correlation studies and case-control studies
IV:	evidence from expert committee reports or opinions and/or clinical experience of respected authorities

We think this is too simplistic. RCTs vary in quality from excellent to un-interpretable, and evidence from observation, experience and basic scientific principles may sometimes be compelling in the absence of trials, randomized or otherwise. This point has been neatly illustrated by an ironic meta-analysis of RCTs of the utility of parachutes in dealing with 'gravitational challenge'.[32]

Sometimes RCTs are simply not appropriate: the importance of understanding the research question and the theoretical constructs of the matter under investigation have been emphasized in an analysis of the role of RCTs in the investigation of the benefit of intercessory prayer.[33] There are many examples, and pulse oximetry is one, where appropriate trials have not been done, partly because the size of study needed to unequivocally demonstrate a clear benefit is very large. A very large, expensive prospective study of pulse oximetry was in fact underpowered (at least in terms of showing a difference in survival) and in the end yielded virtually the same findings as a much less expensive review of 2,000 incidents.[30] The absence of a conventional body of evidence to support a particular therapy or technique is not the same thing as evidence that the therapy or technique does not work.[34] EBM requires the use of the best available evidence. We think this implies the need for *triangulation* – the synthesis of evidence from different sources (e.g. RCTs, expert evidence, and qualitative research). It is also important to incorporate information from patients, where relevant, to inform the interpretation of the data with some indication of what it will mean to the lives of the people on the receiving end of the investigation or treatment.

Quantitative and Qualitative Research We propose, therefore, that the value of qualitative research and the limitations of quantitative research have often been underappreciated in healthcare.[30,34] Medicine is founded on observational research, by which patterns of disease were carefully and accurately described. Qualitative research is powerful for generating hypotheses worth testing by quantitative methods, and for understanding life events.[35] For example, quantitative research may give a measure of the degree of pain relief to be expected from perioperative non-steroidal anti-inflammatory drugs, and a numerical estimation of the risk of these agents.[36] It does not tell us whether the risk and benefit associated with these two numbers is acceptable, or when it might be acceptable; qualitative methods can assist in understanding the opinion of groups of people (such as patients). Furthermore, this example illustrates the fundamental fallacy behind much quantitative research in healthcare. In the cited study (like almost all studies of analgesics) pain is represented by a number. In reality pain is an entirely subjective phenomenon, and furthermore it is multi-dimensional. The translation of the experience of pain into numeric form (to allow the use of quantitative statistical methods) is a qualitative exercise.

We think there is no absolute overarching hierarchy of evidence. Hierarchies such as that of Eccles (Table 6.2) are meaningful only in defined contexts (i.e. the evaluation of questions which lend themselves to quantitative research), and only if they are used in conjunction with an evaluation of the quality of each individual study or review (see Table 6.1). In addressing a particular question for research, the best method is the one best suited to answering the question, and this is not always an RCT. We[30,34] (and others[37,38]) think EBM should include qualitative data.[39] Indeed, large collections of fairly structured qualitative information have attributes somewhere in between those of purely qualitative observations and quantitative data. The word quamtitative has been suggested for such data (as 'm' lies between 'l' and 'n' in the alphabet).[40]

These points are entirely consistent with Sackett's definition of EBM. They simply illustrate that EBM is not a matter of the simplistic application of techniques and formulae, but rather implies a considered approach to understanding the state of the art in healthcare.[41]

Meta-analysis

The results of individual trials can usually be summarized in a standardized way by a measurement of treatment effect. This can be presented in many different formats (see Box 6.6). In treatment trials this is usually expressed as a *relative risk* for categorical data, and *means* for continuous data. These are usually shown with 95 per cent confidence limits. Large trials with high power will generally generate narrower confidence intervals (the calculated result is more likely to be correct).

Meta-analysis is a statistical tool used in conjunction with systematic review.[42,43] It is a technique for amalgamating the data from a number of different trials. These trials should be carefully chosen to ensure that their results are comparable (homogeneity). The results of the studies are scaled according to trial size and power. These results are generally presented graphically on a common scale (usually logarithmic to account for wide variation in results) in a 'Forest plot' (Figure 6.1).

The point estimate and 95 per cent confidence intervals for each trial's result (expressed as relative risk, odds ratio or mean difference) is represented as a box with lines. The box size also represents the trial's sample size. Currently, the major problem is that many articles are published with insufficient data to include in a meta-analysis; publishing a significant P value is often viewed as sufficient. The pooled results of the meta-analysis are displayed at the bottom of the Forest plot. If

Box 6.6 Ways of expressing risk

Risk can be expressed in different ways, which can give very different appearances to the same set of data. Consider the following 2 by 2 table:

	Group 1 (morphine)	Group 2 (placebo)
Outcome present (vomiting)	a (4)	b (2)
Outcome absent (no vomiting)	c (6)	d (8)

Risk Ratio (RR, relative risk) This may be used when the groups to be compared are chosen relative to the factor or intervention (i.e. the columns of the table), such as in clinical trials and prospective or observational trials. It is the proportion of patients with a defined outcome (vomiting) after exposure to the risk factor (morphine) divided by the proportion with the outcome in the absence of the factor (placebo).

$$RR = \quad \frac{a/(a+c)}{b/(b+d)} = \quad \frac{4/10}{2/10} \quad = 2.0 \quad \text{i.e. the risk is double in the group who had morphine}$$

Absolute Risk Reduction (ARR) This is the absolute change in risk. A large relative risk may reflect only a small change in absolute risk (for example the risk of breast cancer in patients taking HRT). In the example above, the absolute risk reduction achieved by avoiding morphine would be 20%:

$$ARR = \quad a/(a+c) - b/(b+d) = \quad 40\% - 20\% = \quad \text{20% more vomiting if morphine given}$$

Number Needed to Treat/Harm (NNT, NNH) This reflects the clinical effect; how many patients must be exposed to a treatment/risk factor to change the outcome in one patient. In this example, how many patients must be exposed to morphine to cause one more patient to vomit. In this setting, this is referred to as the Number Needed to Harm. NNT/NNH is the reciprocal of ARR. This cannot be calculated for retrospective case control studies where groups are chosen in reference to the outcome (i.e. the rows of the table). The clinical application of NNT is dependent on the risk-benefit analysis. For instance a NNH of 5 for morphine causing vomiting may be an acceptable rate, whereas a NNH of 5 for a treatment causing more drastic consequences would not be.

$$NNH = \quad 1/ARR = \quad 1/0.20 = \quad 5 \quad \text{i.e. 5 patients must receive morphine to cause one extra patient to vomit}$$

Odds Ratio (OR) In the case where groups are chosen in reference to outcome, the RR will be defined by how many patients are enrolled in each group, and will not reflect the actual effect. OR may be used in these situations.

The 'odds' is defined as the number of patients who fulfil the criteria for a given endpoint (vomiting) divided by those who do not (no vomiting). The OR, then, is the ratio of the odds for an outcome (vomiting) in treated subjects (morphine) to the odds in untreated patients (placebo). The number of patients enrolled as cases or controls will not affect this. Where outcomes are rare, OR and RR may be almost identical.

$$OR = \frac{a/c}{b/d} = \frac{4/6}{2/8} = 2.7 \quad \text{i.e. the odds of vomiting are 2.7x more likely with morphine than with placebo}$$

this result crosses 'unity' (i.e. relative risk = 1), it is concluded that no difference has been shown in the amalgamated results. Differences in trial characteristics (heterogeneity) can confound the results of meta-analysis. To some extent, this can be corrected for statistically, but if there are substantial differences, then comparison using meta-analysis is thought not be appropriate. Meta-analysis is a powerful tool for combining the results of similar trials with the same outcomes to identify differences that small, individual trials may not be powerful enough to demonstrate.

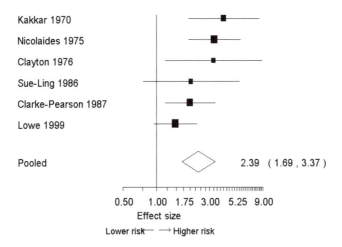

Figure 6.1 Example of a Forest plot[42]

Informed Decision-making by Patients

A focus on the patient is fundamental to modern thinking about quality in healthcare (see Figure 1.1). Perhaps the most obvious manifestation of this focus is to be found in the increased emphasis that has been placed in recent years on informed decision-making and consent. There are sound arguments for this emphasis from psychological (see page 32), ethical (see pages 166–169) and legal perspectives (see pages 149–152).

The Legal Perspective

Many things done to patients would, in other contexts, and the absence of consent, amount to the tort of battery or the crime of assault.[44] The courts permit these things to be done specifically in the context of healthcare and on the proviso that consent is given by the patient.[45]

To a greater or lesser degree consent has always been obtained for medical interventions. It can be argued that the voluntary acquiescence of a patient to a procedure implies consent. Even today this assumption is made about a large number of minor therapeutic manoeuvres. For example, the insertion of an IV catheter or the taking of blood from a vein are normally seen as procedures for which only a simple verbal explanation is required. The fact that a patient sits still, watches the doctor insert the needle and makes no complaint is usually taken as implying consent. Interestingly, there may be a greater onus on healthcare professionals to obtain formal written consent for some of the tests done on blood than there is for taking the blood. For example, in many jurisdictions it would be unlawful to test a patient's blood for evidence of HIV without consent (except in special circumstances). Issues of privacy are also relevant here, and add complexity as the privacy regulations may differ between jurisdictions.

The Bolam Principle and Rogers vs Whittaker The Bolam principle, or test, derives from a classic case known as *Bolam vs Friern Hospital Management Committee*.[46] In this case, the plaintiff had suffered a fractured hip after receiving electro-convulsive therapy without the use of a relaxant drug or appropriate restraint. The defendant argued that he had acted in accordance with common practice. The judge accepted this and ruled that there could be no finding of negligence if the doctor acted in accordance with 'a practice accepted as proper by a responsible body of medical men skilled in that particular art'. It was not necessary to show that the practice was evidence-based, or even that it was in accordance with majority or current opinion, simply that it was in accordance with the practice of some qualified doctors. The judge was following the precedent of an earlier Scottish medical case, *Hunter vs Hanley*, in which that judge had observed,

> '… in the realm of diagnosis and treatment there is ample scope for genuine difference of opinion and one man clearly is not negligent merely because his conclusion differs from that of other professional men, nor because he has displayed less skill or knowledge than others would have shown.'[47]

The Bolam test was applied to medical practice in general but also, more specifically, to informed consent. It amounted to a reasonable doctor test, or custom test. The tide began to turn in the latter half of the twentieth century. For example, in *Edward Wong Finance Co Ltd vs Johnson, Stokes and Master* (in relation to the practice of Hong Kong solicitors), the judge said that the custom test was not conclusive evidence that a practice was prudent.[48] In the medical arena, in South Australia, in *F vs R*, the court accepted that there will be many cases where evidence of professional practice will be decisive, but indicated that:

> '… professions may adopt unreasonable practices. Practices may develop in professions, particularly as to disclosure, not because they serve the interests of the clients, but because they protect the interests or convenience of members of the profession. The court has an obligation to scrutinize professional practices to ensure that they accord with the standard of reasonableness imposed by the law.'[49]

Increasingly, the question is not whether the defendant's conduct conforms with the practices of the profession, but whether it conforms with standards of reasonableness. An Australian case, *Rogers vs Whittaker*,[50] involved an ophthalmologist who failed to disclose to a patient the (very low, 1/14,000) risk of blindness associated with a procedure. Despite evidence that other ophthalmologists would also not have disclosed the risk, the High Court found in favour of the patient. In doing so it established what might be called a 'reasonable patient test'. Commentary on this case sometimes overlooks the fact that the patient had specifically expressed concern about the possibility of blindness. Thus the decision was grounded in an evaluation of the individual patient's needs.

English courts appeared to follow suit in *Bolitho vs City & Hackney Health Authority*.[51] This was a case in which a doctor failed to intubate the trachea of a child who was experiencing respiratory distress. There was evidence that not intubating the trachea might have been clinically justifiable. The comments of the judge appeared to restrict the effect of Bolam. He said:

> '…the judge before accepting a body of opinion as being responsible, reasonable or respectable, will need to be satisfied that, in forming their views, the experts have directed their minds to the question of comparative risks and benefits and have reached a defensible conclusion on the matter.'

He indicated, however, that it would 'very seldom be right for a judge to reach the conclusion that views genuinely held by a competent medical expert are unreasonable'. There is, therefore, some variation between cases and between different countries. However, there is little doubt that the trend has been away from the reasonable doctor test towards the reasonable patient test in respect of informed consent in most parts of the world.

One of the difficulties with a reasonable patient test is that it may be difficult for a doctor to know what a reasonable patient will think after a complication has occurred. There are data to show that a patient's view of reasonableness changes in relation to the amount of information actually disclosed.[52] A patient who has had a complication is likely to become very knowledgeable about that specific complication. The patient may then take a view on what information is reasonable very different from that of a patient who has not experienced the complication. This is a problem because the focus will be on the complication that actually occurred, whereas the possible complications may be many before the event.

This is really about the retrospectroscope again (see page 131). It is currently very difficult for doctors to provide detailed evidence about every possible complication. In reality, neither patients nor the courts expect this. It is perfectly possible to paint a broad-brush picture of likely risks, particularly with respect to risks that are either frequent or serious, and particularly in relation to any concerns expressed by the patient (as in *Rogers vs Whittaker*). A conscientious effort to do this will probably be accepted as reasonable. However, it is our view that it behoves the profession, in striving to achieve a greater degree of informed consent, to move towards endorsed sets of detailed information that could and should be available on the internet or DVDs for patients to view at leisure (see Chapter 12).

Giving patients choice In the opening years of the twenty-first century, most healthcare professionals have accepted the need to disclose to their patients, in some detail, the risks associated with proposed procedures. In fact, there is more to informed consent than disclosure of risk. Risk can only be evaluated in relation to alternatives. If they are to make properly informed decisions, patients need to know the alternatives available to them and the likely consequences of those alternatives

The extent and nature of information that should be provided to a patient does depend on the circumstances and on the available alternatives. In a life-threatening situation, where urgent or immediate action is necessary and there are no reasonable alternatives, it may be enough just to explain what needs to be done, indicate that there are risks, and go ahead. There will be time for the further provision of information and discussion of options after the crisis has been dealt with. In an elective situation, where the indications for a procedure are less than absolute, and when there are options (particularly when one of those options is to do nothing), much more information needs to be provided (Box 6.7).

Competence and capacity These terms are used interchangeably in the context of informed consent. Competence implies the ability to undertake a task, in this case the task of decision making. This requires the ability to understand, assimilate and weigh information and to use the information in making a decision. It also implies the ability to communicate that decision and to articulate any questions or doubts about the decision. However, there is no precisely defined standard of competence. In most countries, the basic assumption is that all patients are competent unless there are reasonable grounds to believe otherwise. Such grounds may include the fact that the patient is too young (a newborn baby for example), is unconscious (on a ventilator for example) or is mentally disordered (which would require formal certification) or intellectually disabled. This all seems straight forward, but becomes more complicated at the margins (for example, in the case of children who are old enough to have a reasonable understanding of proposed treatments, and may not wish to involve their parents).

Cultural issues in informed consent A further dimension to the process of obtaining informed consent relates to the different expectations of people from different cultures. In New Zealand, for example, there is an expectation that health

---

Box 6.7 Angioplasty and cardiac surgery

Many patients undergoing coronary surgery or angioplasty for the treatment of angina imagine that the procedure is being undertaken primarily to improve their life expectancy. Sometimes this will be true, but often there will be little or no prognostic benefit to be obtained from these procedures. It may even be that the effect of the procedure is to reduce the chances of survival. In addition there is a risk of stroke which patients often fear more than the risk of death. The primary indication for many coronary operations or angioplasty procedures is the relief of symptoms. On balance, given the severity of angina, for many patients the risks may be reasonable. However, proper informed consent should make clear to the patient that there are two elements to the decision:

1. the element in relation to life expectancy; and
2. the element in relation to symptoms.

There are certainly patients who, if they clearly understood that a procedure was being undertaken primarily for symptoms, decide to live with the symptoms rather than to take the risks of the procedure.

---

practitioners will follow this country's founding treaty (the Treaty of Waitangi) in respect to members of the indigenous Maori population. What this means in practice is rather loosely defined, but many Maori people believe that decisions should be made by the extended family rather than the individual. This is somewhat in contrast to most non-Maori people in New Zealand who tend to put greater weight on the importance of the autonomy of the individual.

Disclosing Conflicts of Interest[53]

The problems associated with drug and device companies influencing the design and publication of studies have been alluded to on pages 137–143. A yet larger problem lies in the aggressive and highly sophisticated marketing of new 'look-alike' and 'me-too' drugs, with a range of subtle and not-so-subtle inducements to get healthcare professionals to use particular products.[54] In short, the problem is that patients end up unaware that they are taking certain drugs, or being exposed to certain devices, because those prescribing them have been influenced by people or agencies with vested interests. This problem has gained the attention of both the popular media and bodies such as the Australian Competition and Consumer Commission.[55]

> 'There is no such thing as a free lunch. Pharmaceutical companies lavish meals, five-star travel, cash and gifts on doctors for one reason: to encourage them to prescribe their drugs.'[55]

Massive resources are directed towards marketing;[54] we have ourselves been hosted to lavish functions at which we have been encouraged not only to use certain drugs and products in a legitimate way, but to indulge in 'scope-creep' and the 'off-label' use of drugs. A strong argument has been made for a 'genuine commitment to disclosure and transparency in all areas of medical practice'; [53] failure to do this and to be seen to do it will erode the trust upon which the relationship between patients and healthcare professionals depends. Many continuing medical education meetings receive substantial funding from 'the trade' in exchange for prominent exposure of their products and control of dinners and functions at which their products are presented. Ideally each doctor, practice, organization or association should make available (possibly on the internet) a list of benefits received linked to the names of any products they prescribe or use. It has been stated that it is 'impossible to adequately identify, manage or prevent conflicts of interest if doctors, the peak bodies that represent them, and the industry groups with which they deal are not completely open about their interactions'.[53]

As with when things go wrong (see Chapter 8), honesty and transparency is the best policy. It is of note that:[53]

'a recent RCT in the United States of disclosing doctors' financial incentives to patients found that patients' trust in their doctors was unharmed, and their loyalty to their doctor's practice was strengthened.'[56]

Summary

Evidence-based Medicine (EBM)

It is important to base decision making on the best available evidence. However, critical appraisal of both the quality of the research and of its publication is necessary before drawing conclusions. Tools such as systematic review and meta-analysis should be used to assist in decision making, with due consideration of the pitfalls of these techniques. However, many busy practitioners have neither the time nor the expertise to seek out and evaluate the evidence needed for best practice. Increasingly, levels of evidence are being cited (with an important caveat if the studies were funded by a device or drug company) for many therapies which allow practitioners to take a more informed approach to their use. Publications such as the British Medical Journal's 'Clinical Evidence' provide valuable synopses of evidence on many common problems (see Appendix IV).[57] These highlight the continuing paucity of trials on common procedures which are simply accepted as a traditional part of medicine, but which may often be ineffective and occasionally associated with serious adverse events (for example, tonsillectomy, removal of asymptomatic wisdom teeth).[57]

What to Tell Patients

It is beyond the scope of this book to discuss in adequate detail all the possible nuances of informed consent. Suffice to say, that the circumstances range from straight forward to very difficult. In the latter case, much time and empathy is required and consultation with other colleagues is often appropriate. To the greatest extent possible, the health professional should attempt to place him or herself in the role of the patient and to try to understand the situation from that perspective. This is entirely consistent with the notion of patient focused care.

If one takes this approach, it seems clear that most patients will want advice based on 'integrating individual clinical expertise with the best available external clinical evidence from systematic research'.[58] In short, they will want EBM.

Notes

1 Antman, E.M. et al. (1992), 'A Comparison of Results of Meta-Analyses of Randomized Controlled Trials and Recommendations of Clinical Experts. Treatments for Myocardial Infarction', *Journal of the American Medical Association* 268:2, 240–8.
2 Eccles, M., Freemantle, N. and Mason, J. (2001), 'Using Systematic Reviews in Clinical Guideline Development', in Egger, M., Smith, G.D. and Altman, D.G, eds. *Systematic Reviews in Health Care: Meta-Analysis in Context* (London: BMJ Books) pp. 400–18.
3 Sackett, D.L. et al. (1996), 'Evidence Based Medicine: What It Is and What It Isn't', *British Medical Journal* 312:7023, 71–2.
4 Institute of Medicine Committee on Quality of Health Care in America (2001), *Crossing the Quality Chasm: a New Health System for the 21st Century* (Washington DC: National Academies Press).
5 For example, National Health and Medical Research Council of Australia (1999), *National Statement on Ethical Conduct in Research Involving Humans* (Canberra: Commonwealth of Australia) [web document]. Available at: <http://www7.health.gov.au/nhmrc/publications/humans/contents.htm> accessed 8 Jun 2006.
6 Rischbieth, A., Blythe, D., for the Australian and New Zealand Intensive Care Society Clinical Trials Group (ANZICS CTG) (2005), 'Ethical Intensive Care Research: Development of an Ethics Handbook', *Critical Care and Resuscitation* 7:4, 310–21.
7 Matthews, R. (2005), 'Stop Withholding Tried and Tested Treatments', *New Scientist* 9 July 2005, p. 19.
8 Bailar, J.C. and Patterson, K. (1985), 'The Need for a Research Agenda', *New England Journal of Medicine* 312:10, 654–7.
9 Rennie, D. (2002), 'Fourth International Congress on Peer Review in Biomedical Publication', *Journal of the American Medical Association* 287:21, 2759–60.
10 Kavanagh, B.P., Katz, J. and Sandler, A.N. (1994), 'Pain Control After Thoracic Surgery: A Review of Current Techniques', *Anesthesiology* 81:3, 737–59.
11 Huwiler-Muntener, K. et al. (2002), 'Quality of Reporting of Randomized Trials As a Measure of Methodologic Quality', *Journal of the American Medical Association* 287:21, 2801–4.
12 Rodgers, A. et al. (2000), 'Reduction of Postoperative Mortality and Morbidity With Epidural or Spinal Anaesthesia: Results From Overview of Randomised Trials', *British Medical Journal* 321:7275, 1493.
13 Rigg, J.R. et al. (2002), 'Epidural Anaesthesia and Analgesia and Outcome of Major Surgery: A Randomised Trial', *Lancet* 359:9314, 1276–82.
14 Whittington, C.J. et al. (2004), 'Selective Serotonin Reuptake Inhibitors in Childhood Depression: Systematic Review of Published Versus Unpublished Data', *Lancet* 363:9418, 1341–5.

15 Moncrieff, J., Wessely, S. and Hardy, R. (2004), 'Active Placebos Versus Antidepressants for Depression', *Cochrane Database of Systematic Reviews* 2004:1, CD003012.

16 Moncrieff, J. and Kirsch, I. (2005), 'Efficacy of Antidepressants in Adults', *British Medical Journal* 331:7509, 155–7.

17 Begg, C. et al. (1996), 'Improving the Quality of Reporting of Randomized Controlled Trials. The CONSORT statement', *Journal of the American Medical Association* 276:8, 637–9.

18 De Angelis, C. et al. (2004), 'Clinical Trial Registration: a Statement from the International Committee of Medical Journal Editors', *Annals of Internal Medicine* 141(6):477–8.

19 Cronin L. et al. (1995), 'Corticosteroid Treatment for Sepsis: a Critical Appraisal and Meta-Analysis of the Literature', *Critical Care Medicine* 23:8, 1430–9.

20 Bellomo, R. et al. (2000), 'Low-Dose Dopamine in Patients With Early Renal Dysfunction: A Placebo-Controlled Randomised Trial. Australian and New Zealand Intensive Care Society (ANZICS) Clinical Trials Group', *Lancet* 356:9248, 2139–43.

21 SAFE Study Investigators (2004), 'A Comparison of Albumin and Saline for Fluid Resuscitation in the Intensive Care Unit', *New England Journal of Medicine* 350:22, 2247–56.

22 Hill, J.A. (2005), 'In Vino Veritas: Alcohol and Heart Disease', *American Journal of the Medical Sciences* 329:3, 124–35.

23 Rothman, K.J. and Greenland, S. (1998), 'Causation and Causal Influence', in Rothman, K.J. and Greenland, S., eds. *Modern Epidemiology* (Philadelphia: Lippincott Raven).

24 Oxman, A.D. and Guyatt, G.H. (1988), 'Guidelines for Reading Literature Reviews', *Canadian Medical Association Journal* 138:8, 697–703.

25 Benzon, H.T. (1986), 'Epidural Steroid Injections for Low Back Pain and Lumbosacral Radiculopathy', *Pain* 24:3, 277–95.

26 Kepes, E.R. and Duncalf, D. (1985), 'Treatment of Backache with Spinal Injections of Local Anesthetics, Spinal and Systemic Steroids. A Review', *Pain* 22:1, 33–47.

27 Mulrow, C.D. (1987), 'The Medical Review Article: State of the Science', *Annals of Internal Medicine* 106:3, 485–8.

28 Pedersen, T., Duylund Pedersen, B. and Moller A.M. (2003), 'Pulse Oximetry for Perioperative Monitoring', *Cochrane Database of Systematic Reviews* 2003:3, CD002013.

29 Runciman, W.B. et al. (1993), 'The Pulse Oximeter: Applications and Limitations – An Analysis of 2000 Incident Reports', *Anaesthesia and Intensive Care* 21:5, 543–50.

30 Runciman, W.B. (1993), 'Qualitative versus Quantitative Research –Balancing Cost, Yield and Feasibility', *Anaesthesia and Intensive Care* 21:5, 502–5.

31 Runciman, W.B. (2005), 'Iatrogenic Harm and Anaesthesia in Australia', *Anaesthesia and Intensive Care* 33:3, 297–300. We appreciate that this communication is more recent than the Cochrane review in question.

32 Smith, G.C. and Pell, J.P. (2003), 'Parachute Use to Prevent Death and Major Trauma Related to Gravitational Challenge: Systematic Review of Randomised Controlled Trials', *British Medical Journal* 327:7429, 1459–61.

33 Chibnall, J.T., Jeral, J.M. and Cerullo, M.A. (2001), 'Experiments on Distant Intercessory Prayer: God, Science, and the Lesson of Massah', *Archives of Internal Medicine* 161:21, 2529–36.

34 Merry, A.F., Davies, J.M. and Maltby, J.R. (2000), 'Qualitative Research in Health Care', *British Journal of Anaesthesia* 84:5, 552–5.

35 Bernard, C. (1927), *An Introduction to the Study of Experimental Medicine* (New York: MacMillan).

36 Merry, A.F. et al. (2004), 'Clinical Tolerability of Perioperative Tenoxicam in 1001 Patients – a Prospective, Controlled, Double-Blind, Multi-Centre Study, *Pain* 111:3, 313–22.

37 Dixon-Woods, M, and Fitzpatrick, R. (2001), 'Qualitative Research in Systematic Reviews has Established a Place for Itself', *British Medical Journal* 323:7316, 765–6.

38 Dixon-Woods, M. et al. (2005), 'Synthesising Qualittative and Quantitative Evidence: A Review of Possible Methods', *Journal of Helath Services Research and Policy* 10:1, 45–53.

39 Jensen, L.S et al. (2004), 'Evidence-Based Strategies for Preventing Drug Administration Errors During Anaesthesia', *Anaesthesia* 59:5, 493–504.

40 Runciman, W.B (1999), 'Incidents and Accidents in Healthcare: It's Time!', *Journal of Quality and Clinical Practice* 19:1, 1–2.

41 Altman, D.G. and Bland, J.M. (1996), 'Absence of Evidence is Not Evidence of Absence', *Australian Veterinary Journal* 74:4, 311.

42 Edmonds, M.J. et al. (2004), 'Evidence-based Risk Factors for Postoperative Deep Vein Thrombosis', *Australian and New Zealand Journal of Surgery* 74:12, 1082–97.

43 Kakkar, V.V. et al. (1970), 'Deep Vein Thrombosis of the Leg. Is There a "High Risk" Group', *American Journal of Surgery* 120:4, 527–30.

44 Brazier, M. (2003), *Medicines, Patients and the Law*, 3rd edition (London: Penguin).

45 It is worth reflecting on the fact that in other contexts, consent is unlikely to be recognized as a defence for assault.

46 *Bolam vs Friern Hospital Management Committee* (1957), 2 All ER 118 (England).

47 *Hunter vs Hanley* (1955), SC 200 (Scotland).

48 Edward Wong Finance Co Ltd vs Johnson, Stokes and Master (1984), 1 AC 296 (England).

49 *F v R* (1983) 33 SASR 189 (South Australia).

50 *Rogers vs Whittaker* (1992), 175 CLR 479 (Australia).

51 *Bolitho vs City and Hackney Health Authority* (1998), AC 252 (England).

52 Garden, A.L. et al. (1996), 'Anaesthesia Information – What Patients Want to Know', *Anaesthesia and Intensive Care* 24:5, 594–8.

53 Tattersall, M.H.N., Kerridge, I.H. (2006), 'Doctors behaving badly?', *The Medical Journal of Australia* 185:6, 299–300.

54 Angell, M., (2005), *The Truth About the Drug Companies: How They Deceive Us and What To Do About It* (Maryland: Random House).

55 'Stop the gravy train' (editorial) *The Australian* (2006) 7 Aug 8.

56 Pearson, S.D., Kleinman, K., Rusinak, D., Levinson, W. (2006), 'A trial of disclosing physicians' financial incentives to patients', *Arch Intern Med* 166: 623–628.

57 British Medical Journal, *Clinical Evidence* [webpage]. Available at: http://www.clinicalevidence.com accessed 8 Jun 2006.

58 Sackett, D.L. et al. (1997), *Evidence-Based Medicine: How to Practice and Teach EBM* (New York: Churchill Livingstone).

Chapter 7

Ethics, Professional Behaviour and Regulation

Ethics

Medical ethics, bioethics, clinical ethics and professional behaviour are increasingly subjects of debate in the healthcare literature and the lay press. Ethics provides a set of principals for examining the morality of personal and professional behaviour.

Ethics is a field of study concerned with understanding morals, values, judgments, responsibilities and obligations. There are several approaches to ethics. Normative ethicists examine moral questions and values that govern human activity. Meta-ethicists seek to understand moral concepts such as 'right', 'good', 'justice' and 'virtue'. Practical ethicists apply ethical theory to particular areas or problems. Professional ethicists deal with human behaviour and conduct in relation to particular professional groups. The latter two are of particular relevance to healthcare.

The 'four principle' approach to ethics, made famous by Beauchamp and Childress,[1] provides a sound starting point for the analysis of ethical problems in healthcare. The principles are: respect for autonomy, non-maleficence, beneficence and justice. Applying these principles is unfortunately not always straightforward, and one's take on any given situation will differ depending on which school of ethics one belongs to. For example, a utilitarian's[2] interpretation of the net balance of these principles in a particular situation might well differ from the interpretation of a virtue ethicist[3,4] or that of a deontologist.[5] Even within a single school, individuals may differ in their analysis of the same set of facts. Furthermore, it is a mistake to assume that these principles cover all the bases. Hursthouse has pointed out that they amount to virtues, and there are many other virtues that might also need to be considered, such as truthfulness.[3]

Medical Ethics

The field of medical ethics has origins which predate Hippocrates, but it is generally accepted that the Hippocratic Oath gave doctors their first code of ethical practice. A code of practice requires members of a professional group to adhere to a set of rules or desired behaviours. The Hippocratic Oath required physicians to recognize their limitations, not to prescribe deadly drugs, procure abortions, harm patients or have sexual relations with them, and to keep confidential information imparted by patients.[6]

Over the centuries, patients' interests have remained paramount, and the mantra *do no harm* is as important now as it was then. However, views of acceptable behaviour have changed. For example, many societies now condone, or even demand, abortion, a procedure that was previously a crime. The idea that a code of ethics should reflect the values of the society one lives in is embodied in the theory of cultural relativism. This theory is highly controversial at best. The importance of critically evaluating as an individual the moral basis of practices currently accepted within a culture, before simply accepting them, is well illustrated by the behaviour of some doctors in Nazi Germany, who were operating within the rules of their society at the time.

A number of ethical statements were made after the atrocities committed by these Nazi doctors were disclosed at the 1946 Nuremberg Medical Trials (e.g. the Nuremburg Tribunal's pronouncement on informed consent in 1947[7]). These inspired the creation of the World Medical Association and the publication of the Declaration of Geneva in 1948.[8] The Geneva rules, designed to protect the victims of wars, were necessary because the Nazi doctors in Auschwitz had all but abandoned their pledge to do no harm. Their role in legitimizing the killing of people such as the mentally retarded and 'sexual deviants', under the guise of medical necessity, was a key factor in 'normalizing' the genocidal activities of the death camps. It is noteworthy that the USA denied rights accepted at Nuremberg to those captured in Afghanistan after 'September 11', apparently on the basis that they are not legitimate prisoners of war (although the President of the US had 'declared war' on terrorism). Attempts have been made to justify what appears to be the torture of these captives. It has been suggested that physicians of the US military have used and/or made available confidential medical information to facilitate the planning and conduct of torture. This was described as a 'national shame' in an editorial.[9]

The Declaration of Helsinki, which covers rules governing medical research involving humans, was published in 1964.[10] The Declaration may be summarized by the opening sentence of its first paragraph: 'Medical research is subject to ethical standards that promote respect for all human beings and protect their health and rights' (the subject of research ethics is dealt with on pages 137 and 138, and on page 160). Apart from this Declaration and some ethical debates clustered around the beginning and end of life, ethics was not often accorded more than token importance in relation to clinical practice until the late 1990s. Today, increased attention to ethics and professional conduct by governments and regulatory authorities is beginning to impact on the healthcare professions through their professional associations and educational institutions, several of which have published codes of ethical practice (see Appendix V for an example of a code of ethics).[11,12,13] Even politicians are pointing out that inadequate regard for ethical behaviour will progressively erode the status of the medical profession.[14] The events at Guantanemo Bay are particularly worrying because the examples of complicity in torture appear not to have been isolated, covert acts by individual members of the medical profession; rather, they appear to have been officially sanctioned within whatever 'system' was in place.

Bioethics

The development of bioethics in the 1970s as a separate field of applied ethics was a response to a growing need to examine the values implicated in rapidly expanding developments in scientific medicine and healthcare. Technology, specialization and unprecedented advances in science give rise to situations requiring biomedical scientists to re-examine their moral and social responsibilities and obligations. Society is having great difficulty in keeping pace with the ethical implications of advances in areas such as DNA technology, organ donation from living donors, stem cell research and cloning, to name only a few contentious areas. As one dilemma appears to have been resolved another comes along, or a previously apparently resolved dilemma reappears because of changed social, clinical or political circumstances.

Clinical Ethics

Clinical ethics deals with the moral and ethical issues that arise in everyday clinical practice. Ethical dilemmas are becoming a fact of life for healthcare workers; some of the conflicting considerations commonly encountered are listed in Table 7.1. For example, technology can now keep people alive who would otherwise die. This may imply great expense and prolonged, often complex, care. The term 'extraordinary measures' has been coined to describe interventions of this type. The decision to use or withdraw such measures to keep the patient alive may be difficult, especially when the patient is unable to contribute to the discussion and has given no advance directive. Who should make this decision?

Table 7.1   Some of the potentially conflicting considerations commonly encountered by clinicians making ethical decisions

Access	Timeliness	Justice	Risk
Efficiency	Rights	Compensation	Safety
Choice	Autonomy	Retribution	Values
Standardization	Variability	Evidence	Blame
Acceptability	Vulnerability	Effectiveness	Culture
Appropriateness	Complexity	Privacy	Competence
Rationing	Conflict	Disclosure	Accountability
Cost	Mediation	Confidentiality	Privilege

What constitutes extraordinary measures? Conflict may arise between those who want everything done even when treatment is futile, and those who see excessive medical zeal as causing more harm than good. These conflicts may involve any combination of patients, carers, treating teams, and family members. A decision may have implications for other patients, and may involve consideration of all the factors in the left-hand column in Table 7.1, as well as some in the other columns. The late Pope John Paul II indicated that enteral feeding via a tube does not constitute an extraordinary measure, thereby (in theory at least) committing thousands of Catholics to a vegetative existence, and the societies in which they live to enormous ongoing costs which could be spent elsewhere in healthcare.[15] Who should control access to life-saving and life-prolonging equipment such as neonatal intensive care cribs? Are there any conditions or circumstances under which one patient is to be judged more worthy than another? Such questions are now commonplace and there are no ready answers. Some frameworks for healthcare professionals facing ethical decisions are provided below.

Research Ethics

The application of ethical principles to research is important in order to protect the rights and welfare of research participants, including human volunteers. The justification for research is to contribute to knowledge to the benefit of humanity and the researcher's community. It follows that the integrity of the research should be seen as a core ethical principle. Respect for persons requires individuals to be treated as autonomous agents. It follows that individuals with diminished autonomy are entitled to extra protection. This is of particular importance in research, for example, in intensive care, where many of the patients are not in a position to make informed decisions. All organizations which conduct research must have access to a human research ethics committee which should be compliant with the national guidelines in the relevant country.[16,17]

Professional Behaviour

Professionalism is the basis for the relationship between clinicians and society. Health professionals have privileges bestowed upon them by society, not only because of their specialized skills and knowledge, but also because of a social contract between them and society. This contract, which may in varying degrees be implicit or explicit, obliges them to use their skills for curing and healing the sick, and not for exploiting their patients or the healthcare system. Edmund Pellegrino, an American medical philosopher states: 'We [patients] must trust that our vulnerability will not be exploited for power, profit, prestige or pleasure'.[18]

In 1983, The World Medical Association reminded doctors to adhere to the Declaration of Geneva, and urged them to make clinical decisions without concern for profit, to be honest with patients, and to expose incompetent and immoral colleagues.[11] However, systems for ensuring that these injunctions are followed are poorly developed and often not used.

In contrast to the so called 'hard science' of healthcare (but see Chapter 6 for reservations about this concept), ethical rules are often seen as 'soft'. It is our impression that many clinicians have a limited interest in ethics, and not much understanding of the subject. Many struggle when faced with difficult ethical decisions. For example, some simply continue unquestioningly with life sustaining treatment, when it is clear that a patient has no prospect of an acceptable quality of life, and that his or her relatives are in agreement that the patient would not want to survive under these circumstances. This abrogation of responsibility is understandable given that the teaching of ethics has been neglected by healthcare educators. Medical educators need to address this deficit.

Clinical Ethics

Decisions in healthcare reflect an integration of practitioners' scientific and technical knowledge, their knowledge of ethics, and their attitude towards the moral worth of the care in question. Clinical encounters are often complex, and conflicting values may have to be considered. Ethical conflicts cannot always be easily resolved and additional tools may be required to manage dilemmas. A number of ethical frameworks have been developed to assist healthcare workers to analyze clinical ethical problems (see Box 7.1 and Appendix VI).

Ethical Frameworks

The ethical framework of Kerridge, Lowe and McPhee[19] is based on a structured set of tasks (Box 7.1). An alternative is the Jonsen model, which examines problems by analyzing four domains: medical indications, patient references, quality of life and contextual features (see Appendix VI). Although these frameworks are useful, there are no generalizations that will lead to definitive answers in all difficult ethical situations. Each case must be considered on its merits, taking into consideration all the elements of these frameworks, some of which may be in conflict with each other.

Conflicts of Values, Beliefs and Interests – Cultural Competence

Healthcare services are delivered by individuals with a wide variety of beliefs and values. Patients from a wide range of social, economic and cultural backgrounds and of different ages and capacity are treated in these health services. Patients and healthcare workers bring their own life experiences as well as their own cultural, religious and linguistic backgrounds to the bedside. The opportunities for misunderstandings and miscommunication are many. It is important for clinicians to be aware of cultural differences and of the importance of respect for people from different backgrounds.

Healthcare workers should provide care to all who need it that respects, honours and supports cultural diversity. The term 'cultural competence' describes the knowledge, skills and attitudes that a healthcare worker needs to provide care in this way. A culturally competent healthcare worker would be sensitive to all aspects of diversity including gender, culture, disability, religion and background. Specific training may be needed to ensure that healthcare workers understand key

Box 7.1 The Ethical Framework of Kerridge, Lowe and McPhee[19]

Clearly state the problem
- Consider the problem with its context and distinguish between ethical problems and other medical, social, cultural, linguistic and legal issues.
- Explore the meaning of value-laden terms, e.g. futility, quality of life.

Get the facts
- Find out as much as you can about the problem through history, examination and relevant investigations.
- Take the time to listen to patients' narratives and understand their personal and cultural biographies (or those of a family member, carer or friend).
- Are there necessary facts that you do not have? If so, search for them.

Consider the fundamental ethical principles
- Autonomy: What is the patient's approach to the problem?
- Beneficence: What benefits can be obtained for the patient?
- Non-maleficence: What are the risks and how can they be avoided?
- Justice: How are the interests of different parties to be balanced (including those of society at large)?
- Confidentiality/privacy: What information is private and does confidentiality need to be limited or breached?
- Veracity: Has the patient and his or her family been honestly informed and is there any reason why the patient cannot know the truth?

Consider how the problem would look from another perspective or using another theory
- Who are the relevant stakeholders? What is their interest? What do they have to lose? How salient are their interests? How powerful are they? How legitimate are they? How urgent are they?
- How would the problem look from an alternative ethical position? For example, consequentialist, rights-based, virtue-based, feminist, communitarian, care-based.

Identify ethical conflicts
Explain why the conflicts occur and how they may be resolved.

Consider the law
- Identify relevant legal concepts and laws and how they might guide management.
- Examine the relationship between clinical ethical decisions and the law.

Make the ethical decision
- Clearly state the clinical ethical decision and justify it, for example by specifying how guiding principles were balanced and why.
- Identify ethically viable options.
- Take responsibility for the decision.
- Document the decision and the rationale for it.
- Communicate the decision and assist relevant stakeholders to determine an action plan.

points about the cultures of the main groups in their region. Interpreters should be available if needed.

In many parts of the world, healthcare professionals will try to accommodate any reasonable wishes of competent people, whether expressed in advance or when they are sick (see Boxes 7.2 and 7.3).

Box 7.2 Respecting a patient's beliefs

Janet, a 15 year old girl with acute lymphocytic leukaemia, had suffered a relapse and failed to respond to chemotherapy. She was anaemic and thrombocytopenic. Janet understood that a transfusion would make her more comfortable, reduce the possibility of life-threatening bleeding, and perhaps allow her to leave hospital. However, she refused transfusion because of her religious beliefs as a Jehovah's Witness. Janet was aware that her illness was life threatening and that she would die very soon. Janet's parents did not disagree. The staff, who were aware that Janet demonstrated clear thinking and was realistic about her condition, abided by her decision.

Janet's case (Box 7.2) demonstrates how religious beliefs can raise ethical dilemmas for staff. In this case there was no conflict between Janet and her parents and because the healthcare team respected Janet's decision making capacity they abided by her decision for no treatment.

The Multidisciplinary Team

The healthcare team is increasingly being recognized as a critical element in safe, ethical care. The concept is that healthcare should be organized around patients, in teams that cross traditional disciplines and hierarchies. Such a team might include nurses, surgeons, anaesthetists, physiotherapists and administrators, grouped together to provide (for example) orthopaedic services to a community. This concept has been extended to calls for a single ethical code that cuts across disciplinary, professional, organizational and political boundaries, rather than a number of codes each emphasizing the professional autonomy of the various team members.[20, 21]

The healthcare system is very complex and involves multiple providers. This fragmentation promotes manipulation and 'gaming' of the system which confers power on some and makes others vulnerable. We need an approach that recognizes healthcare inequities and provides a fair method for making decisions about who will have access to healthcare (justice). Solutions that work in one institution or community may not be appropriate in another. Flexibility and transparency are therefore essential in organizing the delivery of care. The key is to centre the arrangements on the needs of the particular patients treated in a particular place.

A set of five ethical principles, designed for multidisciplinary groups in healthcare, was first published in 1999. These present a moral framework that can be applied in the workplace (see Box 7.4).

Box 7.3 Fulfilling a patient's wishes

Jamie Oatey was a fit 19 year old who went to the pub with a few friends after playing football. It was a rainy night and he was wearing dark clothes. He was crossing the road to get to a bus stop when he paused in the middle, on the white line, to wait for a car coming from the opposite direction. A car struck him from behind. He suffered a massive head injury, but had no other major injuries. He had a fracture of the base of his skull from which cerebrospinal fluid was leaking and the initial CT scan showed a very swollen brain. The neurosurgeons decided to do a craniectomy, which involves removal of a large area of skull to reduce the pressure on the brain. The family indicated they had had discussions on several occasions and all had agreed that none would want to survive in a significantly compromized state. A repeat CT scan on day three revealed areas of dead brain. It was felt unlikely that brain stem death would occur, as the brain was effectively decompressed both by the craniectomy and the large fracture of the base of the skull through which cerebrospinal fluid continued to drain. The perfusion scan showed continued perfusion to parts of the brain. Because his very concerned family was quite adamant that he would not have wished to survive in a compromized state, and because Jamie had previously expressed a desire to be an organ donor, arrangements were made for him to be a 'non beating heart organ donor'. Normally, after brain death criteria are satisfied, the organs are taken while the heart is still beating, and the ventilator is subsequently removed. In his case he was taken to the operating theatre, prepared for the operation, extubated, allowed to die over a period of twenty minutes, and his kidneys were then taken for transplantation into other patients.

The Rights of Healthcare Workers

So far in the discussion it has been assumed that 'the right thing' is for the needs and desires of patients to be given priority, tempered by reasonable judgement that this will not compromise the needs and desires of other patients. In the United States at the moment there is a surge of legislation reflecting 'the increasing tensions between asserting individual religious values and defending patients' rights'.[22] Bills in nearly half of the States are under consideration which would protect the rights of healthcare workers to refuse to participate in anything they found morally repugnant, arguing that 'conscience is the most sacred of all property'.[23] This protection would apply, for example, to pharmacists who refuse to supply the 'morning after' pill or fill prescriptions for contraceptives, healthcare workers who refuse to be involved in invitro fertilization and even, potentially, social workers who refuse to work with family planning units or gay and lesbian patients. It could be argued that people with these beliefs should not be employed in a tax payer-funded healthcare system unless they work in situations in which these services could be supplied by others in a timely and acceptable fashion. The

---

Box 7.4 The principles developed by the Tavistock Group[21]

- Healthcare is a human right.
- The care of individuals is at the centre of healthcare delivery but must be viewed and practised within the overall context of continuing work to generate the greatest possible health gains for groups and populations.
- The responsibilities of the healthcare delivery system include the prevention of illness and alleviation of disability consistent with the aims of the World Health Organization (WHO).
- Cooperation with each other and those served is imperative for those working within the healthcare delivery system.
- All individuals and groups involved in healthcare, whether providing access or services, have the continuing responsibility to help improve its quality.

---

ethics of cultural relativism suggest that there is no basis for challenging the beliefs of other cultures, however objectionable they may seem, and would support this view. However, on this basis, one would be restrained from criticizing behavior that few would condone – for example that of certain doctors in Nazi Germany or, apparently, in Guantanemo Bay. Cultural relativism is not widely accepted in its simplest form.

However, there is a fine line between tolerance of difference and the suspension of one's own moral judgement in matters that clearly could be construed as wrong. Abortion is a classic example of this. Two of the authors trained as doctors in systems in which involvement in an abortion would have led, if discovered, to deregistration and jail. Both changed countries, and overnight found themselves in systems in which abortion was provided on a daily basis, almost on demand, legally. If the law were taken as a reliable guide to ethical behaviour, then clearly the foundations of ethics would vary according to their location in space and time.

The truth is that there is no simple or universal resolution to this ethical problem, or many others. Most healthcare professionals function pragmatically, within the law, with some degree of compromise, and with due regard for the wishes of their patients. Most of the time, this is a reasonable approach. However, none of us should loose sight of the fact that this might not always be so, and that there might be a time to stand on principle.

Ethics Committees

Some hospitals have established multidisciplinary ethics committees to provide a forum for clinicians to raise ethical and legal concerns associated with particular treatments or decisions. These are distinct from research ethics committees which examine the ethical implications of and recommend safeguards for research projects. These clinical ethics committees are advisory and do not tell clinicians what to do, but do make recommendations. These consultations or meetings have yet to include patients on a routine basis, but do attempt to take into account patients' wishes. In addition to providing clinicians with advice on particular cases these committees may also assist with the development of organizational policies on patient care and facilitate staff and patient education about ethical issues.

The Relationship between Patients and Healthcare Professionals

The patient-provider relationship, typified by the doctor-patient relationship, has undergone several changes. In the eighteenth century, when only wealthy patients called the doctor, patients were dominant. Superior in social standing, patients often made the lives of doctors very difficult; smart doctors, in addition to their bed side skills, learnt the art of pleasing. The era of science and technology that would widen the knowledge gap between patients and doctors had yet to arrive. Medical historian Roy Porter observes that the public in the eighteenth century were far from fatalistic about their healthcare.[24] Rather, they were medically literate and expected to be involved in their healthcare and in decisions about treatments. This need for patronage, combined with competition from quacks, kept the status of doctors low until the end of the nineteenth century.

Scientific discoveries gave impetus to medicine by adding to the skills and knowledge of doctors in areas such as physiology and chemistry. No longer were they solely dependent on a black leather bag containing an assortment of untested, mostly ineffective remedies. Scientific advances and the industrial revolution also saw a rapid growth in the number of hospitals and changes to the organization of the medical profession (see Chapter 3). Porter dates the development of medical specialization to the growth of hospitals in the nineteenth century, and sees it as a natural outcome of scientific, institutional and therapeutic developments.[25]

With this growth of hospitals, medicine moved more towards being a complex inter-dependent and impersonal social service.[26] Doctors' knowledge and skills far outpaced those of patients, causing patients to become less assertive and more willing to rely on doctors' views about their ailments. The changing roles of patients and doctors gave birth to the age of medical paternalism. Paternalism in this context refers to overriding the autonomy of patients 'for their own good' (which is consistent with but not necessary for beneficence). Paternalistic relationships between patients and health providers were common for most of the twentieth century. Joseph Collins in a 1927 publication of Harper's Monthly Magazine wrote that every physician should cultivate the art of lying for the benefit of patients, stating that depression, anxiety and loss of hope were just a few conditions that lying could prevent.[27]

A third type of relationship based on shared decision making is now in ascendancy, that of a partnership between doctors and patients. The ethical principle underpinning the focus on partnership is 'respect for autonomy'. This refers to the moral right of patients to have personal preferences and make choices. It can also be interpreted to confer similar rights on healthcare professionals. Respect for autonomy obliges healthcare professionals to provide information relevant to the patient's condition, to probe for and ensure understanding and voluntariness, and to foster good decision making.[28] The goal is to have fully informed patients who have been helped to understand their situation and who make informed decisions without undue influence or coercion.

Patients will differ in the extent to which they wish to be involved in decision making. Not all patients want to make decisions. They may feel too close to their own or a family member's situation, be confused about the options or happy to place their trust in their healthcare provider's knowledge and skills. However, they should be made aware that they can become more involved and seek more information at any stage, should they wish to do so.

Decision Making and Autonomy

The right of patient self-determination is well entrenched both in law and in ethical codes. Respect for patient autonomy now occupies centre stage in medical ethics. In considering patient autonomy one needs to think about truth telling, confidentiality, privacy, disclosure of information and consent. Each is important and all have important implications for healthcare professionals.

Most would agree that *truth telling* is required for all but the minority of (often elderly) patients who indicate clearly that they do not want to be told their diagnosis or prognosis. These patients may be more comfortable with euphemisms, and some clinicians might well conclude that acquiescence with these wishes is ethical. The place of truth telling may also be questioned in relation to young children facing death. It can be very difficult to know what to do for the best with such patients. Each situation will need to be assessed on its individual merits, in consultation with the patient's family. *Confidentiality* is necessary to safeguard privacy and great care should be taken to protect particularly sensitive information, especially that which is not of immediate relevance to the patient's current problem. It is not necessary to record that an elderly patient had a sexually transmitted disease as a young adult when he or she presents with, for example, macular degeneration, or for a biomedical engineer to know a patient's identity or diagnosis when called upon to fix a monitoring device in the operating room. The requirements for confidentiality overlap with those for privacy. As a general principle, information which can identify a patient should not be revealed unless this is necessary for the clinical care of that patient.

Regulations with respect to privacy are complex and vary from jurisdiction to jurisdiction. It is important to be aware of local requirements and to put measures in place to remind people not to reveal identifiers unless consent has been given or it is necessary for patient care.

Consent has been dealt with in some detail on pages 148–153. Nevertheless some healthcare workers remain ambivalent about the provision of informed consent. They tend to provide the following reasons:

Healthcare workers have years of training and are the experts One argument against acknowledging the role patients can play in decision making in healthcare is that they are not experts. A related argument is that *it is impossible to know how much information should be provided to patients*. These arguments rely in part on

---

Box 7.5 Extraordinary measures?

Mavis Brown was a 92 year old lady who had been living in hostel accommodation in an aged care facility. She presented with severe back and groin pain and was acutely unwell with low blood pressure and poor urine output. Investigation revealed that she had a large calculus obstructing the outflow to her right kidney. She was brought in by her relatives who indicated that she had signed an 'advance directive' that she did not wish to have extraordinary measures in the event of a problem which would compromize her quality of life. She was normally a sprightly lady who enjoyed outings with her children and grandchildren. The family was in favour of her being given morphine and allowed to die. However, the surgeon in consultation with an intensive care specialist, felt that it would be worthwhile to remove the staghorn calculus and give her intensive therapy for a few days, as this was a completely correctable problem, and as sepsis from urinary tract infection can nearly always be successfully treated if the cause is removed. It was put to the family that there was a reasonable chance of her returning to a good quality of life if treatment was prompt and aggressive, although it would involve life support machines such as a ventilator for a few days. The family reluctantly agreed with the plan of action to be aggressive, but it was agreed by all in advance that should any complication ensue, such as a stroke, post-operative pneumonia, or renal failure, treatment would be withdrawn and only comfort measures applied. She duly had the procedure, was ventilated for three days and had invasive hemodynamic monitoring, and made a full recovery.

---

the belief that scientific knowledge is certain knowledge and that knowledge grows normally by accumulation and is acquired and stored in a person's mind.[29] Neil McIntyre and Karl Popper pointed out that this belief underpinned professional ethics for most of the twentieth century, culminating in a culture of 'authority'. Some health providers still believe that their authority is undermined when patients question their diagnoses and treatments. This is not a sustainable position in modern healthcare. Furthermore, it is disingenuous to suggest that informed consent implies that the patient must be brought to the same level of understanding as the doctor. In fact, the notion that either the patient or the doctor is ever likely to be fully informed is fallacious. It is impossible for healthcare workers to know everything of relevance to their patients. There are more than 40,000 biomedical journals and the number doubles every 20 years. To keep completely up to date a primary care doctor, for example, would have to read 20 articles a day 365 days a year.[30] It is, however, relatively easy for a doctor to understand and impart, and for a patient to take on board, the key points related to decisions. It is also quite practical for a doctor to respond truthfully to most questions asked by a patient, even if only by admitting that he or she does not know the answer. The adequacy of information should be judged by reference to the person's particular needs (see pages 149 to 151).

Adherents to the authority model may end up denying patients their autonomy twice – first, by deliberately withholding pertinent information and second, by providing information framed in a way that will influence a patient's response. Many patients willingly accept their doctors' recommendations without carefully weighing the risks and benefits.[31,32] Patients can be subtly coerced to have a certain treatment, particularly when clinicians are convinced of the 'rightness' of that treatment. There is a high risk of this when healthcare workers express their clinical opinions about the procedure at the same time as they give information about the risks and benefits. For example, if a surgeon recommends an arthroscopy of the knee, many patients are likely to interpret this as implying that they actually need the procedure. Their take on the situation might be rather different if the surgeon said that an arthroscopy was a possibility, but that the option to do nothing was also reasonable. Respect for autonomy requires that the patient's values and desires guide treatment choices, not the healthcare worker's. This implies that factual information should be provided in a value-free manner.

Many patients do not want to make decisions about their treatment A third argument often given against autonomy is that many patients do not want to make decisions, particularly when their condition is life threatening or involves a painful treatment. This is natural because patients may have different levels of education and comprehension, and different degrees of aversion to having to make such decisions. They may also be very young or very old, sick, vulnerable and not functioning at their best. Some patients choose not to exercise autonomy, and this is reasonable, but it does not negate the principle that autonomy is important. Patients can only choose to relinquish autonomy if they have it in the first place. Some patients may want to relinquish autonomy for some things and not others; relinquishment of autonomy should not be interpreted to mean that a patient does not want interactive conversations. Discussions, explanations and the answering of questions are still necessary and can preserve a substantial degree of autonomy for even those patients who do not want to make decisions in relation to their treatment.

Ethical issues are never simple. In the end autonomy is only a virtue, and only one of many virtues. It is almost as disingenuous to over-emphasize autonomy as to deny its importance. This is in fact a fourth way of undermining the value of informed consent. It amounts to disengaging from the human interaction with one's patients and acting like an autonomy-providing automaton. No system of ethics should rest its analysis on a single principle or virtue.. Clearly non-maleficence, beneficence and justice must also be considered in our evaluation of how much to tell a patient, and how to frame the information. Some ethicists might add charity and compassion to the list. Some cultures place less emphasis on the autonomy of the individual and more on the importance of the group – the extended family, tribe or society as a whole (see pages 151-152 and 187 - 188). Perhaps an honest commitment to doing the right thing would be the best guide, but such a commitment must be based on a thorough understanding of the principles at stake, of the particular circumstances and, wherever possible, of the wishes of the patient.

Box 7.6 A natural death

Miss Leape was a 44 year old aerobics instructor. She was very fit, had been a vegetarian for many years, and did not smoke or drink. She was having some trouble reading the small print in the newspaper, and went to an optometrist to have her eyes checked. He confirmed that she needed reading glasses, but also found a melanoma on her retina. She went to her usual naturopath, who made some dietary recommendations and suggested that she should drink only distilled water. The naturopath suggested she go to an ophthalmologist, who was asked to photograph the melanoma regularly to track its progress. He pleaded with the patient and her naturopath to agree to the conventional treatment of the removal of the eye, as the condition was almost definitely completely curable at that stage, but would be fatal if left alone. He agreed to see her weekly with a view to escalating the pressure to have the operation. On the third visit, however, it became quite apparent that the patient and the naturopath were determined to pursue their course of action but wanted him to track the progress of the melanoma by taking photographs. He regretfully declined to do this as he felt he could not be involved in the case. He did try to contact the patient on two further occasions, but she did not agree to attend his rooms. He subsequently heard from a colleague that she had died from melanoma secondaries in her brain.

Reporting Unethical Practice

A salient feature of the many enquiries about patient harm caused by the actions of individuals is that people knew or were concerned about the activities of these individuals but failed to report their concerns at the time. In the infamous case of Harold Shipman, who is believed to have murdered over 200 patients between 1975–2000, there were early signs of his aberrant behaviour (see Box 4.4). The enquiry into these deaths, conducted by Dame Janet Smith, identified a number of times when his behaviour should have been reported and checked.[33] For example, Shipman ingratiated himself with the manager of the pharmacy next to his practice and she frequently supplied him with ampoules of diamorphine in circumstances which should instead have led to questions. Similarly, many expressed concern about a Dr. Patel in Queensland, Australia, who, it is alleged, was responsible for the deaths of several patients, but no action was taken (see Box 7.8).

The hidden culture People who work in healthcare soon discover there are two ways of doing things; the official way and the unofficial way. Hospital policies and guidelines set out the correct procedures but in reality many are not followed because the rules of a 'hidden culture' operate. The hidden culture refers to the way things are actually done rather than the way things ought to be done. This has also been described as the difference between 'sacred' (or officially condoned) knowledge and 'profane' (or hidden-culture) knowledge. A good example of this is the gap between the knowledge of medical and nursing students about ethical practice and the ethical practice they sometimes see on the wards. They may know and understand the main components of informed consent but when they visit wards they routinely see junior doctors obtaining consent from patients under circumstances in which the patients are obviously not fully informed, if only because the person obtaining the consent does not have the experience or knowledge to answer questions about the proposed procedure or treatment. Students soon learn to follow the accepted practices, even though they may know that these contravene hospital policy. One study of 108 final year medical students showed that nearly half reported that they had been placed in clinical situations in which they felt pressured to act unethically.[34] Sixty-one per cent said they had frequently witnessed a clinical teacher acting unethically. This study also highlighted the lack of discussion around ethical problems and the failure to resolve these issues when they arise.

The disdain that some staff have for organizational guidelines and protocols is also a symptom of the hidden culture. Most healthcare workers know that hospitals are awash with rules and regulations that are routinely ignored or violated without repercussions. In most instances, failure to follow a rule does not result in an injury to patients, but there are also times when it does.

If a junior member of a medical team is uncomfortable with the actions of a more senior clinician it is very difficult for him or her to report the senior because maintaining the confidence of more experienced clinicians is very important. Progression up the medical hierarchy depends on favourable reports based on informal and formal feedback and subjective and objective assessments about competence and commitment (see page 72).

This dependence of junior staff on senior clinicians also influences other practices that may be harmful to patients, such as reluctance to disclose inexperience which can expose patients to increased risk of an adverse event. Junior doctors who have been working long hours and feel fatigued may also be reluctant to advise their supervisors of this for fear of receiving an unfavourable report for being seen as 'lacking in commitment'.

The difficulty for junior staff and healthcare students is that, with no accepted structure for reporting such matters, they are often unsure of the right way to respond when they see unethical behaviour. They know they should do something, but what? 'Whistleblowers' tend to have a very hard time. Although many countries have introduced legislation to protect those who act in good faith, this legislation is not necessarily effective. The four Australian nurses who made allegations of sub-standard care at Campbelltown and Camden hospitals in New South Wales and the doctor who disclosed the high death rate from paediatric cardiac surgery at the Royal Bristol Infirmary were all severely criticized and ostracized from their organizations and professional bodies (at least in their immediate environment). The problem for these whistleblowers was the absence of a culture that valued patient safety.[35,36] When organizational and professional agendas dominate the workplace, it is almost impossible to speak out with impunity. Nevertheless, if the legitimacy of doing so was generally accepted

Box 7.7 The end of the line

Mrs. Ada Smith was an 87 year old widow who presented with pneumonia after having had a flu-like illness for three days. She lived alone in a small cottage. Her husband had died six months previously. They had lived in the same cottage for over 60 years. She had been depressed since her husband died, had not been eating well, had lost weight and had several falls. Her family believed strongly that the time had come for her to be looked after in an aged care facility. She was the subject of a medical emergency team call when the oxygen saturation in her blood fell below 90 per cent. When spoken to and examined, it was clear that she was struggling, was unable to cough up her infected sputum, and had severe pleuritic pain. A blood gas test revealed that her breathing was failing. It was indicated to the patient that she would require a period in the intensive care unit with an endotracheal tube and a ventilator to help clear her secretions and support her breathing whilst she was very unwell. She indicated that unless she could be guaranteed that she could return home well enough to continue living on her own, she should not be treated. This led to a discussion around the bedside with the patient and her family. It became quite clear that she was vehemently opposed to moving from her cottage, and that her eyesight (macular degeneration) had got much worse over the last few months. She was willing to regard the pneumonia as her terminal illness. It was agreed to leave her in the ward but continue conventional therapy, including morphine for the pleuritic pain, even though this had the potential to further compromise her breathing. She died 12 hours later.

because all healthcare professionals had been adequately exposed to the elements of safety and quality (see pages 240–243), then the technique of graded assertiveness (see page 232) would provide a way forward.

Identifying and dealing with incompetent or impaired healthcare workers All healthcare workers make errors; several chapters in this book outline the systemic nature of error and show how the design of services inevitably means mistakes will occur. Competent people learn from their errors and adjust their practice to avoid making similar mistakes in the future (see Chapter 9). The best initial response to a concern about a clinician's performance is one based on a systems approach, in which errors are viewed as flaws in the system rather than the person. However, there are times when the problem is the inadequate performance of a person. The presence of poorly performing individuals within the workforce may itself be seen as a manifestation of flaws in the system, such as inadequate credentialling, failure to check references, or failure to follow up on complaints and concerns raised by staff (see Box 7.8).

Healthcare workers, like the rest of the population, are susceptible to both acute and chronic diseases. They also age and may become out of touch with modern treatments and techniques. Under these circumstances, they require

---

Box 7.8 The Bundaberg Hospital scandal[37]

In 2003 Dr. Jayant Patel was appointed as a surgical medical officer at Bundaberg Hospital and subsequently promoted to Director of Surgery. Over the following two years, he operated on about 1,000 patients, of whom 88 died and 14 suffered serious complications. A clinical review found that Dr Patel directly contributed to the deaths of 8 patients and may have exhibited an unacceptable level of care in another 8 patients who died. Dr. Patel lacked many of the attributes of a competent surgeon.

All this may not have happened had the 2003 registration process of Dr. Patel by the Queensland Medical Board been more rigorous. An in-depth review would have uncovered the facts that Dr. Patel had been placed on probation for three years in 1983 for 'gross negligence' in his practice at Rochester Hospital in New York State, that in 2000 the Oregon Board of Medical Examiners in the United States restricted the scope of his surgery, and that in 2001, under threat of having his licence revoked in New York State, he instead obtained permission to surrender his licence to practise. Repeated complaints by senior nursing staff, including some in writing, fell on deaf ears, and it was only when a letter from the nursing staff was tabled in Queensland Parliament, that the matter came out into the open. Dr. Patel left the country unimpeded.

---

sympathy and help. Many licensing and professional bodies have established programs to manage impaired health professionals. Despite this, those in the professions are often slow to refer or report their colleagues to these bodies. Healthcare workers have an obligation to ensure that only competent and capable people treat patients. Meeting this obligation requires the reporting of incompetent people. In many cases, training and education will be sufficient to ensure that these people regain the knowledge and skills needed to practise safely. However, some individuals will need to stop treating patients.

There are many models for managing poorly performing, incompetent or impaired healthcare workers. One model used by the health system in New South Wales in Australia relies on categorizing these issues into one of three levels.

- Level 1 covers clinicians' practice, performance or patient outcomes which deviate from normal expectations or from those of their peers, but where there have been no adverse outcomes to patients. This would require the local health service or hospital to conduct a formal review of the clinicians' clinical performance.
- Level 2 covers matters that require investigation by a public health organization. More than one event causing significant morbidity or mortality may typically be involved, indicating a pattern of practice which raises issues about the knowledge and skills of the individual.
- Level 3 covers clinicians who are considered dangerous, with a substantial gap in knowledge and skills, serious impairment or evidence of recklessness.

Although such processes are essential, the vast majority of iatrogenic harm is not caused by a few 'bad eggs', but by large numbers of clinicians whose practice is generally of a high standard. Many such clinicians have areas of sporadic (or even consistent) non compliance with accepted basic standards of practice. An example would be a highly skilled orthopaedic surgeon who did not regard thrombo-embolism prophylaxis as necessary after a knee replacement, in spite of overwhelming evidence to the contrary. Addressing this type of problem will require healthcare to move away from authority-based idiosyncratic practice towards evidence-based standardized practice. Ideally this should be underpinned by regulation, as in other high risk industries.

Regulation

A key purpose of regulation is the abatement or control of risks to society. In the context of this book regulation can be considered to comprise the mechanisms or processes of clinical and corporate governance aimed at safeguarding and improving safety and quality. Traditionally, professionals have 'self-regulated'. However, a number of high-profile cases have clearly demonstrated instances of the abject failure of whatever self-regulatory processes were, or were thought to have been, in place[38,39] (See pages 37, 90, 173). Self-regulation is therefore perceived by many as inadequate (see Box 7.9).

Box 7.9 Perceived problems with self-regulation[40]

Health professionals may:

- demand and be given unreasonable levels of professional autonomy, and resist adherence to checklists and protocols;
- be reluctant to demonstrate accountability and resist monitoring of performance, practice and outcomes;
- discourage trainees, with varying degrees of subtlety, from seeking assistance after hours;
- lack transparency in their own practices, accept sub-optimal performance by colleagues, and fail to draw attention to inadequacies in the system and adverse events within their practices;
- lack patient-centredness and covertly or overtly impose their views, practices and plans on their patients; or
- routinely give inadequate information when obtaining consent and fail to disclose, when an adverse event occurs, that a problem was iatrogenic.

There is no doubt that it has been, and still is, possible to practise clinical medicine in an idiosyncratic manner and largely escape scrutiny or regulation. Medical investigation and treatment do have to be tailored to the needs, desires and co-morbidities of individual patients, but there appears to be an attitude, on the part of some at least, that adherence to standard evidence-based, system-wide protocols is never worthwhile or is even undesirable. Many hospitals, for their part, continue to allow huge variations in practice, fail to ensure adequate staffing and supervision after hours, and make do with poorly orientated part time locum or agency staff with little commitment to making the system work. Corporate violations are rife, and many waiting times ridiculous. The result is that many patients do not receive best practice care and things go wrong far too often.

We propose that one of the reasons for the pervasiveness of these problems lies in the piecemeal, ineffective regulation of healthcare. The term regulation, to many health professionals, evokes the image of enforcing a set of rules. However, this is just one end of the spectrum of regulation, the 'hard' end; regulation actually includes a range of strategies from 'soft' to 'hard' (see Figure 7.1).

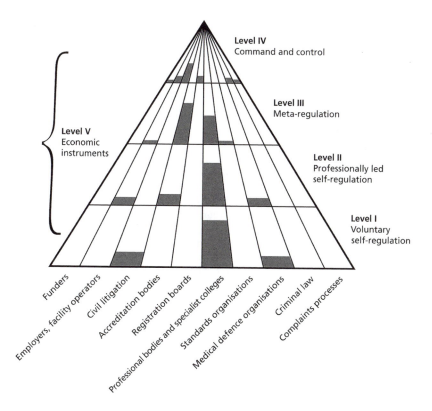

Figure 7.1 **The 'regulatory pyramid'** Shaded areas show the extent of involvement of various organizations[41]

The concept of *responsive regulation* implies the use of strategies appropriate to the situation and context, starting wherever possible, at the 'soft' end of the spectrum (the bottom of the pyramid in Figure 7.1). This approach tends to be more effective than beginning at the 'hard end', but it needs to be underpinned by a genuine prospect of meaningful sanctions for persistent non-compliance with the rules.[41]

There are at least ten types of organizations which play some regulatory role at one or more of the five levels of regulation within healthcare (see Figure 7.1). No one type of organization spans all five levels, and cross-communication between these organizations is generally sporadic or non existent. There are few clinical standards, and virtually no systematic checks on compliance with those standards that do exist. Even if persistent non-compliers were to be identified, a fundamental prerequisite for regulation is often missing, that of inexorable escalation of sanctions. A more detailed discussion of the sorts of activities that do and should take place at these various levels of regulation in healthcare will be provided in Chapter 11 (see pages 262–265).

Notes

1   Beauchamp, T.L. and Childress, J.F. (2001), *Principles of Biomedical Ethics*, 5th edition (New York: Oxford University Press).
2   Classical utilitarianism is based on three propositions: actions should be judged by their consequences; in assessing these consequences all that matters is the amount of happiness or unhappiness that is created; and each person's happiness is of equal value (i.e. one's own happiness is no more important than anyone else's). It is often referred to as the pursuit of the greatest happiness for the greatest number of people. Classical utilitarianism is sometimes called act-utilitarianism, because each individual act is judged on its merits. A more recent modification of the theory is called rule-utilitarianism. In this, one evaluates the consequence of the application of a rule (e.g. that one should never lie) universally rather than only in the context of an individual set of circumstances. More sophisticated versions of utilitarianism have been developed to refine the underlying principles to cope with particularly problematic moral issues.
3   Hursthouse, R. (1999), *On Virtue Ethics* (Oxford: Oxford University Press).
4   Aristotle related morality to character, judged in relation to virtues (in effect, good character traits). Virtues include things such as courage, honesty, generosity, truthfulness and compassion. Some virtues are associated with divine law, including faith, hope and charity. Modern virtue ethics is centred on character rather than actions.
5   Deos means duty; deontologists believe that ethics depends on identifying the right set of duties (or rules) to follow. Kant's hypothetical imperatives are illustrated by concepts such as: to loose weight, go on a diet. His categorical imperative is an absolute rule, such as never lie. The test of whether an imperative is categorical is to ask whether or not it can be made universal. Rules such as this underpin deontology. Unlike rule-utilitarians, deontologists approach the establishment of rules from perspectives other than consequentialism alone.
6   Hippocrates (400 BCE), 'The Oath', translated by Adams, F., available at: http://classics.mit.edu/Hippocrates/hippooath.html accessed 11 Jun 2006.

7   'The Nuremberg Code (1947)', in Mitscherlich, A. and Mielke, F. (1949), *Doctors of Infamy: the Story of the Nazi Medical Crimes* (New York: Henry Schuman) pp. xxiii-xxv.

8   *Declaration of Geneva (1948)*, adopted by the General Assembly of the World Medical Association, Geneva, Switzerland, September 1948.

9   Okie, S. (2005), 'Glimpses of Guantanamo – Medical Ethics and the War on Terror', *New England Journal of Medicine* 353:24, 2529–34.

10 World Medical Assembly, *Declaration of Helsinki (1964)*, adopted by the 18th World Medical Assembly, Helsinki, Finland, June 1964, amended by the 29th World Medical Assembly, Tokyo, Japan, October 1975 and the 35th World Medical Assembly, Venice, Italy, October 1983. See: World Medical Organization (1996), 'Declaration of Helsinki', *British Medical Journal* 313:7070, 1448–9.

11 World Medical Association, *World Medical Association Code of Medical Ethics,* adopted by the 3rd General Assembly of the World Medical Association, London, England, October 1949 and amended by the 22nd World Medical Assembly, Sydney, Australia, August 1968 and the 35th World Medical Assembly, Venice, Italy, October 1983. Available at: http://www.wma.net/e/policy/c8.htm accessed 11 Jun 2006.

12 American Medical Association, Council on Ethical and Judicial Affairs (2005), *Code of Medical Ethics – Current Opinions with Annotations, 2004–2005* (Chicago: American Medical Association) [web document], available at: http://www.ama-assn.org/ama/pub/category/2498.html accessed 11 Jun 2006.

13 American Nurses Association (2005), *Code of Ethics for Nurses with Interpretive Statements,* The Center for Ethics and Human Rights [web document]. Available at: http://nursingworld.org/ethics/code/protected_nwcoe303.htm accessed 11 Jun 2006.

14 Australian Health Minister Tony Abbott: Metherell, M. (2005), 'Doctors Need to Take Hard Look at Ethics', *Sydney Morning Herald* 30 May.

15 Pope John Paul II (2004), *Address of John Paul II to the Participants in the International Congress on 'Life-Sustaining Treatments and Vegetative State: Scientific Advances and Ethical Dilemmas'* 20 Mar. Available at: http://www.vatican.va/holy_father/john_paul_ii/speeches/2004/march/documents/hf_jpii_spe_20040320_congress-fiamc_en.html accessed 11 Jun 2006.

16 Van der Weyden, M.B. (2006), 'Preventing and Processing Research Misconduct: A New Australian Code for Responsible Research', *Medical Journal of Australia* 184:9, 430–1.

17 National Health and Medical Research Council, Australia (1999), *National Statement on Ethical Conduct in Research Involving Humans* (Canberra: Commonwealth of Australia) <http://www7.health.gov.au/nhmrc/publications/humans/contents.htm> accessed 11 Jun 2006.

18 Pellegrino, E.D. and Thomasma, D.C. (1993), *The Virtues in Medical Practice* (New York: Oxford University Press).

19 Kerridge, I., Lowe, M. and McPhee, J. (1998), *Ethics and Law for the Health Professions* (Katoomba, New South Wales: Social Science Press).

20 Berwick, D. et al. (1997), 'An Ethical Code for Everybody in Health Care', *British Medical Journal* 315:7123, 1633–4.

21 Smith, R., Hiatt, H. and Berwick, D. (1999), 'Shared Ethical Principles for Everybody in Health Care: a Working Draft from the Tavistock Group', *British Medical Journal* 318:7178, 248–51.

22 Stein, R. (2006), 'Proposals Pit Religious Values Against Patient Rights', *Washington Post* 2 Feb.

23 Stein, R. (2006), 'Health Workers' Choice Debated. Proposals Back Right Not To Treat', *Washington Post* 30 Jan, p.A01.

24 Porter, R. (2001), *Bodies Politic: Disease, Death and Doctors in Britain, 1650–1900* (London: Reaktion Books).

25 Porter, R. (1997), *The Greatest Benefit to Mankind: A Medical History of Humanity from Antiquity to the Present* (London: Harper Collins).

26 Knowles, J.H. (1965), *Hospitals, Doctors, and the Public Interest* (Cambridge, Massachusetts: Harvard University Press).

27 Collins, J. (1927), 'Should doctors tell the truth?', *Harper's Monthly Magazine* 155, 320–6.

28 Gawande, A. (1999), 'Whose Body is it, Anyway? What Doctors Should Do When Patients Make Bad Decisions', *The New Yorker* Oct 4, 84–91.

29 McIntyre, N. and Popper, K. (1983), 'The Critical Attitude in Medicine: the Need for a New Ethics', *British Medical Journal* 287:6409, 1919–23.

30 Wyatt, J. (1991), 'Use and Sources of Medical Knowledge', *Lancet* 338:8779, 1368–73.

31 Siminoff, L.A. and Fetting, J.H. (1991), 'Factors Affecting Treatment Decisions for a Life Threatening Illness: the Case of Medical Treatment of Breast Cancer', *Social Science and Medicine* 32:7, 813–8.

32 Roling, G.T. et al. (1977), 'An Appraisal of Patients' Reactions to "Informed Consent" for Peroral Endoscopy', *Gastrointestinal Endoscopy* 24:2, 69–70.

33 The Shipman 1 (2002), *First Report: Death Disguised* (London: The Stationery Office).

34 Hicks, L.K. et al. (2001), 'Understanding the Clinical Dilemmas That Shape Medical Students' Ethical Development: Questionnaire Survey and Focus Group Study', *British Medical Journal* 322:7288, 709–10.

35 Van der Weyden, M. (2004), 'The "Cam" Affair: an Isolated Incident or Destined to be Repeated?', *Medical Journal of Australia* 180:3, 100–1.

36 Bolsin, S.N. (1998), 'Professional Misconduct: The Bristol Case', *Medical Journal of Australia* 169:7, 369–72.

37 Van Der Weyden, M.B. (2005), 'The Bundaberg Hospital Scandal: The Need For Reform in Queensland and Beyond', *Medical Journal of Australia* 183:6, 284–5.

38 Faunce, T.A. and Bolsin, S.N. (2004), 'Three Australian Whistle-Blowing Sagas: Lessons for Internal and External Regulation', *Medical Journal of Australia* 181:1, 44–7.

39 Irvine, D. (2004), 'Health Service Reforms in the United Kingdom After Bristol', *Medical Journal of Australia* 181:1, 28–9.

40 Watterson, L., personal communication.

41 Adapted from Braithwaite, J., Healy, J. and Dwan, K. (2005), *The Governance of Health Safety and Quality* (Canberra: Commonwealth of Australia).

Chapter 8

When Things Go Wrong:
Looking After the People Involved

Background

The uncertainty of medicine and the poor design of the healthcare system create many opportunities for things to go wrong. Major disruptions to routine services are quite common. Harm to patients is frequent (see Chapter 2). Healthcare professionals have to manage the consequences of the unintended effects and inefficiencies of the system in which they work, even when they themselves may be amongst those inconvenienced or harmed.

The key to looking after the people involved when things go wrong is good communication. If patients and their families and friends are clearly and honestly informed about things that have gone wrong, and regularly updated on the plans to deal with these problems, it should be possible to maintain trust. The establishment of trust begins at the first contact with a patient. Trust depends on ongoing open and appropriate communication. Trust greatly enhances the ability of all concerned to manage the consequences of a serious adverse event, should one occur. For example, if the patient has been told that he or she has been colonized with an opportunistic organism, and warned that this may lead to further problems, it becomes much easier to discuss these problems (e.g. the development of an abscess or bacterial endocarditis) when they arise.

The consequences of an adverse event are analogous to those of a severe head injury. After a head injury, the damage caused by the initial event is known as the primary injury; this damage is added to by subsequent events (such as hypoxia and hypotension) which cause secondary injury. The primary injury is a *fait accompli*, but the extent of the secondary damage is, to a substantial extent, in the hands of the medical team. A major effort, therefore, should be directed towards minimizing the secondary harm. After an adverse event in healthcare, secondary factors can cause as much or more harm as the initial event. This secondary harm may be the result of poor communication, lack of empathy, or failure to provide support where it is needed. As with head injury, the extent of secondary damage is in the hands of the team.

Some members of the health care team may fear that complete honesty after an adverse event will increase the chances of litigation or complaint.[1] On the contrary, the value of open communication at the time that harm occurs in protecting against litigation is a recurring theme in the literature. For a patient, adequate timely disclosure can make all the difference to coming to terms with the consequences of a medical error. The desire for information, and frustration with not getting it, are commonly cited as reasons for litigation. There is no way of knowing when any particular patient will bring an action against a health professional, but it does seem that failure to provide information increases the chances that this will happen.[1] In Australia there is now a standard for 'open disclosure' after adverse events in healthcare.[2]

The Immediate Response

When an adverse event occurs in healthcare there must be an immediate response by the team (see Box 8.1). Early meetings will be needed between the affected patients (and their families and friends) and the professionals responsible for their care (see Box 8.2). After this, follow up will be necessary to provide for ongoing care of the people and for dealing with any issues arising from the event (see *respond, record, disclose* and *support* in Figure 1.5, and Boxes 8.1 and 8.4). For a comprehensive review on breaking bad news see Ptacek and colleagues.[3]

Box 8.1 The immediate response (see Figure 1.5)

- *Secure* the situation (*respond*):
  - make sure the patient is safe; and
  - make sure that no-one else is likely to be harmed.
- *Record* what happened, what was done, and what is to be done.
- *Plan*:
  - the initial contact with the patient and/or family and friends;
  - who will break the bad news and what they will say (*disclose*); and
  - the early meetings (who, when, where).
- *Support:*
  - the primary victim (the patient); and
  - the secondary victim (staff members involved).

Secure the Situation

The first step is to ensure that the patient is as safe as possible. This might entail transfer by an appropriate team to a tertiary facility. The next important step is to make sure that no-one else can be harmed. The possibility that there may be some fault in equipment, gas supply or drug batch must be considered. If the problem has occurred in an operating room or resuscitation room and there is any possibility that it has been caused by one of these problems, then the next case should be deferred, or undertaken in a new room, until the room in which the event occurred has been thoroughly checked. All equipment and drugs should be isolated for later examination if there is any chance that they may be implicated. Whatever the cause, if the adverse event has been serious it is very important not to proceed with the next case until the immediate aftermath of the problem has been dealt with. In particular, if staff have been traumatized by the event (which is likely), it is important that people are found to support them and that they are relieved from normal duties and freed up to deal with the immediate problems of the injured patient and then to look after their own welfare.

Record What Happened, What was Done and What is to be Done

Detailed documentation is essential, and should be undertaken immediately if possible. If many people arrive to assist with a crisis, it may be well worth allocating this task to one person. Documentation may be critical for the ongoing care of the patient; it will be of inestimable value in any subsequent analysis of root causes; and it will be of great service to the patient, the staff and the hospital in any downstream enquiries or proceedings.

Sometimes, especially in an evolving emergency, immediate documentation is not possible. In this case, it should be undertaken as early as possible. When done later it is important to document the time the note was made as well as the time and date of the event. Nothing should be deleted or removed from the record. Any alterations should be clear, dated and signed as such. If something comes to light to negate or alter a previous opinion, this should be indicated by way of a new note, appropriately timed and dated. Avoid gratuitous criticism of others.

Only facts should be recorded. Opinions may subsequently prove to be incorrect, and have considerable potential to be misleading and unhelpful. If it is felt essential for the ongoing management of the patient for an opinion to be recorded, then it needs to be clearly identified as such.[4]

Plan the Initial Contact with the Patient and/or Family and Friends

Planning should start at this stage. Breaking bad news is never easy; it can be done well, but without forethought and planning there is a high chance that it will be done badly. For some clinicians, because of the nature of their work, the need to break bad news will occur frequently, and experience will lead over time to a well-refined approach. For many, the situation will be as unfamiliar as it is unhappy. The settings will vary enormously, but the principles apply as much in a tertiary hospital as they do to a general practice, or a community based psychiatric service. Whatever the circumstances, planning is the key to minimizing the secondary harm that can so easily occur during this process.

A series of meetings will usually be needed. At this point, thought should be given to who should break the bad news and what exactly should be said and what should not be said. Planning is not a one-off event, but an ongoing process, and there will be time to consider the subsequent meetings later.

Who Should be Told First?

Depending on the circumstances, bad news may need to be given to several people. There is no doubt that the patient, if alive, has a right to know what has happened, but he or she may not be in a position to receive information, at least at the outset. He or she may be on a ventilator, brain damaged, dead or just very ill.

The others who need to know what has happened may or may not be related to the patient. Clinicians have long understood the need for a 'next of kin' or 'significant other' to be identified in the documentation of every patient, so it is usually not difficult to know where to start.

The Initial Contact

It is generally agreed that details of bad news should not usually be delivered over the telephone. If the initial contact has to be over the telephone, it should perhaps be made by a person not immediately involved in the incident, who can truthfully say that he or she does not have any first-hand details of the problem, but has been asked to telephone and ask the family to come into the hospital. This may allow more time for the medical situation to be stabilized and for those involved to plan. It may well be appropriate to reveal that things are bad, or even that the patient has not survived, especially if asked, but at least it will be possible to defer a detailed and prolonged discussion to a more appropriate time and setting, without compromising honesty or appearing to be unfeeling. It will often be a good idea to suggest that the contacted person should bring a friend or relative to provide support and perhaps deal with practical matters such as driving and finding parking. Ideally, arrangements should be made to meet at an easily found rendezvous, from which an escort can be provided to the intended place of meeting.

The First Meeting

The group of healthcare professionals attending the first meeting should be kept small so as not to intimidate those who are to be informed of what went wrong. On the other hand it is seldom wise for anyone to do this alone. At least one other person should be present to monitor and possibly moderate the proceedings, and to provide corroboration if there is any later dispute over what was said.

Bad news should be broken by a senior clinician who should introduce him or herself, and then start by foreshadowing that there will be bad news, and expressing regret and empathy. It is important that the initial news be kept simple and limited to facts. Opinions, if subsequently found to be erroneous, will be difficult to retract at a later stage.

These first meetings may have to be kept relatively short. Friends and relatives may need time to come to grips with the situation and may be unable to absorb detailed information at short notice. It should be indicated that there can be a series of meetings over several hours or days, so that it will be possible for all the necessary issues to be covered over this period.

After the bad news has been given, a more definitive meeting should be suggested and planned. The family should be asked to invite people they would like to attend that meeting. It may be necessary to set the time of the meeting after they have had the opportunity to contact key people and organize their own commitments.

Once it is clear who will attend, and when, more planning is needed. This is the time to decide who will lead the discussions at the second meeting and who will provide support for the clinician directly involved in the event.

The Subsequent Meetings

Ongoing planning is essential (Box 8.2). Flexibility may be needed to accommodate developing concerns, changes in the patient's condition, or the emergence of new information such as the results of tests.

Box 8.2 A checklist for planning meetings for handling bad news[3,4,5]

- Venue and timing.
- Who should be there?
- Conduct of the meetings:
  - communication;
  - trust;
  - empathy;
  - respect;
  - listening;
  - soliciting questions;
  - cultural sensitivity; and
  - recognizing and dealing with emotional responses.
- The agenda:
  - acknowledgement of the problem;
  - expression of regret – saying sorry;
  - a resume of events so far;
  - the rationale for the treatment/procedure/investigation;
  - what went wrong and what immediate steps were taken; and
  - what is planned
- Summary and invitation for questions.
- Identifying people and means for ongoing questions and support.
- Follow up – planning the next steps.

Venue and Timing

Meetings should be timed so that the most important people can get there. The room should be set up for the purpose. It should have comfortable furniture and be private. There should be no physical barriers (such as tables) between the people who are trying to communicate with each other. There should be a telephone to allow those being interviewed to make calls easily, and without any need to pay for them. The meeting should, as far as possible, be free from interruptions. Allow plenty of time. If some of those who attend have to keep their pagers or mobile telephones on, because of possible urgent calls, they should indicate this and apologize in advance for any interruptions. However it is much to be preferred that pagers and phones are managed by a person (such as a secretary or junior doctor) who is outside the meeting and can intervene only if a truly urgent situation arises. This is a good example of the need to place a very high priority on managing the aftermath of an adverse event. Subliminal messages can be very powerful.

Who Should be There?

The people invited by the patient or family might include friends, a trusted community or religious leader, a lawyer, or an independent doctor. In some cultures there may be a request for the senior clinician to address a large group of people (for example, the extended family), and in these circumstances it may be necessary to find a large room.

Conduct of the Meetings

The leader of the group representing the hospital staff should be pre-arranged. This should usually be the senior consultant involved in the event. If for some reason this is not possible or seems inadvisable, an experienced and senior colleague should take this role, and an explanation should be provided for this approach. Patients want to hear from the clinicians actually involved, so even if they are unable to lead the process, every effort should be made for them to take part.

The leader should start with introductions, shaking hands with the relevant people and (in most cultures) making eye contact. The introductions should indicate the roles of each member of the group.

The leader should then proceed to an update of the news. It is highly desirable to use patients' names. For example, he or she might say:

> 'I am afraid that I have to tell you that things have become more serious. John has taken a turn for the worse. We are trying to do everything to rectify the situation but the outlook is not good.'

Or the news might be:

> 'I am sorry to say that we do not have John's post-mortem results yet, so we can't tell you anything new, but we expect to hear something later today'.

Communication As always, communication is the key to the whole process. Where necessary, interpreters should be organized and used appropriately. The patient and/or family have to feel that their views are being taken seriously and that they have the ability to influence the course of events. They should get the opportunity to have input into decisions and they should be asked about their desires and wishes.[6] Good communication at this stage will be remembered with gratitude.

Box 8.3 An airway disaster

Charles Grieves was a 42 year old, long-term unemployed father of two young children. He was a heavy smoker and drinker, and had previously been admitted to hospital for asthma and respiratory tract infections during winter. He was brought into the emergency department by his wife at 11pm, acutely unwell, with an oxygen saturation on pulse oximetry of 87 per cent. He had resisted coming to hospital all day and was not happy about being there. As he was desaturating, confused and tachycardic, a medical emergency team (MET) was called who gave him oxygen by mask and transferred him immediately to the intensive care unit. The intensive care unit was staffed that night by a relatively junior doctor. The consultant had just gone home having been at the hospital all evening. The junior doctor was on the medical emergency team, and was also looking after the small intensive care unit. On arrival in intensive care, the patient was struggling, incoherent and progressively desaturating. The young doctor put a needle in a vein, gave some sedative, and tried to intubate the patient's trachea. The patient obstructed completely and the doctor was unable to place an endotracheal tube. He attempted to ventilate the lungs, using a bag and mask. The patient had a cardiac arrest and external cardiac massage was started.

An anaesthetist had been called as soon as the patient arrived in ICU, but only arrived ten minutes after the first attempt at intubation, because he had been in the operating theatre with a patient. He was also unable to place an endotracheal tube, but was successful in inserting a laryngeal mask. After 20 minutes of external cardiac massage and ventilation by mask the patient was eventually stabilized, and intubation achieved at this stage.

The anaesthetist had to go back to the operating room and the young doctor had two more MET calls in the next hour. In the chaos, the patient's relatives were not called. The patient's wife came in to the hospital at 8am to find her husband on a ventilator and unconscious. The consultant who had arrived for the day's work sat down with the wife and with the junior doctor and explained what had happened. He indicated the likelihood of a poor neurological outcome. He arranged for the family to come in after the ward round at midday to have a discussion. An extended family arrived. These people were initially very angry, particularly as the wife had not been called in the middle of the night. However, they were also aware that the hospital was short-staffed, and the wife told the rest of the group that the doctor had been very upset and had clearly had a bad night.

It was agreed to meet the following morning at 9 o'clock. At 5am the patient became hypertensive and brachycardic and his pupils became fixed and dilated. It was clear that there had been swelling of the brain which had resulted in brain death. The wife was called and told that the patient had taken a significant turn for the worse. It was agreed that the meeting would proceed as scheduled at 9 o'clock with the extended family. At this meeting the family was told the man had suffered brain death as a result of a prolonged arrest consequent on the failure to secure an airway. The consultant expressed profound regret and apologized, and offered to summon the junior doctor who had been involved (he had finished his stint of night-duty and was at home). The extended family attended when the ventilator was removed and subsequently, at midday, another meeting was held. At this the family thanked the medical and nursing staff for having done their best, indicated that they would be talking to their local politician about the inadequate staffing at the hospital, a well-known problem, and indicated that they would not be pursuing the hospital itself or any of the staff.

Poor communication will simply add to the pain of people who are already trying to deal with a terrible situation, and in addition can sow the seeds for subsequent complaints and even litigation. Important information and explanations should be repeated at least twice, on separate occasions, and feedback sought to determine that those concerned have understood what has been said. The words used must be appropriate to the listener. Jargon should be avoided. Medical terms, if used at all, should be explained. There should be pauses to make sure that everyone understands what is being said. Diagrams may be useful, and so may x-rays or other images. For example, showing a perfusion scan which demonstrates that there is no blood flow to the brain may be more convincing than simply saying that clinical tests are indicative of brain death.

Friends and relatives are a big help in this process. They can contribute to the discussion, ask questions which might otherwise not be asked, and assist with subsequent recall of what was said.

Trust The patient and/or family should be reassured that they will be kept informed and will be consulted before any important decisions are made. There must be explicit ongoing recognition of their autonomy (although they will almost invariably take most of the advice given to them). Ongoing respect for autonomy is extremely important because the patient has been harmed by a person and system in which he or she placed considerable trust, and on which he or she may now be dependent for on-going care. An invitation should be given for a second opinion to be obtained, if wanted. It should be emphasized that decisions are not set in stone, and that discussions can continue and plans can be revised on a daily or even hourly basis as events unfold.

Empathy It has been said that 'a physician need not fully share in a patient's hopes or fears to respect, learn about and respond to them'.[7] It is important to respond empathically to the emotional reactions of patients and their relatives. Empathizing has been described as 'making a connection with the patient and experiencing his or her emotions as an extension of your own, and communicating an understanding of his or her position and feelings'.[8]

Respect Appropriate respect should be displayed to the patient and the patient's family or friends by one's behaviour and choice of words. If there is a person of authority, such as a matriarch, patriarch, or community leader, this should be acknowledged by addressing him or her directly from time to time. Patients may have had unrealistic expectations and may easily misinterpret actions, words, or even body language. It must be remembered that they are in a strange environment and even if their views and conclusions seem quite disconnected from actual events, they should be listened to carefully, and not immediately contradicted. There will be plenty of time to clarify the situation.

Listening It is important to observe the patient or family members' emotions and, if unsure, ask about their feelings or thoughts. It is important to listen to what they say, even though the relevance of their comments to the particular situation at hand may not be immediately obvious.

Soliciting questions Questions should be invited, and it should be made clear early on that contact numbers will be provided at the end of the interview so that those present can seek reassurance or clarification at a later time or date about anything that may come to mind.

Cultural sensitivity As always, culturally sensitivity is essential. Behaviour which could possibly be construed as displaying bias, prejudice or discrimination must be avoided.[9] Impatience and intolerance should not be displayed by people co-ordinating visitors at the bedside, even when large groups of supporters or members of extended families are involved. Liaison officers and interpreters belonging to the appropriate ethnic group can provide invaluable advice as to issues which should be addressed and those which may be inappropriate. A strong argument can be made for special attention to be paid to the requirements of members of indigenous peoples. This is usually only an issue when such people are in a minority – when indigenous people are in a majority there is generally no argument.

New Zealand provides an interesting example of a country grappling with these challenges. In New Zealand, the rights of Maori are enshrined in law through the Treaty of Waitangi, the country's founding document. This emphasis does not diminish the rights of other cultural groups, but makes explicit the special situation of those for whom this country is their only ancestral home. It is not unreasonable to expect healthcare professionals to make an effort to learn something of the language and customs of minority groups of the area in which they work, precisely because these people are not foreign, even though they may not be dominant. By contrast, people from distant lands who are seldom seen in a particular country might have to be pragmatic and fit in with local customs (although, obviously, they still deserve to be treated with respect and understanding). In New Zealand few doctors speak Maori and almost all (if not all) Maori speak fluent English, but many healthcare workers have taken part in courses on the Treaty and on aspects of Maori culture, often held in traditional meeting houses (or marae). For example, most would know that the head is sacred to Maori (an issue for anaesthetists who must handle the heads of their patients), and that sitting on a patient's bed may give offence. More importantly they would also know that the extended family (called the whanau) is extremely important for many Maori. Autonomy of the individual is a European construct; for traditional Maori, decision making involves the wider family. Respect for the Maori language is paid in other ways; many meetings are opened with a brief address in Maori, and the Maori language, as one of the two official languages of New Zealand, is incorporated into many official documents and on many signs in hospitals (and other public places).

No doubt these measures fall short of what could be done, but they illustrate some of the possibilities. Ideally one would involve Maori healthcare workers in every aspect of the care of Maori patients, and certainly in dealing with the aftermath of an adverse event. In practice Maori are seriously under-represented in the healthcare workforce. Hospitals in New Zealand have therefore appointed Maori liaison staff to fill this gap, at least for circumstances in which the needs for direct involvement in the team by Maori are greatest. The University of Auckland has an active policy of promoting the training of Maori doctors. The Ministry of Health has an official mandate to address inequities in healthcare outcomes with specific reference to Maori. It is not our brief to enter the complex discussion of the pros and cons of affirmative action, but rather to illustrate the complexity of the issues surrounding indigenous populations in healthcare, and the extent to which these issues pervade the layers of healthcare illustrated in Figure 1.1.

Respect for indigenous people is not just a matter of courtesy. On all healthcare measures, minority indigenous people fare worse than the rest of the population in the USA, Canada, Australia and New Zealand (at least). Part of this problem is alienation, which leads to less utilization of healthcare services even when access is not difficult for other reasons. Respect is a very important part of overcoming this barrier to the provision of high quality healthcare to people whose need for it is considerable. Respect paid at a time of emotional pain, after an adverse event, is particularly important. Failure to do this may well compound the secondary damage arising from the aftermath of an adverse event, and lead to withdrawal of a patient or indeed an entire extended family from future participation in the healthcare system.

Recognizing and dealing with emotional responses The normal range of responses to bad news include silence, disbelief, denial, tearfulness and anger. It is often worth acknowledging these responses and pointing out that they are normal, and that there may be feelings of guilt or of anger towards other family members or towards health care professionals. It is most important to remain calm and not respond to angry or insulting behaviour on the part of relatives. Responding in kind is likely to escalate the tension and can even lead to violence. This is not the time for 'zero tolerance'.

The Agenda

It is worth preparing a formal agenda for these meetings, even if this is not explicitly tabled. Some flexibility may be needed in covering the items on the agenda, particularly in relation to order, but a prepared agenda makes it more likely that all the important points will be dealt with.

Acknowledgement of the problem After the introductions it is important that the spokesperson again acknowledge the fact that there has been a problem and briefly outline the nature of the problem.

Expression of regret – saying sorry The acknowledgement of the problem should be followed by an expression of regret. Saying sorry does not imply liability, and is important for those involved to demonstrate their concern and show empathy.

A resume of events so far It is useful to indicate to everyone present that one is going to go back over old ground and summarize how the patient came to be in hospital, and what their main problems were then.

The rationale for the treatment/procedure/investigation The rationale for the treatment, procedure or investigation which preceded or led to the adverse event should be revisited in some detail, because it is common for those involved to ask: 'What if an alternative course of action had been taken?' or 'What if we had insisted that someone be called earlier?' The better the communication before the event, the easier this part of the discussion will be now.

What went wrong and what immediate steps were taken Some explanation will have been given at the first meeting of what went wrong. More detail can be provided now, sticking to the facts and not offering opinions. The steps taken to deal with the problem should be explained. For example, if the patient's trachea has been intubated and ventilation of the lungs begun, the reasons for this should be outlined and the relatives forewarned about the tubes, monitors and machines implicit in this form of therapy. They should be told if the patient has been sedated.

What is planned A brief outline should be given of plans for the remainder of that day or night and for what is anticipated in the ensuing days. At this stage it is worthwhile setting up the next meeting or series of meetings. It may be convenient, for example, to set a meeting for each day after the ward round, when the results of any tests or consultations will be available and the day's plans can be discussed. It should be emphasized again that major steps will not be taken without consultation.

Summary and Invitation for Questions

At the end of each meeting a brief summary should be given, and those present should again be invited to ask questions. They should be reminded that they probably will not have taken in all the information and will need to come back for clarification.

Identifying People and Means for Ongoing Questions and Support

It is a good idea for the person leading the discussion to provide the family with his or her mobile phone or pager number and invite anyone to make contact at any stage. In our experience this is very rarely abused. A great deal of reassurance and support can be given with simple answers to questions about concerns which may otherwise cause protracted and unnecessary worry. It is a good idea to nominate a single person on the medical team to handle all questions, and to counsel the family against seeking opinions from many different staff members. This approach leads to mixed messages, with some people trying to be optimistic and cheer the family up, and others giving conservative responses which may be found depressing. It may also be appropriate to ask the family, if large, to nominate a representative to facilitate communication. Help with logistical matters (see below) should be arranged, by way of a social worker or patient advocate, for example.

Following Up – Planning the Next Steps

Having set up a process of regular meetings, it is essential to retain a strong focus on ongoing communication as events unfold. An extra phone call from a senior specialist at a critical time can make all the difference to conveying a sense of personal attention and care.

Box 8.4 Following up – people and issues

- The patient and their family and/or friends.
- The staff and their family and/or friends.
- The unit/hospital/facility – administrative matters.
- Publicity and the media.
- Handling complaints and litigation.
- Taking steps to prevent a recurrence – the safety and quality agenda.

The Patient and their Family and/or Friends

It is often useful to appoint a senior nurse or social worker to co-ordinate day-to-day logistics, in addition to the person nominated for communication. It may be appropriate to provide accommodation in or near the hospital. Consideration should be given to matters such as transport and car-parking, out-of-pocket expenses, and letters or certificates to employers or officials in relation to welfare or other forms of support.

For certain problems, such as awareness under anaesthesia, it may be appropriate to involve a psychologist or psychiatrist. The anaesthetist should consider personally introducing this specialist to the patient; an introduction of this type is likely to convey a strong sense of professionalism and concern on the anaesthetist's part.[4]

If a breadwinner has been harmed, immediate financial help may be required. If disability is likely to be ongoing, facilities to cope with this may be needed. Alterations to the home, the car or the workplace may make an enormous difference to a patient. Additional nursing in the home, or respite care, can also facilitate progress. Early involvement of a social worker and relevant organizations should be arranged (see Box 8.6).

Box 8.5 A torrential, fatal bleed

Samantha O'Brien was a 17 year old girl who had been the front seat passenger of a car which had run into a trailer parked, without lights, on the side of a country road. The driver was unharmed, but she suffered extensive leg and pelvic injuries. She went on to get severe lung problems ('adult respiratory distress syndrome') as a consequence of her serious injuries and blood loss, and was, for two weeks, ventilated on 100 per cent oxygen. She suffered a number of complications along the way, including septicaemia from a central venous line infection. During her six weeks in intensive care her family spent most of the time at her bedside and was exceptionally worried and engaged in her progress. There was excellent communication on a daily basis between members of the staff and the family, which was well liked by all the staff.

After six weeks, it was indicated that Samantha was being weaned off the ventilator and it was planned on the Monday morning to remove her tracheostomy tube. She was spending time in the courtyard out in the sunshine. In the early hours of Saturday morning her tracheostomy tube became dislodged. The registrar in the intensive care unit decided to replace it so as to follow through the plan to remove the tube on the Monday morning. He sedated Samantha and inserted a new tube.

However, there was considerable scar tissue around the tracheostomy site and in doing so he ruptured a major artery which had become involved in the scar tissue. Samantha suffered a torrential bleed and in spite of senior surgical and medical staff being summoned immediately, and all possible steps taken to try to resuscitate her, she died on the way to the cardio-thoracic operating theatre. The family arrived very soon thereafter. The senior intensive care specialist and cardiac surgeon who had been summoned broke the bad news. Everyone was devastated and support mechanisms were put into place for the doctor who had tried to change the tube. The father, although shattered by the event, attended part of a debriefing meeting to express, on behalf of the family, his support to the staff involved and thanks for their care.. Debriefing was required for that nightshift on the intensive care unit as well for the two subsequent dayshifts.

Medico-legal matters If the family wishes to make a complaint or consider litigation then they should be given advice on how to go about this. In some countries (e.g. New Zealand) the provision of such advice is a legal requirement. Protracted, adversarial medico-legal proceedings can be very damaging to all concerned, not least those laying the complaints. Being helpful, avoiding any appearance of defensiveness and facilitating access to high quality advice may reduce hostility and mitigate the inevitable unpleasantness of legal proceedings if these do eventuate. There are many creative ways of helping families work through difficult positions (see Box 8.6) and non-adversarial options are much more likely to be chosen in a supportive atmosphere than in a defensive one.

Box 8.6 A creative response to a catastrophe

Mrs. Young, a 69 year old patient with Type 2 diabetes, who was overweight and hypertensive, was admitted with a urinary tract infection. Overnight she became confused and started trying to climb out of bed. The bedrails were raised. At 5 o'clock in the morning she was found lying on the floor. With the assistance of the family and several nurses she was placed back into the bed. At 8 o'clock in the morning she suffered a respiratory arrest and the arrest team was called. The anaesthetist on the team noted that Mrs Young did not move when her trachea was intubated with no sedation.

She was transferred, intubated and ventilated, to a tertiary referral hospital. The suspicion of quadriplegia was confirmed. This was a catastrophic situation and had medico-legal proceedings been drawn out it is quite likely that she would have died before they were completed. The tort would have died with her. However, the insurers for the State Government established from the family that her burning desire was to spend the rest of her days with close access to her four grandchildren.

Her house was modified, all the relatives received training, and she survived eight years as a quadriplegic being nursed by the family with some assistance from district nurses. The family expressed their appreciation for the prompt and appropriate measures taken to ameliorate the disaster.

Out-of-pocket expenses directly related to an adverse event should certainly be met (see below). Fees for taking care of the immediate medical sequelae when a patient has been harmed should be discussed early. The principle should be to waive those fees related to erroneous procedures or to the costs of dealing with the immediate aftermath of the erroneous event where the error is obvious and the needs are apparent. Under these circumstances it is appropriate from every perspective for the patient to be promptly and explicitly relieved of this worry. Unfortunately, there may often be some lack of clarity over what it will or will not be appropriate to cover. For example, after cardiac surgery a variable period of time in intensive care is normal, and this might be expected to be prolonged in a proportion of high risk cases. It may not be reasonable to waive the entire cost of this care simply because of some minor technical problem in a complicated operation, particularly if the patient has been warned of this risk. Conversely there will be cases in which the fact that an error has caused the need for additional care is obvious – as in Jessica Santillan's case, for example, in which incompatible organs were implanted (see Box 1.1). In either situation, early discussion based on a clear statement that expenses will be waived to the extent reasonable will go a long way towards alleviating concern and resentment.

For minor problems (although the patient may not regard them as minor), arrangements should be made for the harm to be assessed and an offer to meet all reasonable expenses should be made by the healthcare facility. Dental damage, for example, makes up 30 per cent of all claims related to anaesthesia, but only 1 per cent of the cost.[10]

Discussion over the extent of liability for major long term consequences, such as paraplegia, should of course be deferred, and most patients would understand that this is a matter which cannot reasonably be settled without proper legal process.

The Staff and their Family and/or Friends It goes without saying that the healthcare professionals involved in any adverse event should consult their indemnity organizations at the earliest opportunity (even in the middle of the night), and keep them informed of all developments. Many of the lawyers working for these organizations have become very well informed on the merits of treating injured patients honestly and appropriately, and may even assist in this process, perhaps with advice behind the scenes.

Having done that, it is highly desirable for a reasonably senior person to arrange for the person/s involved to be rostered off clinical duties – partly to allow them to arrange the necessary interviews and handle the paperwork, but also, importantly, to allow them time to reflect and to come to grips with what has happened. They should be offered some immediate support. When a patient has been harmed the experience for the healthcare professional/s is a traumatic one, with the vast majority suffering profound feelings of guilt and remorse. Support is needed in talking to the patient and/or relatives, as the long standing culture has been not to reveal errors to colleagues or to those harmed.[11-13] A suitable sympathetic colleague should be identified to seek out the person/s involved and offer a kind word and emotional and logistical support. It may not be a good idea to give the person time off work, because this can be interpreted as a loss of trust, but efforts should certainly be made, discreetly if need be, to ensure that the person works in a supportive environment.

Each case should be treated on its own merits, but it is important to realize that healthcare professionals, understandably, do not cope very well with problems of this nature, and often go on to be quite profoundly disturbed for a long period of time – sometimes for the rest of their lives. Moreover, they will often not spontaneously talk the matter through with either a colleague or a family member.[11-13] It is well worth seeking the person out to see how things are going and have a chat over a cup or coffee, or a drink after work. If appropriate, a consultation with a suitably qualified psychologist or psychiatrist of the person's choice can be suggested.

If litigation follows, then the staff member will be exposed to a prolonged experience that can become very unpleasant. Again, a real effort should be made to offer ongoing support.[11,12]

The unit/hospital/facility – administrative matters There is increasing recognition of the importance of a coordinated, well-organized and consistent response to the patient and family after an adverse event, which should come from the unit or healthcare facility as a whole. The tendency in the past to let a single health professional sort the matter out, with only his or her medical defence organization to help, has been associated with feelings of abandonment and betrayal of trust on the part of patients and families. Any healthcare institution should have protocols established and in regular use to ensure that bad news is broken appropriately. The protocols should cover:

- expressions of regret;
- an apology;
- the immediate steps needed to look after and support the patient and family;
- the avenues to be made available to answer any questions;
- the arrangements for meeting out of pocket expenses such as accommodation and transport;
- the arrangements for compensation for minor problems;
- the provision of information in relation to the patient's right to complain, and about the appropriate first steps if he or she wishes to bring a legal action against the staff or institution (see below);
- the relevant people to deal with the initial legal processes over major problems;
- the arrangements for relieving affected staff from their immediate clinical responsibilities;
- the arrangements for providing support to the affected staff;
- the incident forms, mortality reports and other paper work to be completed while things are fresh in everyone's minds;
- procedures to follow if a patient has died (contacting the coroner, leaving catheters, tubes and equipment in place etc); and
- channels of communication (statements provided for the media, if they inquire, or for authorities such as the coroner should always be checked carefully for completeness and accuracy by a nominated senior clinician and the facility's press liaison officer).

In some healthcare facilities, senior clinicians have undertaken training in communication and human factors. These people's role in helping with the planning and conduct of processes following an adverse event should be embedded into the protocol.

Proper processes for handling the aftermath of harm to patients is an essential part of institutional risk management, and in many hospitals, risk management staff take a pro-active, coordinating role. Investment in these processes will save cost by limiting secondary harm to patients and family, reducing harm to staff, facilitating equitable and efficient medico-legal consequences, and protecting the reputations of the institution and its employees. It follows that clinicians involved in any significant adverse event should be required to inform the hospital administration through their line managers as early as possible, so that these processes can be activated in good time.

Publicity and the media As in the case of Jessica Santillan (Box 1.1), an adverse event may generate major interest from the media. A great deal of skill is required in interacting with the media, and much may be at stake for all concerned. Larger institutions often employ specialist staff to deal with the media. If such a staff member is not available, it may be wise to seek advice from another institution or a consultant in the field.

Handling complaints and litigation If the patient and family and/or friends wish to make a complaint they should be directed towards the person who normally handles such matters; all organizations have formal complaint handling mechanisms. This person may be able to provide advice on issues such as which legal firms are experienced and proficient in handling medico-legal matters. In the UK there is an organization called Action against Medical Accidents (AvMA) which provides support and advice to those who have suffered or been affected by iatrogenic harm (see page 87).[14]

Taking steps to prevent a recurrence – the safety and quality agenda People who have been harmed, and their friends and relatives, are often particularly concerned that a similar thing should not be allowed to happen again. The facts that the matter is to be subjected to a thorough investigation, that the findings and recommendations will be entered into a database, and that steps will be taken to try to prevent such a thing from happening again should be made known to the patient and families or friends early on. In the event of an enquiry or root cause analysis (see Chapter 9), it should be indicated that the key findings and recommendations will be passed on to the patient, family and friends.

Summary

When a serious adverse event has occurred, it should not be 'business as usual'. Once the primary harm has been dealt with, colleagues and line managers must immediately swing into action to prevent secondary damage both to those harmed, and to those involved in the incident and care of the patient. It may be necessary to defer routine work. Extra staff may be needed to help with looking after the patient and family, to support staff who may have been traumatized by the event, and to assist with the follow-up, documentation, notification of relevant people, and other administrative matters. Ongoing communication with the patient and/or family is of the utmost importance. They must be assured that the causes of the event will be investigated, and that changes will be introduced to prevent a similar thing from happening again.

Notes

1   Vincent, C., Stanhope, N. and Crowley-Murphy, M. (1999), 'Reasons for Not Reporting Adverse Incidents: an Empirical Study', *Journal of Evaluation in Clinical Practice* 5:1, 13–21.

2   Australian Council for Safety and Quality in Health Care (2003), *Open Disclosure Standard: a National Standard for Open Communication in Public and Private Hospitals, Following an Adverse Event in Health Care* (Canberra: Commonwealth Department of Health and Ageing).

3   Ptacek, J.T. and Eberhardt, T.L. (1996), 'Breaking Bad News: a Review of the Literature', *Journal of the American Medical Association* 276:6, 496–502.

4   Bacon, A.K. et al. (2005), 'Crisis Management During Anaesthesia: Recovering From a Crisis', *Quality and Safety in Health Care* 14:3, e25.

5   Baile, W.F. et al. (2000), 'SPIKES – A Six-Step Protocol for Delivering Bad News: Application to the Patient With Cancer', *The Oncologist* 5:4, 302–11.

6   Baylis, F. (1997), 'Errors in Medicine: Nurturing Truthfulness', *Journal of Clinical Ethics* 8:4, 336–40.

7   Back, A.L. et al. (2003), 'Teaching Communication Skills to Medical Oncology Fellows', *Journal of Clinical Oncology* 21:12, 2433–6.

8   Dias, L. et al. (2003), 'Breaking Bad News: a Patient's Perspective', *The Oncologist* 8:6, 587–96.

9   Genao, I. et al. (2003), 'Building the Case for Cultural Competence', *American Journal of Medical Sciences* 326:3, 136–40.

10 Runciman, W.B. (2005), 'Iatrogenic Harm and Anaesthesia in Australia', *Anaesthesia and Intensive Care* 33:3, 297–300.

Chapter 9

When Things Go Wrong: Preventing a Recurrence

In Chapter 8 we outlined how to take care of patients and staff when something has gone wrong. In this chapter we turn our attention to managing the event and preventing the same thing from happening again. The frameworks for risk management and the continuous improvement of quality in healthcare shown in Figures 1.5 and 2.1 provide a sound basis for this undertaking, and are followed in this chapter.

In the section on identifying the risks in healthcare we have used the Advanced Incident Management System (AIMS)[1] as a template. This system was developed in Australia and provides a comprehensive approach to the reporting of incidents and the tracking of the processes which follow, and is consistent with the frameworks shown in Figures 1.5 and 1.6.[2]

In the section on evaluating, analyzing and treating the risks in healthcare we have used the structured approach to Root Cause Analysis (RCA) developed by James Bagian as our template.[3,4,5] This approach is used by The Veterans Administration (VA) National Center for Patient Safety (NCPS), for the investigation of serious adverse events, and has been adapted for use, nationwide in several countries including Denmark and Australia. There are other systems for reporting, tracking and analyzing incidents and adverse events.[6,7,8] We chose AIMS and the VA system as examples because they both recognize and accommodate the multiplicity of factors that contribute to or cause things that go wrong in healthcare, and both try to systematically identify and address inadequacies in the system.

The story of the awake paralysis of Mrs. Jones, described in Box 4.6 on page 103, is used to illustrate many of the points made in this chapter, and should be reviewed now.

A Systems Approach (see 'Understand the Context', Figure 2.1)

The orientation in AIMS and the VA approach is towards the system, not the person. The theory underlying both is based on the model of organizational accidents outlined in Chapter 5, and assumes that underlying most iatrogenic harm is the failure of one or more (usually several) links in a chain of contributory factors or root causes (see Figure 5.2).[9] A fundamental principle underpinning the collection of information about incidents and for RCA is that the contributing factors, or root causes, of things that go wrong are often to be found in parts of the system far removed from the scene of the event.[5] It follows that a failure to identify and address these root causes will leave the scene set for a recurrence of similar events.

Box 9.1 Awake paralysis – again and again and again

The case of Mrs. Jones was described in Box 4.6, in which she was inadvertently paralyzed whilst awake and waiting for an operation.[10] The anaesthetist was, in effect, found to have been negligent, although it was not deemed necessary to refer the matter to any disciplinary or regulatory authority. Changes in practice proposed by the anaesthetist included the use of different sized syringes, taking care not to carry muscle relaxants out of the operating room, and reading labels out loud when administering drugs. These were deemed adequate responses to the problem on his part. The systemic response was to disseminate the report produced by the Health Disability Commissioner (HDC) for educational purposes.

However, during the three years between the incident and the final report, within the same city, at least three more drug errors were made by anaesthetists in which a muscle relaxant was given instead of another drug, with the result that three more patients were subjected to the experience of awake paralysis, an experience described by the HDC's adviser as 'extremely harrowing'. In one case the patient was left unattended and might well have died had the nurse in the adjacent recovery area not noticed his distress and provided emergency artificial ventilation.

The AIMS database records several errors leading to awake paralysis of patients every year.[11] We now know that the medical defence organizations in Australia have been made aware of more than ten such cases each year,[12] but their usual practice is not to disseminate this information. It seems reasonable to assume that these are genuine errors – anaesthetists do not usually set out to give their patients harrowing experiences. Therefore it would seem appropriate to examine the circumstances under which they occur and to take steps to error-proof the system, rather than focus on the alleged failings of each successive practitioner in falling into the same trap as his or her predecessors, and expose yet more patients to the same problem.

If several essentially identical adverse events occur within a reasonably short time, this is strongly suggestive that something more than simple negligence is at play (see Box 9.1). The possibility of one doctor being particularly error-prone is plausible, but if the same error is also being made by other doctors, then it is likely that factors within the system are creating circumstances in which that particular error is likely to occur. Further recurrences will only be prevented if weaknesses at all levels are identified and addressed. Ideally this should be done the first time a serious event occurs; however the healthcare system has typically been slow in introducing systemic changes, even to well documented problems. At the time of Mrs. Jones's event there was substantial empirical evidence (including locally relevant evidence[13]) in the peer-reviewed literature to show that drug administration error is an endemic problem in anaesthesia, as it is in healthcare generally.[11,14] There was every reason in this case both to suspect that factors within the system had contributed to the problem and to initiate a root cause analysis to identify them.

Reporting When Things Go Wrong (see 'Identifying the Risks', Figure 2.1)

Comprehensive documentation in the medical record is essential after any adverse event in healthcare, but this does not in itself reduce the risk of that event recurring. If safety is to be improved, incidents need to be reported, the reports analyzed, and appropriate changes identified and implemented (see Figure 1.5). Aggregation of data collected as a routine whenever adverse events (or near misses) occur will provide an indication of what is going wrong at any particular time in any particular institution. This information is the starting point for improving the system. These data can be used to monitor progress over time and to identify new and unexpected problems which may arise out of change.[1] It is also possible to make some comparisons between units or practices on the basis of data of this type. Of course, incident reporting does not include a numerator or denominator, and this limitation must be understood. Nevertheless, practical information can be obtained that can inform and energize the process of quality improvement in healthcare. Incident reporting supplements and complements the collection of more traditional, denominator-based indices of performance, and often surpasses these methods in its potential to promote improvements in safety. It is particularly suited to characterizing the low frequency events which make up most of the things that go wrong in healthcare.[1,15]

Every healthcare organization should have an ongoing system for incident reporting and for acting on the data collected in this way. Data from other sources should also be collected and aggregated (see Table 2.5). Where possible, many institutions should pool data to develop databases large enough to permit meaningful analysis of information about uncommon events. We believe that the facility should also exist for healthcare professionals to submit reports anonymously for inclusion in a database controlled by the professional body responsible for their area of practice, such as a specialist college. This will bring together information specific to each discipline from a far greater number of reports than would be provided within any single institution. For example, the AIMS-Anaesthesia collection in Australia now has well over 10,000 anonymous incident reports from which over 120 peer-reviewed articles have been published.[16] Many safety initiatives have been carried out by the College of Anaesthetists in response to well over 100 recommendations arising from these publications.[17] The development of the International Standards for a Safe Practice of Anaesthesia[18] was heavily influenced by information from this data-base[19,20] and there is strong inferential evidence that there has been a major impact on patient safety.[21]

Ideally, all incidents should be reported. Incidents include adverse events (incidents in which a patient was harmed), near misses (incidents in which there was a potential for a bad outcome, but a bad outcome did not actually occur) and sentinel events (serious adverse events which should never be allowed to happen) (see Appendix I). Hospitals which receive public funding in Australia and America are required to report sentinel events. A list of these is provided on page 49.

Anonymity

In order to obtain as much information about as many events as possible, provision for anonymous reports should be part of any comprehensive incident reporting system. Anonymity allows information to be collected which otherwise would not become available. Anonymous reports should supplement other mechanisms for collecting or recording information, and should not replace or compromise them.[22] Personal identification (PIN) numbers can be used to provide feedback on aggregated data to individuals while retaining their anonymity.

However, in the vast majority of cases, the individuals involved are happy to provide details of their identity and of the local circumstances relevant to the incident. There are occasions when specific information of this type is very useful in improving the system. For example, it should be possible to identify a faulty piece of equipment simply, quickly and directly, so that it can be repaired or replaced as soon as possible. A report that says Dr Smith had a problem with an infusion pump in theatre 2 on Wednesday carries more weight than one which has been de-identified to the point that the person place and time cannot be identified. It also facilitates the process of going back to Dr Smith for more details. This type of information should be collected in parallel with the anonymously collected data. In the UK, local reports have identifiers, but the information sent to the central database at the National Patient Safety Agency is de-identified.[6]

Notifying and Capturing Basic Information

After an adverse event, once the patient has been made secure and the medical record completed (see Figure 1.5 and page 181), it is important to report the basic facts and notify the relevant people (see Box 9.3), so that the event can be followed up. This should be a formal requirement within any organization, and is called 'notification'. Ideally notification will be to a line manager or a designated patient safety or risk management officer, but this may vary according to the institution and the setting. For example, in a community-based practice the people to notify may be quite different from those in a hospital. Ideally, one step should be all that is required of the clinical staff and triage should occur before senior line managers are informed (see below).

In some jurisdictions, all reporting is now directly to a call centre staffed by operators with access to and training in AIMS.[23] This facilitates many aspects of the process, notably standardization of data collection, which allows the generation of reliable summary reports from aggregated data.

Box 9.2 Basic information

- What happened.
- Who was involved.
- When did it happen.
- Where did it happen.
- The severity of the actual or potential harm.
- The likelihood of recurrence.
- The consequences.

Triage – The Link between Incident Reporting and Action

In a properly set up system, large numbers of incident reports will be generated every week.[24] The resources required for an in-depth analysis of any incident should be aimed at addressing the most serious risks faced by an organization. Therefore it is essential to conduct some form of triage to separate those incidents which warrant such analysis from those which can be dealt with more simply.

A trained patient safety officer should examine the notification report and determine the actual or potential severity of the incident, and its likelihood of recurrence. On this basis a severity assessment code (SAC) should be allocated (see Appendix VII). The SAC is used to determine who should be notified (Box 9.3), whether more detailed information should be obtained, and whether a root cause analysis should be done.

Follow-Up

Once notified, the people listed in Box 9.3 should take whatever steps are deemed necessary. For many incidents, this will be all that is required. Some reporting systems have space on the notification form (electronic or paper) for documenting the steps to be taken, and for documenting when these have been taken (see Figure 9.1). For example, if a patient has suffered a rare reaction to a drug used for the right indication and given in the right way, the only practical step that can be taken locally to promote safety may be notification, via the institution's pharmacy, to the national adverse drug reaction reporting body. Likewise, if an infusion pump ceased to function, all that has to happen is for it to be replaced or repaired. However, if someone was harmed, if there was potential for serious harm, or if the incident was thought to be particularly instructive, then it may be appropriate to obtain further information and undertake a more detailed analysis of the event with a view to identifying actions to improve safety.

Box 9.3   Examples of people who may be sent a copy of the notification after a severity assessment code (SAC) has been allocated to an incident

- The line manager and/or head of department.
- The risk manager and/or medical defence organization if litigation is a possibility.
- The patient advocate or adviser for a potential complaint.
- The pharmacy and/or national drug reporting body for a medication incident.
- A biomedical engineer and/or national devices reporting body for a problem with a device or equipment.
- Building and engineering services for an infrastructure problem.
- The infection control team for an infection control problem.
- The occupational health and safety claims manager if a staff member has been harmed or put at serious risk.
- The hospital insurer if a visitor or a contractor has been harmed or there is damage or loss to plant or equipment.
- The media liaison officer if adverse publicity is possible.
- The police if an absconder could harm him or herself, or anyone else, or if it is thought that a criminal offence has been committed.

Confidentiality and Statutory Immunity

If further information is to be gathered, there are great advantages in doing this under conditions of strict confidentiality or statutory immunity. Under these conditions, those supplying information are less likely to be inhibited by fear of adverse consequences within the workplace, through the media, or in the courts. This means that more detailed, varied and potentially useful information can be obtained than a simple outline of the basic facts. In particular, opinions as well as facts can be sought and obtained. Opinions will of course need to be identified as such and evaluated on their merits, but may at times provide exceedingly useful leads to the initiatives needed to solve a difficult problem. It is also vitally important that unsubstantiated opinion does not become the source of slander, particularly in hospitals where the wide dissemination of often grossly inaccurate and potentially damaging gossip is usually the rule rather than the exception. Even facts are best kept confidential until a proper understanding has been developed of how or whether they contributed to a complicated event.

The provisions for statutory immunity in countries that have them generally apply only to information collected solely for the purposes of improving quality and safety. It is very important to understand the locally applicable arrangements, and follow them meticulously, if immunity is to be safeguarded. In general, separate processes are needed if information is required for any other purpose. The protection applies only to the information gathered in such an investigation,

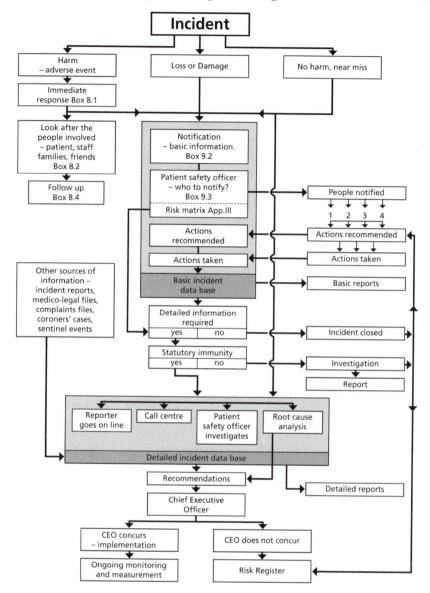

Figure 9.1 A flow diagram of actions that may be taken after an incident

and does not in any way limit the potential for a parallel process to inquire into any alleged malfeasance.

It is necessary to determine whether it is likely there has been any inappropriate or unacceptable behaviour on the part of anyone involved before starting an investigation under the protection of statutory immunity. If it is likely, then a separate investigation for the purposes of discipline or performance management may need to be instigated, with due regard for the legal rights of all involved. The patient and relatives should be informed that such an investigation is underway. If there has been no inappropriate behaviour, as is usually the case, the more desirable process of gathering further information and opinions in a confidential manner can begin.

A good example of how to do this preliminary triage is provided by the process developed and used successfully by the VA in the USA,[3] which has now been adopted Australia-wide. Four questions are asked. An affirmative answer to any question will shift the focus from a protected investigation to one in which the information collected may be used against the individual whose behaviour is suspect. The questions are:

- Was the problem the result of a deliberately unsafe act?
- Was the problem the result of a criminal act?
- Was patient abuse of any kind involved?
- Were any staff involved impaired by drug or alcohol use?

Arrangements vary greatly between countries. In the United Kingdom, for example, there is no provision for statutory immunity. The practice has been for the employee to be suspended from duty pending investigation in most (80 per cent) serious patient safety incidents. An audit into this process concluded that this suspension was nearly always inappropriate and that more effective handling of the proceedings would save the NHS £14 million per year.[25] To improve this process an 'incident decision tree' based on Reason's 'culpability tree' was developed to provide guidance on whether suspension should be considered. This tree involves a series of structured questions about the individual's actions, motives and behaviour at the time of the incident.[26] The questions cover four tests in sequence. These are:

- Deliberate harm test.
- Incapacity test.
- Foresight test.
- Substitution test..

The first two overlap with the VA questions listed above. The foresight test examines whether protocols were available, were reasonable, and were adhered to. The substitution test assesses how a peer might have dealt with the situation.

There is a strong argument for the general approach underpinned by these two sets of questions. It is consistent with the 'just culture' philosophy which has been advanced by Marx.[27] The objective is to improve patient safety. This will almost always be achieved more efficiently by investigations in which the allocation of blame is not at stake. Most legal processes required for a finding of fault against an individual seldom elucidate the underlying contributing factors, and add considerable cost, time and emotional trauma to any investigation. This will seldom be worthwhile. More importantly, in a blame-oriented process the focus is highly likely to move away from an examination of system deficiencies towards the proof or disproof of guilt in an individual, and this will be detrimental to the improvement of patient safety.

There are limits to the extent to which one can reliably determine culpability in relation to an event on its face appearances, without a detailed investigation, even if everyone is telling the truth (see Chapter 5). To make matters worse, the relatively infrequent situations in which malfeasance has been a factor contributing to harm to a patient are the very ones in which the truth may be hard to find. A detailed investigation will often be necessary if a truly credible judgement of blameworthiness is to be made. There is considerable empirical and theoretical evidence to suggest that very few cases of harm to patients in healthcare are the result of serious individual wrongdoing. It follows that the best value for all concerned (notably the public) is likely to be obtained by a pragmatic approach to triage which will allow the greatest proportion possible of the available resource to be directed towards pursuing improvements in the system rather than trying to find scapegoats.

Capturing Detailed Information

Detailed information may be gathered on forms using tick boxes or free narrative, or both. Each approach has advantages and disadvantages. One disadvantage of relying on free narrative is that complete sets of information are unlikely to be proffered spontaneously. This implies that attempts at subsequent analysis, particularly using techniques for 'data mining', will be compromised by missing data. On the other hand tick boxes used on their own will usually provide insufficient detail for a useful analysis of a complex incident. The tendency is for multiple forms to evolve to cater for the range of possible events. Very different information is needed in each case for falls, drug errors, pressure ulcers, needle sticks, infections, and so on.

There are various proprietary systems for collecting incident reporting data, and each has its strengths and weaknesses. AIMS uses a series of intuitive, cascading on-screen questions to populate the various components of the underlying information model (see Figure 1.6 and Appendix VIII). As with the preliminary notification, this more detailed information can be collected in a number of ways. The person directly involved can go on-line and enter answers to the interactive questions directly. However, it is better, for consistency, for a trained member of staff to interview the person reporting the incident face-to-face or over the telephone, asking questions from prompts on the computer screen, and entering the answers on-line immediately. It may at times be necessary for further enquiries to be made later about aspects of the incident which remain unclear after this process has been completed. Ideally, the system should allow ongoing tracking and recording of what is being done about the incident, so that reporters and others, such as line managers, can follow up what is being planned or has been done in response to the report.[1]

Root Cause or Systems Analysis

If an event is allocated a SAC in the most serious category (see Appendix VII), a formal RCA should be undertaken to identify measures which reduce the chances of recurrence.

The Resources Required for Root Cause Analysis

An in-depth RCA requires considerable resources. In VA hospitals, provision is made for nation-wide training of facilitators who are required to attend a three-day course. In Australia, this has been compressed into a two-day course in some jurisdictions. RCA is undertaken by a multidisciplinary team (typically of half-a-dozen members) which meets for half a day every week for four to six weeks. This team requires administrative support and space to work. Tools have been developed for RCA, including sophisticated computer software.

Although a fairly thorough analysis using the RCA framework can be conducted by individual clinicians, researchers or risk managers, it is best to use a multidisciplinary team for serious incidents. The team approach has value for teaching as well as for thorough investigation of latent factors within the system. It is particularly effective as a vehicle for introducing systems thinking to hospital staff. Recruiting a wide range of staff to work in RCA teams has been found to be a potent influence for promoting the culture change which has been identified by many authorities as a priority for improving patient safety.[28] However, it is vital to ensure that people within the system do not use the process to 'point score' or undermine any staff member. Penalties for disclosing information to anyone outside the RCA investigation are of great value in this regard. Certain forms of legislation for statutory immunity for approved quality improvement processes provide such penalties. Such legislative arrangements vary considerably, and it is important to understand the law pertaining to one's own jurisdiction to ensure that the correct processes are followed meticulously.

The Team

The RCA team should be made up of individuals closely involved with the processes and systems under review, but not actually involved in the event. If RCA were to be undertaken in the case of Mrs. Jones, one might expect the team to include an anaesthetist, a nurse from the holding area, a pharmacist, a surgeon and an operating room manager. Anyone who might add value should be included.

RCA teams have benefited from the insights of orderlies, architects, psychologists, engineers and many other people who may have expertise not usually found in doctors and nurses. For pragmatic reasons, the team should be limited to five or six people.

The team should be facilitated (not necessarily led) by a person who has received formal training in RCA. The facilitator is responsible for training the team. This training will inevitably be limited, but should include sufficient information for the members to understand the objectives of RCA and to appreciate the importance of focusing on the wider system and on factors which may have predisposed to the event. Written material will be useful for this purpose. The facilitator also has an important role in monitoring and guiding the process as the RCA proceeds. It is not necessary for the facilitator to have expertise directly related to the event. The expertise related to the event resides in the members of the team; the particular expertise brought to the team by the facilitator lies in RCA – something many health professionals know little about. The distinction between being an expert in surgery (for example) and being an expert in quality and safety in healthcare is not always apparent to clinicians, and may need to be politely explained by the facilitator.

Individuals co-opted to the team need to be allocated time for this task. Typically the team will meet weekly, for two to three hours at a time, over a period of five or six weeks.

How does the Patient Fit in?

In a patient-centred approach to quality one might ask whether the patient should be part of the RCA team. As with the health professionals actually involved in the event, the answer must be 'no', in the interests of objectivity and in order to ensure that information collected solely for the RCA remains confidential. Lay people may be included on the team, but they should be chosen for their expertise in relation to the incident, or in order to obtain the perspective of a consumer. On the other hand, it is very important that the patient and his or her family be kept apprized of the process that is being carried out. Regular communication should occur between the patient, the health professionals involved in the incident and a member of the RCA team. It is important for patients to feel that their problem is being taken seriously, and that people care enough to tell them what is happening.

Finding out What Happened

All approaches to RCA involve establishing, as far as possible, exactly what happened. The first step is to review the documents related to the incident. These may include the medical record, incident form, hospital policy documents and letters from the patient and the health professionals involved in the incident. It is also important to review the literature and search incident databases for similar events. There is no point in 're-inventing the wheel', and a proper understanding of established knowledge in relation to the incident is essential.

There is a reasonably well developed literature on the topic of drug administration error in anaesthesia. It seems that this was either not accessed or not given sufficient weight by the expert advisors to the HDC in the case of Mrs. Jones. Some of the suggestions were sensible, but one, that Dr. Aders would use different syringe sizes to distinguish his drugs in the future, is not supported by the weight of evidence in the literature. Also, several simple evidence-based strategies were not suggested which perhaps should have been – that he should always check the syringe with a second person, for example.[29] Similarly, systems-orientated solutions described in the literature might also have been suggested, such as the use of pre-filled syringes, at least for drugs known to be associated with a high risk of error.[11, 29]

Ideally, the team should visit the site of the event. It is often very helpful to see for oneself the environment, equipment and surroundings associated with an incident. The team should talk to staff who work in the area, take photographs, make sketches, and try to recreate in their minds exactly what happened.

A list should be made of people to be interviewed. This will of course include all those actually involved with the incident (including the patient or his or her family), and anyone else who could shed light on what happened. Once the list has been completed, the interviews need to be conducted.

The event flow chart

The flow chart (Figure 9.2) is a key tool in process improvement. It provides a common understanding of what happened. It reduces the likelihood of different interpretations of the same event (at least within the team). It is useful for developing problem statements and preliminary causal statements, from which a cause and effect diagram can be developed.

A flow chart provides a diagrammatic outline of the 'story' and defines what happened chronologically. Speculation should be avoided in making flow charts; it is important to keep to what actually occurred. Narrative and annotations should be used for the fine detail. It is best to start simply, and then build up the detail by repeatedly asking the question 'why?'.

The VA system provides software to allow an event flow chart to be constructed, documenting the time-course of events. This can then be expanded and annotated as the process continues. However, it is possible to achieve the same thing using paper and pens. Sticky labels are useful for this exercise.

Problem Statement (see 'Identify the Risks', Figure 2.1)

Once one has defined and documented what happened it should be possible to write a clear statement of the problem to be addressed. The wording of this 'Problem Statement' is very important. Effective prevention begins with agreeing on a definition of the problem to be avoided.

For example, if in the morning I find I cannot start my car and I define the problem as 'my car won't start', the probability is that I will become fixated on getting it started. If on the other hand I define the problem as 'I need to get to work by 7.30am', I open up a much wider range of solutions to this more fundamental problem. These solutions might include walking to work, taking a bus or getting a taxi. There is a similar difference, for example, in preventing awake paralysis specifically and preventing drug administration error more generally. Certain monitors allow the detection of this condition, and their use may well reduce its occurrence even if the wrong drug is given.[30] If there are two or more problems (as in this example), each deserves a statement, and the statements can then be prioritized. The aim in writing the problem statement is not to finesse a solution, but rather to think more deeply about the precise nature of the problem at hand.

Contributory Factors or Root Causes (see 'Evaluate the Risks', Figure 2.1)

The next step is to identify as many contributory factors or root causes as possible. Several techniques may be helpful. The first is brainstorming: getting each member of the team to suggest anything that comes to mind. At this stage, quantity is more important than quality, and every idea should be recorded. The sorts of factors which may influence patient safety have been outlined at the top of Figure 1.6 and include:

- *Environmental factors* Insufficient priority given to safety issues; a long-standing blame culture; legal pressures against open discussion to learn from adverse events.
- *Organizational factors* Inadequate staffing levels; poor or absent policies; a culture in which productivity takes priority over safety (an attitude of 'press on regardless'); high workload and fatigue; limited access to essential equipment; inadequate administrative support, leading to reduced time with patients.
- *Team staff factors* Poor supervision of junior staff; poor communication between professional groups; juniors discouraged from seeking assistance.
- *Individual staff factors* Lack of knowledge or experience; long term fatigue and stress; having to 'multi-task'.
- *Task factors* Lack of clear protocols and guidelines; non-availability or delay in obtaining test results; task poorly defined.
- *Patient factors* Distressed patients; communication and cultural barriers between patients and staff; multiple co-morbidities.

A second technique is to refer to the flow chart and ask the question 'What was this caused by' for each stage or event. In the case of Mrs. Jones one would ask why patients were transferred to the holding area before receiving a pre-medication, why sedation was needed in the holding area, why the syringes were not obviously distinguishable, why awake paralysis actually occurred when the wrong drug was given, and so on. In the VA, Triage Cards™ are used as a third method of identifying contributory causes.[4] Questions on flip-charts are arranged in groups to facilitate the process of eliciting key points about different aspects of the system.

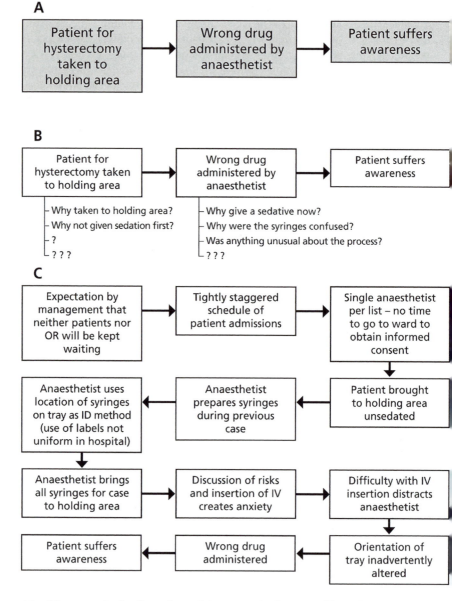

A) First steps in the flow chart of the events in the case of Mrs. Jones.
B) Documenting the process of questions about each event.
C) Expanding the chart on the basis of the answers.

Figure 9.2 An event flow chart

Examples of triage questions used by the VA system to identify contributing factors are:

- *Communication* Was the patient correctly identified? Was information from patient assessments shared by members of the treatment team on a timely basis?
- *Environment* Was the work environment designed for its function? Had there been an environmental risk assessment?
- *Equipment* Was equipment designed for its intended purpose? Had a documented safety review been performed on the equipment?
- *Barriers* What barriers and controls were involved in this? Were they designed to protect patients, staff, equipment, or environment?
- *Rules, policies and procedures* Was there an overall management plan for addressing risk and assigning responsibility for risk? Had a previous audit been done for a similar event, were the causes identified, and were effective interventions developed and implemented on a timely basis?
- *Fatigue/scheduling* Were the levels of vibration, noise, and other environmental conditions appropriate? Did personnel have adequate sleep?

As contributory factors are identified, they should be documented. In the first instance this is probably best done by annotating the flow chart (Figure 9.3). Once a good number have been identified, and no more are readily forthcoming, a cause and effect diagram should be constructed.

Cause and effect diagrams A cause and effect diagram supplements the flow chart and assists with probing further into why an event happened (Figure 9.4). It extends the identified sequence of causal events and diminishes the likelihood of attribution to a single error or 'smoking gun'. It should begin with one or two problem statements, and show how these may have been caused by (a few) actions and (many) latent conditions in the system. The cause and effect diagram is useful to distinguish conditions (about which it is often possible to do something) from actions (which tend to be more difficult to prevent).

Root Cause Statements

The final step in the process of identifying why the incident occurred is the development of root cause statements. As with problem statements, the way these are written is very important, and can make a great deal of difference to the identification of effective actions. In the VA process there are five rules for writing root cause statements.

- The 'cause and effect' relationship must be explicit and understandable.
- Negative value judgments should be avoided.
- Each human error must have a preceding cause.
- Each procedural deviation must have a preceding cause.
- Failure to act is only causal when there was a pre-existing duty to act.

C

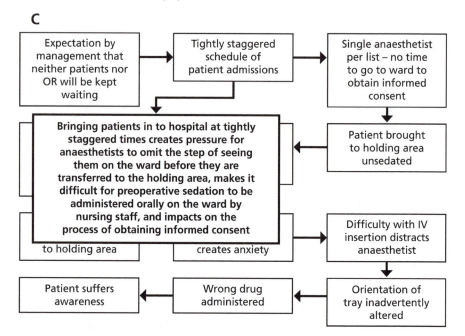

Figure 9.3 Excerpt from Figure 9.2 with the addition of a clearly articulated contributory factor to the flow diagram

These rules are designed to ensure that the outcome of the RCA is useful. In each of the examples below there is no obvious solution to the first (poorly written) statement, but it is possible to understand how one might do something about the second (more explicitly written statement), which identifies aspects of the system which, if not addressed, would increase the likelihood of a recurrence of the incident.

The 'cause and effect' relationship must be explicit and understandable. First statement: 'Dr. Aders should not have administered intravenous sedation to a patient in the holding area of the operating room (OR).' Second statement: 'The arrangement of bringing patients in to hospital at tightly staggered times creates pressure for anaesthetists to omit the step of seeing them on the ward before they are transferred to the holding area in the operating room suite, and makes it difficult for preoperative sedation to be administered orally on the ward by nursing staff.' Also, 'the holding area is not set up with the pre-requisite drug drawers, labels, and monitoring equipment to administer intravenous drugs safely, so anaesthetists who wish to give IV drugs in this area must draw them up in the OR and bring them into the holding area'.

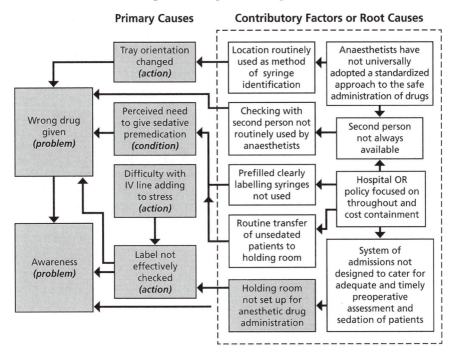

Figure 9.4 A cause and effect diagram

Negative value judgments should be avoided First statement: 'Dr. Aders' system for syringe identification was inadequate'. Second statement: 'Anaesthetists in our institution do not routinely put labels on all syringes, which creates the potential for confusion if other methods of drug identification fail'.

Each human error must have a preceding cause First statement: 'Dr. Aders gave the wrong drug'. Second statement: 'The use of position on the tray by some anaesthetists in our institution to distinguish between syringes may lead to the selection of the wrong syringe when the orientation of the tray is inadvertently altered.'

Each procedural deviation must have a preceding cause First statement: 'Dr. Aders did not check the identity of the drug before injecting it'. Second statement: 'Because of pressure to proceed, and the anxiety of the patient (which had been aggravated by difficulties in inserting an IV line), Dr. Aders omitted his usual checks of the syringe.'

Failure to act is only causal when there was a pre-existing duty to act First statement: 'The nurse did not monitor the patient after the intravenous sedation was administered'. Second statement: 'There is no established protocol in the holding area for nurses to monitor patients after the injection of intravenous sedation'.

Preventing a Recurrence – Recommendations (see 'Treat the Risks', Figure 2.1)

The outcome of an RCA should be a recommendation. There are three possible responses to a risk once it has been identified.

* Eliminate it: requires action.
* Control it: requires action (which may include insuring against the risk).
* Accept it.

Each of these responses may be legitimate, but the choice should be informed and made actively, and the reasons for it documented and communicated to those affected by the risk. The RCA team's recommendation should begin with this high level of choice, and the CEO should keep these three options in mind when responding to the team's recommendations. A recommendation for action should:

* address a root cause of the problem;
* be specific and concrete;
* be easily understood;
* be possible to implement;
* define the person/s responsible for its implementation; and
* define an implementation timeline.

In the end, it is *action* that makes systems safer (see page 249). Certain types of action are more likely to be effective than others. On this basis, actions may be designated as 'strong', 'intermediate' or 'weak' (Table 9.1). Actions should make clear who will do what, and when,

Table 9.1 Examples of actions which might be recommended after an RCA

Strong	Intermediate	Weak
Changes to plant or equipment	Increased staffing	Checklists
Simplification of process	Double checks	Warning signs
Standardization of process	Redundancy	New procedures or policies
Forcing functions	Better records	Memoranda

Before the team finalizes its recommendations, information about similar events should be reviewed. The sources of such information are listed in Table 2.5. If the information from all these sources is systematically collected in one comprehensive system using a common classification, an excellent overview of what is going wrong can be obtained[1] (see Figure 1.5). There are proposals for national or even international repositories of such data, with all the information classified using an agreed international patient safety classification.[2,31]

Engaging Senior Management (see 'Communicate and Consult', Figure 1.5)

The allocation of substantial resources to RCA will only be worthwhile if the process results in clear recommendations and if senior management is committed to responding to these recommendations. This commitment includes a preparedness to allocate time to busy staff to conduct an in-depth RCA, support each step of the process, and provide an appropriate response to the output of the analysis. Time should be allocated for the team to present its recommendations to the CEO, including adequate time for discussion. In the VA system, there is a requirement for the recommendations from RCA to either be 'concurred with' by the CEO, in which case they must be funded and implemented, or 'not concurred with', in which case the reasons must be part of a document which is made public (see Figure 9.1). This is a very important mechanism for gaining genuine co-operation between workers at the 'coal-face' and senior management. An inadequate response to the report of an RCA team undermines the whole process and weakens the culture of safety. For example, in the case of Mrs. Jones, the hospital's medical advisory committee requested a report from an anaesthetist. The report contained a number of recommendations intended to reduce the likelihood of a recurrence of such an event, but it generated no response – not even a formal decision to reject its recommendations.

The Soft Systems Methodology

The main difficulty encountered with the RCA process, and with strategies arising from analyzing incident reports, has been in achieving the necessary changes in attitude and cooperation to implement the recommendations. An approach called 'soft systems methodology' comprises a structured, step by step approach based on a framework for bringing together and involving a range of stakeholders to overcome barriers and facilitate the implementation of corrective strategies. This approach recognizes that implementation strategies are often unsuccessful because they do not take account of the complex socio-technical systems in which the problems are embedded.

Currently, there are four common approaches to problem resolution; the first involves manipulating the *local politics* to gain influence and resources, often at the expense of others. The second is based on *economic reasoning*, where everything is considered in terms of productivity and efficiency, ignoring what drives behaviour change in individuals. The third approach is the *bio-medical* or *scientific* one which tends to consider the problem in abstract terms and artificially isolate it from the local political and social context. The fourth is a *managerial* or *business* approach which tends to use tools imported from industry such as re-structuring and re-engineering. The problems with each of these approaches are outlined in more detail in Appendix IX.

The soft systems methodology proposes 'that the core characteristics of the solution to deep seated healthcare problems are: a structured, multi-faceted approach; engagement of a wide range of stake holders; encouragement and opportunity for those involved to learn together; understanding the nature of complex systems and how people behave within them; an appreciation of what culture is, what it does, and how it might be changed; the alignment of system wide, organizational, institutional and individual interests in goals; explicit statements about the rules people are playing under; a recognition that connections people make – their relationships with others – are at the heart of complex systems; and to grasp that the system is always emergent – that there are no definitive outcomes or resolutions'.[32]

The core characteristics of solutions to deep seated healthcare problems and a flow chart of the 16 stages of the soft system methodology solution have been provided as Appendix IX. Clearly this is a comprehensive process, which can only be undertaken for important problems, but it explicitly recognizes that healthcare problems are deeply embedded in a complex socio-technical system which is remarkably hard to change.

Measuring the Effectiveness of an Action (see 'Monitor and Review', Figure 2.1)

The outcome of any intervention to improve safety should be monitored because it may not be effective and because *revenge effects* may occur. Revenge effects are unexpected and undesirable consequences of actions intended to improve safety in any organization (see the 'blocked filter' problem in Box 4.5).[33] Another example of a revenge effect is to be found in relation to screening for prostatic cancer, which may result in some men suffering serious side effects from treatment they did not need, because their cancer would not have manifested during their lifetime. It is not always easy to measure the outcome of an action. Ideally, a measure should:

- indicate the effectiveness of an action, not document its completion;
- be quantifiable with a numerator and a denominator;
- have a defined sampling strategy over a defined time period; and
- have realistic goals (100 per cent elimination of a problem is usually impossible).

Conventional measurement may not be possible for low frequency events, where ongoing surveillance with incident monitoring may be the only option.[21,34] In any event, the issue of measurement and ongoing monitoring should be explicitly addressed in the recommendations from every RCA.

Identifying and Responding to Additional Risks

A thorough RCA will often identify risks that had previously not been noticed. In the analysis of the case of Mrs. Jones, it becomes clear that the process by which assessment by the anaesthetist is carried out at the last minute in the holding area, and the similar way in which informed consent for anaesthesia is obtained, are both inadequate. Although neither of these deficiencies in the system created an incident on this occasion, the risks are obvious. An extension of the analysis into these risks might produce a recommendation for routine pre-admission clinics to be held by anaesthetists several days ahead of time. This is a proposal that could also address several of the contributory factors related to the event that actually occurred – patients would be less anxious, the need for discussion immediately before the operation would be limited and the need to give sedation in the holding area could be eliminated.

It can be seen that recommendations may arise from a thorough RCA which deal with problems at levels of the system far removed from the 'smoking gun'. Who would think, on first examining the facts, that one effective response to a wrong-drug error would be to set up pre-admission clinics for anaesthesia?

Conclusion

In responding to an incident, after attending to those affected it is important to report the facts and then take systematic measures to prevent the recurrence of a similar event. Through reporting, everyone's individual experiences can be aggregated to form a collective pool of information which can be used to devise preventive and corrective strategies to make the healthcare system safer. For serious events, RCA is appropriate.

RCA is a comprehensive, systems-based response to an adverse event or near-miss, designed to identify actions capable of improving the safety of patients and reducing risk for the organization. RCA is not easy, and requires resources. It should identify as many contributory factors or root causes as possible. A thorough RCA should result in recommendations which will improve the safety of the system, not only in respect of events which actually occurred, but often in respect of other (previously unidentified) risks as well. RCA is a very important mechanism for recruiting healthcare professionals and other healthcare workers to systems thinking, for changing individual behaviour, and ultimately for developing a culture of safety within healthcare.[35]

Notes

1   Runciman, W.B. (2002), 'Lessons from the Australian Patient Safety Foundation: Setting Up a National Patient Safety Surveillance System – Is This the Right Model?', *Quality and Safety in Health Care* 11:3, 246–51.

2   Runciman, W.B. et al. (2006), 'An Integrated Framework For Safety, Quality and Risk Management: An Information and Incident Management System Based On a Universal Classification', *Quality and Safety in Health Care* 15:Suppl I, i82-i90.

3   VA National Center for Patient Safety (2002), *VHA National Patient Safety Improvement Handbook* (Washington DC: Department of Veterans Affairs, Veterans Health Administration). Available at: <http://www.va.gov/ncps/Pubs/NCPShb.pdf> accessed 26 Jun 2006.

4   VA National Center for Patient Safety, *Triage Cards*[TM], available at: http://www.va.gov/ncps/CogAids/Triage/index.html accessed 26 Jun 2006.

5   Bagian, J. et al. (2002), *Root Cause Analysis Tools*, VA National Center for Patient Safety [web resource], available at: http://www.va.gov/ncps/CogAids/RCA/index.html accessed 26 Jun 2006.

6   National Patient Safety Agency. *National Reporting Goes Live* [web page] http://www.npsa.nhs.uk/health/reporting/background accessed 26 June 2006.

7   Scobie, S. and Thomson, R. (2005), *Building a Memory: Preventing Harm, Reducing Risks and Improving Patient Safety* (London: National Patient Safety Agency). Available at: www.npsa.nhs.uk/site/media/documents/1269_PSO_Report_FINAL.pdf accessed 26 Jun 2006.

8   Vincent, C. (2003), 'Understanding and Responding to Adverse Events', *New England Journal of Medicine* 348:11, 1051–6.

9   Reason, J. (2000), 'Human Error: Models and Management', *British Medical Journal* 320:7237, 768–70.

10 Health and Disability Commissioner (2004), *Case 02HDC05291. Anaesthetist. Error in Administration of Anaesthetic,* Health and Disability Commissioner of New Zealand, Auckland.

11 Bergman, I.J., Kluger, M.T. and Short, T.G. (2002), 'Awareness During General Anaesthesia: A Review of 81 Cases from the Anaesthetic Incident Monitoring Study', *Anaesthesia* 57:6, 549–56.

12 Aders, A. and Aders, H. (2005), 'Anaesthesia Adverse Incident Reports: An Australian Study of 1,231 Outcomes', *Anaesthesia and Intensive Care* 33:3, 336–44.

13 Merry, A.F. and Peck, D.J. (1995), 'Anaesthetists, Errors in Drug Administration and the Law', *New Zealand Medical Journal* 108:1000, 185–7.

14 Currie, M. et al. (1993), 'The "Wrong Drug" Problem in Anaesthesia: An Analysis of 2,000 Incident Reports', *Anaesthesia and Intensive Care* 21:5, 596–601.

15 Runciman, W.B, Edmonds, M.J. and Pradhan, M. (2002), 'Setting Priorities For Patient Safety', *Quality and Safety in Health Care* 11:3, 224–9.

16 Australian Patient Safety Foundation (2005), *Published Articles on Patient Safety* [Web document], available at: http://www.apsf.net.au/ accessed 26 Jun 2006.

17 Runciman, W.B. et al. (1993), 'System Failure: An Analysis of 2,000 Incident Reports', *Anaesthesia and Intensive Care* 21:5, 684–95.

18 International Task Force on Anaesthesia Safety (Australia, Runciman; Canada, Duncan; Finland, Tammisto; France, Desmonts; Germany, Stoeckel; Japan, Ikeda; Netherlands, Booi; UK, Hanning; USA, Eichhorn & Gravenstein) (1993), 'International Standards for a Safe Practice of Anaesthesia', *European Journal of Anaesthesiology* 10:7Suppl., 12–5.

19 Runciman, W.B. (1993), 'Commentary on Equipment Recommendations', *European Journal of Anaesthesiology* 10:7 Suppl., 16–8.

20 Runciman, W.B. (1993), 'Risk Assessment in the Formulation of Anaesthesia Safety Standards', *European Journal of Anaesthesiology* 10:7 Suppl., 26–32.

21 Runciman, W.B. (2005), 'Iatrogenic Harm and Anaesthesia in Australia', *Anaesthesia and Intensive Care* 33:3, 297–300.

22 Runciman, B., Merry, A. and Smith, A.M. (2001), 'Improving Patients' Safety By Gathering Information. Anonymous Reporting Has An Important Role', *British Medical Journal* 323:7308, 298.

23 All incident reporting via AIMS in South Australia is now via a call centre.

24 Between 300 and 400 incidents were being reported each week per million population in the Australian states of New South Wales and South Australia in June 2006.

25 National Audit Office (2003), *The Management of Suspensions Of Clinical Staff in NHS Hospital and Ambulance Trusts in England* (London: The Stationery Office).

26 National Patient Safety Agency (2004), *Incident Decision Tree* [website], National Patient Safety Agency, United Kingdom, available at: http://www.npsa.nhs.uk/ health/resources/incident_decision_tree accessed 26 Jun 2006.

27 Marx, D. (2001), *Patient Safety and the "Just Culture": a Primer for Health Care Executives* (New York: Columbia University), available at: <http://www.mers-tm.net/index.html> accessed 26 Jun 2006.

28 Kaplan, H.S. and Rabin Fastman, B. (2003), 'Organization of Event Reporting Data For Sense Making and System Improvement', *Quality and Safety in Health Care* 12: Suppl. 2, ii68–ii72.

29 Jensen, L.S. et al. (2004), 'Evidence-Based Strategies for Preventing Drug Administration Errors During Anaesthesia', *Anaesthesia* 59:5, 493–504.

30 Myles, P.S. et al. (2004), 'Bispectral Index Monitoring To Prevent Awareness During Anaesthesia: the B-Aware Randomised Controlled Trial', *Lancet* 363:9423, 1757–63.

31 Clinton, H.R. and Obama, B. (2006, 'Making Patient Safety the Centerpiece of Medical Liability Reform', *New England Journal of Medicine* 354:21, 2205–8.

32 Braithwaite, J. et al. (2002), 'Introducing Soft Systems Methodology Plus (SSM+): Why We Need It and What It Can Contribute', *Australian Health Review* 25:2, 191–8.

33 Tenner, E. (1997), *Why Things Bite Back: Technology and the Revenge of Unintended Consequences* (New York: Vintage Books).

34 Runciman, W.B. (1993), 'Qualitative versus Quantitative Research – Balancing Cost, Yield and Feasibility', *Anaesthesia and Intensive Care* 21:5, 502–5.

35 Carroll JS, Rudolph JW, Hatakenaka S. (2002), 'Learning from Experience in High-Hazard Organizations', *Research in Organizational Behaviour* 24, 87–137.

Chapter 10

Getting the Best Out of People

At the very heart of healthcare lie the people for whom the system exists – the patients, together with those who apply their skills and knowledge to treat them, the individual clinicians. In the next two chapters we will consider how to get the best out of people and the system, starting from the centre of Figure 1.1 and working outwards. Of course, any division into layers is artificial – the people are part of the system, and the system is in the end no more than all the people who work within it, the technology they use, and the infrastructure with which they work. All are inextricably inter-related. Effective and ethical people will promote a good system; a good system will attract (and even produce) effective and ethical people.

Healthcare consists of a series of personal interactions between those receiving the care and those delivering it. Within these interactions many active errors occur, springing traps set by the latent factors (or 'resident pathogens'), which are manifestations of the dysfunctional aspects of the environment and organization of healthcare (see Figure 1.6 and Chapter 3). Here, at the 'sharp end', where the core business of healthcare is carried out, an enormous influence can be exerted to ensure that the right thing is done, and that it is done in a manner that is safe, effective and acceptable to the patient. Here, every day, millions of potential errors and system failures are detected and prevented from turning into adverse events.

There are great advantages in fully engaging and involving patients in the pursuit of their own safety and in ensuring they get the best care. Mutual understanding and co-operation between patients and their carers will greatly facilitate this.

Getting the Best Out of Patients

Patients, by definition, have healthcare needs that should be addressed. However it is all too easy to focus on these needs and forget that they are people. They are individuals, and should be treated in the context of their wishes, desires, fears and hopes, which will have been moulded by their cultures, past experiences, problems, attitudes and beliefs. This implies developing a unique relationship with each one. Relationships begin with an introduction and develop over time. It should go without saying that people should be polite and pleasant, and shake hands and hold eye contact where appropriate. Listening is important. Treating the patients as though they are not really there when discussing them or their condition is not a good way to establish or maintain rapport (see Box 10.1). It is vital that senior nurses and doctors act as good role models in this respect. The traditional teaching ward round, with 20 people standing around whilst a patient is discussed and examined, does little to foster respect for the privacy and autonomy of individual patients.

Box 10.1 Presenting a recently admitted patient at the evening handover round

'This is an obese 24 year old girl, who is a single mother with a past history of drug abuse (her friends, worried by her response to ecstasy at a party, had taken her to the emergency department 4 years previously), who has presented with a vaginal discharge and lower abdominal pain. She smokes, in spite of a history of asthma. We don't really know where she's been or what she has been up to. She was pretty uncooperative when I tried to do a vaginal examination so I think someone else should have a go. I have sent a septic screen off and started broad spectrum antibiotics in case she's picked up something nasty'.

This is not the best way of presenting a new patient who has been admitted with what turned out to be acute appendicitis, especially when her mother and father are sitting just outside the room, within earshot.

Continuity of care is highly desirable. It is increasingly difficult to provide, but is appreciated. Even in a busy intensive care unit, for example, patients and relatives appreciate seeing the same faces from one day to the next, and developing relationships with those who hold their lives in their hands – or perhaps the lives of their loved ones. We have already addressed the importance of understanding the concerns and risks perceived by individual patients (see pages 30–36), of properly informing patients (see pages 166–169), of obtaining consent for procedures (see pages 148–153), and of cultural awareness and sensitivity on the part of those interacting with patients (see pages 161–163, and 187–188). This requires more than a passing acquaintance. An argument for a designated case manager for each patient will be made below (see page 231).

Patients represent an enormous resource for monitoring their own treatment and progress and ensuring that the right things happen. However, for patients to do this, they must understand what the plans are and how things are to be done (see Box 10.2). This is partly a matter of providing information, but it is also a matter of changing attitudes. The tradition has been for passivity to be encouraged; the all-knowing doctor decides what should be done, the infallible nurse carries out the instructions, and the helpless recipient submits 'patiently'. It is in reaction to this model that some have advocated abandoning the term 'patient' in favor of labels such as 'consumer' or 'client' which imply a much more engaged role.

The information that might assist patients and their families in monitoring their own care ranges from the mundane, such as how often their blood pressure and blood sugar are to be monitored, to the more complex, such as the details of their planned surgery and anaesthesia. This information can be provided in a wide variety of ways. It can take the form of the product information insert in the drug packet, supplemented by some simple advice from the pharmacist, or of a short pamphlet on the disease to be treated. Patients can be directed to informative websites or other sources of information (see Appendix IV and X). In Australia, a 'ten tips' guide for patients has been made widely available (see Box 10.3).[1]

Box 10.2 The patient as a force for safety

One of the authors of this book was admitted to a major teaching hospital for surgical repair of a fractured tibia and fibula. The surgeon outlined the options for preventing deep venous thrombosis, which could lead to pulmonary embolus and possible death. It was agreed that an anticoagulant should be used, as a daily subcutaneous injection.

On the first postoperative day, the patient, although quite sedated by pain killers, noticed that he had not been given such an injection. He politely asked a nurse why this was so. He explained that he was quite happy to be guided by his doctors if they had changed their minds and decided he would be better off without the injections, but he wanted to be sure that a mistake had not been made.

The nurse checked, and sure enough, the junior doctors had simply forgotten to prescribe the drug. Not all patients would have the knowledge to identify a failure of this sort, but it would not take much time to provide them and their families with enough information to allow them to monitor their own care. One could easily say something like: 'We will give you an injection under the skin of your tummy every day. This will be an anticoagulant to prevent blood clots in your leg which can dislodge, be carried to lungs, and cause problems. If for some reason you don't get these injections, please let us know – they are really important.'

Informed *consent* should usually be more than informed *assent*. Perhaps 'informed *choice*' would be a better term. The process should allow patients to ensure that all their options are considered, and to weigh up the benefits and risks of all sensible alternatives, including in most cases the alternative of doing nothing. Guidance from clinicians is essential, but in the end it is the patient who should decide what he or she wants and does not want.[2]

Patients, collectively, can also make valuable contributions at other levels of the healthcare system. Many are well placed to act as consumer representatives on the committees of specialist colleges, healthcare facilities, accreditation bodies and registration boards. The value of consumer input is being progressively recognized, and much credit should be given to those consumers who have driven major initiatives.[3]

Volunteers, many of whom are past or current patients, also make an enormous contribution to healthcare. Many hospitals have strong volunteer organizations whose contributions range from staffing health promotion units and running cafeterias to managing visitors in intensive care units.

Box 10.3 Ten tips for patients for safer healthcare[1]

1. Be actively involved in your own healthcare.
2. Speak up if you have any questions or concerns.
3. Learn more about your condition or treatments by asking your doctor or nurse and by using other reliable sources of information.
4. Keep a list of all the medicines you are taking.
5. Make sure you understand the medicines you are taking.
6. Make sure you get the results of any test or procedure.
7. Talk to your doctor or other healthcare professional about your options if you need to go into hospital.
8. Make sure you understand what will happen if you need surgery or a procedure.
9. Make sure you, your doctor and your surgeon all agree on exactly what will be done during the operation.
10. Before you leave hospital, ask your doctor or other healthcare professional to explain the treatment plan you will use at home.

Getting the Best Out of Individual Clinicians

As emphasized above, healthcare consists of a series of interactions between patients and clinicians. These will be of high quality and low risk if patients are engaged and clinicians are competent, knowledgeable, well motivated and up-to-date with the latest skills and evidence in the areas in which they practise. This starts with basic education and training but needs a life-time commitment to continuing professional development (CPD).[4] This should be tailored to the needs of individual healthcare professionals in response to changes in their roles and in the nature of healthcare. Conscientious attention to CPD will satisfy the desire to provide optimal care for patients, honor ethical and contractual obligations to employers and society, and provide ongoing job satisfaction. The form that CPD takes may be moulded by regulation and guided and facilitated by clinical governance.

Using the word in its broadest sense, any activity aimed at the abatement of risk may be called *regulation*.[5] Regulation optimizes the interactions between patients and healthcare professionals, either directly or through measures to ensure that infrastructure and technology are adequate for the interactions to occur safely and effectively. Regulation is not just about enforcing a set of rules. It spans a range of strategies from 'soft' to 'hard' (see Figure 10.1). *Responsive regulation* implies the use of strategies appropriate to the situation and context, starting wherever possible, at the 'soft' end of the spectrum, and is well suited to application in healthcare.[5] The facilitation and organization of these strategies comes under the heading of *clinical governance* and will be dealt with when teams are discussed.

Voluntary Self-regulation (Figure 7.1: Level I)

Voluntary self-regulation sits as the foundation or base of the regulatory pyramid shown in Figure 7.1. The other layers shown in this figure are more likely to be effective if this foundation is sound. Imposed regulation is seldom effective if those who are regulated are not appropriately motivated, or do not believe in the value of the process. Voluntary self-regulation is progressively becoming more focused. Personal reading, attendance at meetings, and participation in ward rounds are all part of CPD. Informal teaching at the bedside, in small groups (with the patient's permission), or reviewing cases in larger groups away from patients, can contribute effectively to needs-based education, both for those taught and for those doing the teaching. Teaching involves thinking, reflection, and preparation, and is itself an effective form of self-education. Opportunistic learning and teaching of this sort become a way of life for many healthcare professionals.

Self-regulation includes some more structured safety and quality activities. To date, most CPD has been based on objectives thought to be generally desirable, like attending conferences or reading journals. However, the trend is now towards more personalized approaches, based on identifying and addressing the needs of each individual. Taking on a portfolio related to safety and quality is an excellent way of developing and maintaining a focus for CPD, and is likely to be more effective than simply ticking boxes in a points-based scheme. Nearly everyone has an innate flair for and particular interest in certain aspects of their professional practice and this provides an excellent way of structuring such an interest. It can provide the basis for contributing to journal clubs and participating in tutorial programmes for students, trainees and other staff. Participating in quality improvement projects, conducting or assisting research activities, and being involved in developing guidelines, pathways and protocols are all ways of making important contributions to progressively adopting structured evidence-based approaches as part of everyday practice.

For new areas and for areas in which there have been recent major advances, attendance at courses and training sessions is an important way of bringing oneself up to date. As indicated at the beginning of this book, safety has only been widely recognized as a major issue for the last five years, and other aspects of quality such as the need to reduce variation in clinical practice, for the last 10–15 years. Integration of safety and quality into undergraduate courses has been slow and many healthcare professionals have not had many opportunities for being exposed to systematic expositions on these subjects.

However, postgraduate opportunities for education in these areas are now plentiful. Medical defence organizations have started running sessions on communication and risk management and attendance may earn a reduction in premiums. Root cause analysis (RCA) training is now sponsored by Health Departments in some centres (see Chapter 9). Thousands of healthcare professionals have attended these courses, which provide relevant education,

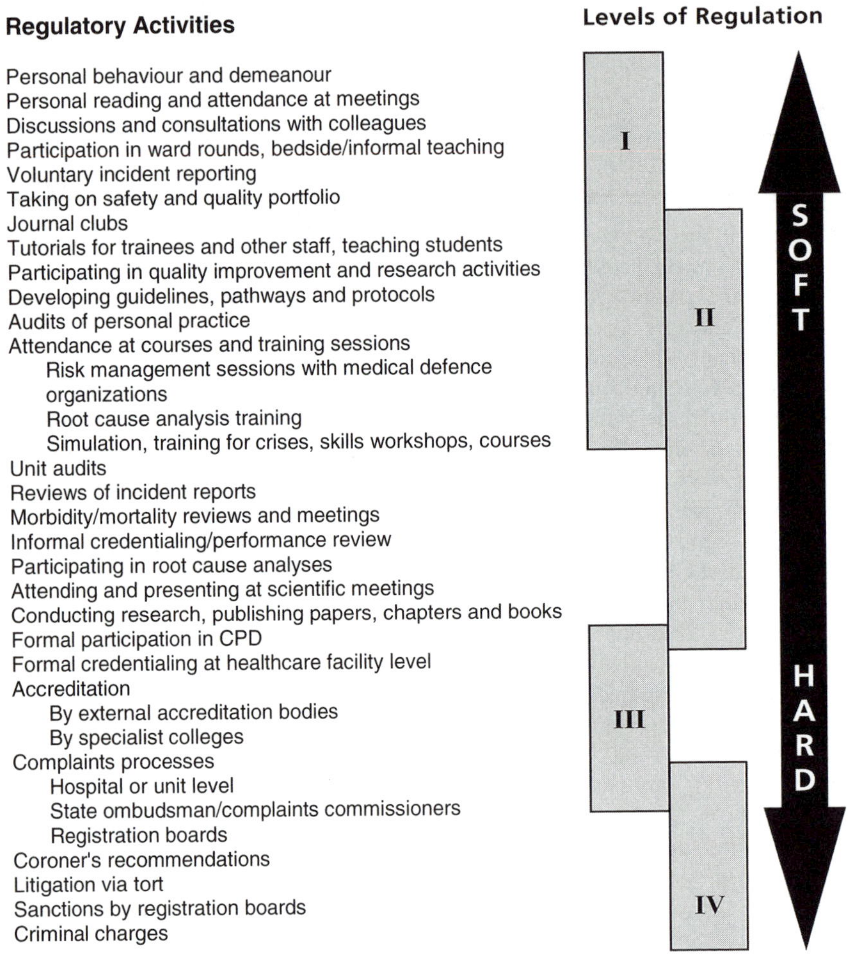

Regulatory Activities   **Levels of Regulation**

Personal behaviour and demeanour
Personal reading and attendance at meetings
Discussions and consultations with colleagues
Participation in ward rounds, bedside/informal teaching
Voluntary incident reporting
Taking on safety and quality portfolio
Journal clubs
Tutorials for trainees and other staff, teaching students
Participating in quality improvement and research activities
Developing guidelines, pathways and protocols
Audits of personal practice
Attendance at courses and training sessions
    Risk management sessions with medical defence
    organizations
    Root cause analysis training
    Simulation, training for crises, skills workshops, courses
Unit audits
Reviews of incident reports
Morbidity/mortality reviews and meetings
Informal credentialing/performance review
Participating in root cause analyses
Attending and presenting at scientific meetings
Conducting research, publishing papers, chapters and books
Formal participation in CPD
Formal credentialing at healthcare facility level
Accreditation
    By external accreditation bodies
    By specialist colleges
Complaints processes
    Hospital or unit level
    State ombudsman/complaints commissioners
    Registration boards
Coroner's recommendations
Litigation via tort
Sanctions by registration boards
Criminal charges

Figure 10.1   Regulation, from the 'soft' to the 'hard' end of the spectrum
I-IV refer to the levels of regulation shown in Figure 7.1 (page 175).
I: Voluntary self-regulation; II: Professionally-led self-regulation;
III: Meta-regulation; IV: 'Command and Control'; V: This involves
the use of financial levers, which can range from soft to hard.[5] See
text, pages 225-229.

and recruit members of the existing workforce to systems thinking and direct
involvement in producing change.

Finally, a form of voluntary self-regulation which is quite developed in some
areas of healthcare involves members of a group actively looking after each

other. Individuals with extra experience or skills will identify those who are inexperienced or unskilled and spontaneously provide teaching, assistance and support in the work place. This is represented by the concept of a community of practice, and is a form of informal 'grass-roots' mutual supervision and support.

Professionally-led Self-regulation (Figure 7.1: Level II)

The range of activities within the purview of professionally-led self-regulation is shown in Figure 10.1; there is an overlap with personal self-regulation. Many of these activities would be required for a department to be accredited by a specialist college as suitable for training specialists. The vast majority of the resources, time and effort for carrying out these activities are provided by the healthcare professionals themselves, as part of personal and peer-oriented continuing medical education and professional development.

Many clinicians devote an enormous amount of time and energy to the activities of their specialist colleges or craft groups. These include accrediting hospitals for training, providing ongoing medical education, organizing scientific meetings, mentoring and educating trainees, acting as examiners, and a host of other activities. Most of this work is voluntary; it produces no financial gain to those who undertake it. Many employers support these activities by providing time away from clinical work, but many clinicians are partly or completely self-employed, and participation does cost them money through lost opportunities for private practice.

Awareness of the elements of safety and quality postdates the basic education of many healthcare professionals, so there is an argument for encouraging all to attend courses and training sessions in these areas. These include risk management sessions, RCA training and simulation. Simulation is dealt with further at the end of this chapter.

Meta-regulation (Figure 7.1: Level III)

Meta-regulation is the process by which an external agency ensures that self-regulation is effectively carried out and that basic standards with respect to structure, process and outcome are adhered to by an organization or facility. Credentialling and accreditation are examples of meta-regulation (see Box 10.4).[6,7]

Individual clinicians may be involved in meta-regulation in various ways: they may be interviewed as part of an accreditation process; they may act as surveyors for accreditation bodies; they may collect information for clinical indicators; or they may take part in the review of peers and their performance. If meta-regulation is seen to be constructive, and to result in improvements to infrastructure, equipment and procedures, individuals will engage in the process. If it is perceived to be primarily an exercise in ticking boxes on a form very little will be achieved.

Box 10.4 Credentialling[6]

Credentialling is the formal process of assessing a professional healthcare provider's credentials in relation to his or her professional role. Recommendations are made to an institution's governing body following a determination of what the particular professional healthcare provider may or may not do in a facility. Credentialling is a function of the requirements of the organization in which an individual works, as well as his or her competencies. Therefore it may at times be appropriate not to credential someone to undertake a procedure even if he or she is able to do so. Credentialling may range from certified competence to use an item of equipment to recognition of the ability to carry out invasive high risk procedures.

'Command and Control' (Figure 7.1: Level IV)

If self-regulation and meta-regulation are effective, there should be little need for anything else. All the evidence suggests that the vast majority of things which go wrong in healthcare involve clinicians who are well motivated and trying to do the right thing. Unfortunately there are exceptions, and it is important that these are identified and dealt with if confidence in the health professions is to be maintained. Voluntary and professional self-regulation are threatened, to the detriment of both patients and clinicians, if professionals permit incompetence or negligence to go unheeded.

There are often early signs that a practitioner is not coping, is behaving differently, or has aspects of his or her practice which peers may regard as unsatisfactory or idiosyncratic. Common causes of these problems are major extrinsic life-stressors, such as relationship problems, illness, or alcohol or drug abuse, and early intervention is clearly best. In many jurisdictions a small group of senior respected clinicians is maintained, to whom practitioners who are unwell or otherwise at risk can be referred, in confidence. This approach can often be effective, but if the referred practitioners do not respond to advice or their transgressions are serious they should be dealt with more formally by a healthcare authority or registration board (see page 265). It is most important that steps are taken early to ensure that patients are not put at risk (see page 172–174).

There are many ways in which problems with individual clinicians can come to light. At the local level, peers may draw attention to a problem, or a complaint may be laid by a patient to a head of department or to the chief executive officer of the healthcare facility. Many problems can be dealt with at this level. Most healthcare facilities have complaints officers or patient advocates who can take the matter up, investigate it, take the necessary steps to put things right and provide an apology and feedback.[8] More serious problems can be referred to officials such as a state ombudsman or complaints commissioner or directly to a registration board. There are an increasing number of mechanisms in various jurisdictions by which registration boards will have attention drawn to problems with a practitioner. Civil and criminal litigation must be reported to registration authorities in most countries. Reports may also arise from coronial enquiries.

Sanctions may also be applied to poor practitioners by civil litigation (including actions for exemplary damages) or, ultimately, by criminal charges (see pages 90–91). By the time these measures are required, it is a fair guess that much damage will have been done to patients, other clinicians and the system as a whole. The criminal law is a particularly poor means of regulating clinical practice (see page 91). It should be reserved for the rare cases of genuinely blameworthy behaviour.

Economic Instruments in Regulation (Figure 7.1: Level V)

Financial levers can be used for improving safety and quality. Unfortunately, many of the economic incentives in healthcare are at present perverse in their effect (see page 75–77), and encourage practices which, at the system wide level, do not pass muster from an ethical perspective. This is an important problem, and needs to be addressed. However, it is not obvious how healthcare should be structured to promote safety and quality. Current system-wide strategies often lead either to over-servicing or under-servicing (see page 77). Direct financial incentives to conform with safety and quality standards seem to be the only viable possibility, and these are being trialed in some areas.[9] It is important that doctors and professional bodies not dissociate themselves from an understanding of and involvement in healthcare economics.

The threat of litigation does exert some influence on everyday practice, and probably encourages compliance by hospitals and individual clinicians with guidelines such as those for the use of oximeters and capnographs during anaesthesia. Some insurance companies offer discounts for low-claim track records, or for compliance with predefined standards of best practice.

Getting it Right from the Bottom Up – for Individual Clinicians

As indicated at the beginning of this chapter, individuals cannot be considered in isolation from 'the system'. Individual clinicians can keep themselves up to date, hone their skills, contribute to all the activities listed at levels I, II and III in Figure 10.1, and still be seriously constrained by the working conditions, administrative arrangements and limited resources in the system in which they work. We have provided many examples in Chapter 3 of how deficiencies in the system may frustrate the best intentions. An example is given in Box 10.5 in which poor quality care (or almost no care) was virtually inevitable because a hospital was gridlocked, and patients and healthcare professionals were trapped in a dysfunctional system.

Box 10.5 A failed admission[10]

Mrs. Mater got up to get a drink of water at midnight, at 86 years of age, and fell onto a pail and mop that had been left out, badly lacerating her leg. She activated her personal duress alarm, and an ambulance crew took her to the Emergency Department of a large teaching hospital. Her son, a consultant at the hospital, was overseas. She was admitted under the plastic surgery unit, after a 4 hour wait, as it was decided that the wound should undergo formal debridement and skin grafting. She was admitted by a surgical intern and was fasted, awaiting the availability of an operating theatre. On the morning of the following day, some 30 hours after her admission, she was offered breakfast. She queried this and phoned her son who was in the USA. Despite knowing 'the system' he was unable to locate any member of the covering team or to determine the identity of the plastic surgical registrar who was supposed to be looking after her. The ward staff could not help as they were busy and she was an outlying patient.

The switchboard operator managed to locate two plastic surgical registrars, but both denied being on call. A direct call to the duty anaesthetist revealed that there was little prospect of a case of that low priority being dealt before 10pm, at which stage it would be deferred to the following day, for which there was already a huge backlog. The son declined an offer to jump the queue, because there were higher priority cases waiting, but did ask the duty anaesthetist to arrange to have an intravenous line inserted, as his mother had had nothing to eat or drink for 36 hours.

He contacted a plastic surgeon at a private hospital and arranged for her transfer. As she was about to be transferred by the ambulance team, the plastic surgery team (registrar, resident and intern) arrived to sort out the backlog in their work. They had all been tied up in the operating theatre, with major trauma cases, in breach of the guidelines for working hours. Their pagers had been held by a theatre nurse who had left them unattended while assisting in an additional theatre which had been opened to help with the overload. The plastic surgical team on the next shift was not responsible for the patients admitted on the previous shift, and did not have Mrs. Mater on their books. They called the son (in the middle of the night in the USA) and apologized. But he, they and the patient understood that they were all victims of the system (or lack of system)(see also page 262).

The debridement and skin grafting were carried out uneventfully at 4pm that afternoon under local anaesthetic at the private hospital.

The reality is that, for the foreseeable future, individual clinicians will have to safeguard their patients and do their best to provide high quality care in spite of the inadequacies of the system. How can they best do this? Ten tips for healthcare professionals and workers follow (see Box 10.6).

10.6 Ten tips for clinicians for safer care

1. Know your patients, listen, assess and reassess. Appoint a case manager.
2. Know your limits, do not overstretch.
3. Simplify and standardize.
4. Teach, train, learn and get involved.
5. Communicate and document.
6. Be a champion for safety, high quality care and ethical behaviour.
7. Practise graded assertiveness.
8. Find and use the fixers.
9. Learn from your mistakes and from system failures.
10. Follow through.

---

1. *Know your patients, listen, assess and reassess* whenever in doubt or whenever anything goes wrong. Listen to the patient and listen to their friends and relatives. Listen to other staff from all disciplines and at all levels. Some really unlikely, implausible things can occur and one can look very silly when a patient is harmed because these were dismissed. Reassess the situation by checking the history previously taken, updating the history, examining the patient and looking at any test results. Compare these to previous clinical findings and results, and consider the possibility that notes and diagnoses made so far could be erroneous. Consciously avoid fixation errors (see page 116). Ideally, members of a team or practice should designate one clinician to be the *case manager* responsible for oversight of the progress of any particular patient. The patient should know who this person is, and be able to contact him or her. Other members of the team can check with this person to see if things are on track. For hospitalized patients, this contact should be maintained post discharge, in case there are residual problems. This approach addresses the problem of diffused responsibility and makes it possible for at least one person to know the whole picture in relation to each patient.

2. *Know your limits; do not overstretch* Seek help when you need it. Seek help when you think you might need it. Seek help when you are not sure if you need it or not. Try to make sure that the person or persons helping you have the requisite knowledge and skills and will complement your efforts in a crisis. Do not accept the 'see one, do one, teach one' tradition. Decide what you are able to do and request the appropriate degree of help or supervision for anything that exceeds your ability or experience.

3. *Simplify and standardize* Get involved in simplifying and standardizing protocols and processes relevant to the problems at hand. Collate these into a unit handbook which should be made available in hard copy and on the intranet. No matter how mundane a process (in fact, especially if a process is mundane), it should be standardized. Standardization for standardization's sake is a good thing. Standardization makes it possible for anyone involved in

the process (including the patient) to detect a potential problem, and perhaps intercept it and make sure that things stay on track. Use checklists, protocols, and care pathways meticulously whenever they are available.[11] Question why other people are not using them. Document your (presumably valid) reasons for deviating from them when this is appropriate. Ask other people to do so. Explain that this documentation is necessary to prevent the next practitioner from doing the wrong thing.

4. *Teach, train, learn and get involved* The many ways in which this can be done have been dealt with earlier in this chapter (see Figure 10.1 and pages 225-227).

5. *Communicate and document* everything, including who has said what to patients and their friends or relatives. Make sure that verbal orders are also written down, and make sure that written orders are also communicated verbally. There is no harm in telling a supervisor what you have asked a more junior person to do or in telling a junior what you have asked a supervisor to do. Keep the patient 'in the loop'. This is particularly important during handover at the change of shifts. Use a structured document if one exists and try to encourage your unit or team to develop one if not.

6. *Be a champion for safety, high quality care, and ethical behaviour* Anticipate and identify risk and do not tolerate unethical behaviours or practices. Always speak up if you think something is wrong. Question tests and procedures which will not achieve something positive for the patient, or which involve risks which the patient may not know about and which may outweigh their potential benefit. Involve the patients and or their friends and relatives in all decisions about their care.

7. *Practise graded assertiveness* Do not be afraid to question the clinical or professional conduct of anyone, no matter how senior. Practise *progressive graded assertiveness*:[12]

    - Quietly ask an innocent question about why something is planned.
    - Start to query its risks and benefits.
    - Point out that you are concerned about a particular aspect of the plan.
    - Point out that you are not sure that you find the proposed plan acceptable.
    - Ask for further justification and request another opinion.
    - Indicate that it is not acceptable and that you are not prepared to be involved.
    - Indicate that you are not prepared to stand by and see it happen.

8. *Find and use opinion-leaders* Seek out good clinical leadership and people with experience and wisdom. Use them as sounding boards and recruit their

support if you find you are in conflict with a person or a practice that is planned (even if it is accepted as routine in that particular unit or team).

9. *Learn from your mistakes and from system failures* Make sure you learn from your own mistakes and from system failures you encounter, and give others the greatest chance of doing so. This can only happen if the information is put into a pool where it can be accessed and analyzed by others. This involves reporting incidents in reasonable detail, following them up, and trying to make sure that appropriate attention has been paid to them.

10. *Follow through* When you think something unacceptable has happened, make sure that you let the appropriate senior person know and leave them in no doubt that you want to see that particular problem followed up. Later on, make sure that the problem has indeed been properly investigated, and that the necessary steps have been taken to deal with it, or that reasons have been documented as to why it can not be dealt with at present.

Getting the Best Out of Teams, Units and Departments – Clinical Governance

Clinical governance is the process by which clinicians organize themselves, or are organized by colleagues with clinical credentials, with the aim of ensuring that patients receive safe, high quality care. Of the dimensions of quality shown in Figure 1.1, safety, effectiveness, acceptability and appropriateness are clearly within the remit of clinical governance. This is also true for access, timeliness and efficiency, but when it comes to these dimensions of healthcare, the aims of clinical governance are often in conflict with those of healthcare administrators and funders.

Waiting times are often inordinately long, compromising access and timeliness. Constraints on resources and personnel have, in many areas, reached the point where inefficiency rather than efficiency has been the result (see Box 10.5). Clinicians may have notional responsibility for clinical care, but in practice they are seldom given the necessary control over resources to allow them to provide the quantity and standard of care that is needed. It is exceptionally frustrating to find oneself accountable for the treatment of a life-threatening emergency and to be confronted with inadequate staffing, equipment and procedures. This is made worse if a person with no such clinical responsibility has failed to provide them, or worse, has declined to provide them.

There is no doubt that clinicians, administrators and funders can become desensitized to circumstances and practices which, in terms of risk and inconvenience to patients, would be unacceptable in other areas of human endeavor. Corporate violations often become routine (see Box 3.1 and Chapter 5). This phenomenon has been termed the 'normalization of deviance'; even the public has become used to having experiences when they are unwell they would not tolerate at the local library or when registering their dog.

There are, of course, notable exceptions, and in the last five years considerable effort has gone into trying to make patient flows more efficient and into creating multidisciplinary teams to work on the interface between clinical and corporate governance. There are both major centres and rural hospitals that have made exemplary progress in this regard.

This discussion cycles back to the point about the value of voluntary self-regulation. Highly trained, well-motivated individuals will try to do the right thing if empowered to do so. Their training should encompass the financial side of healthcare as well as the principles of safety and quality. There is no simple formula, but the one clear message is that the best-trained people in the system (the senior clinicians) need to engage in the financial implications of healthcare, not simply from the perspective of regarding their 'patch' of healthcare as a business, but from the perspective of the public good. What is more, they need to be encouraged and empowered in this endeavor.

What can Clinicians do to Organize Things?

The arrangements with respect to clinical governance vary from those in which clinicians have to organize themselves informally (as happens in some small family practices or specialist groups) to highly structured, relatively hierarchical systems in academic or clinical departments. A common arrangement is for individuals to volunteer for, or be asked to take responsibility for, particular safety and quality 'portfolios' (see Box 10.7).

In some countries, many clinicians whose income is virtually all made in the private sector do some sessions in the public sector simply in order to participate in some of the activities listed in Figure 10.1. Their doing this is a form of self-governance; the desirability of the arrangement which permits isolated private practice in the first place is another question. In the USA much private practice is institutionalized, and practitioners tend to be in either one institution or another. Some of the most famous medical institutions in the USA are private, and are often linked to prestigious (in some cases Ivy League) private universities. Clinical governance in these institutions may be exemplary – several lead the way in establishing guidelines in many areas of practice, but, at the other end of the spectrum, lie departments and hospitals in which attitudes are more *laissez faire*.

Clinical governance includes making sure that the facilities and time are available for people to undertake CPD and contribute to the tasks listed in Figure 10.1 Some people may prefer to do more clinical work, and devote relatively little time to these tasks. Others may go through periods in their career in which they devote a great deal of time to these activities, and need some of their clinical duties to be covered by colleagues. It is very demanding to become involved in standards organizations, to conve national scientific meetings, or sit on major committees of specialist colleges or government departments.

It is highly desirable that the time spent on clinical work, research, teaching and administration be valued equally. Few current systems provide direct payment for the latter activities, except through relatively modest grants or teaching contracts. Individuals may be paid for these activities through salary, or by income sharing arrangements in which the group as a whole agrees that they are a legitimate part of the overall enterprise of healthcare. As is so often the case, the best results are obtained from the willing engagement of the individuals concerned in making the right thing happen. These include those responsible for administration of healthcare; many managers accept that a commitment to quality is an overhead of the business of healthcare – as it is in any industry.

Box 10.7 Typical tasks and portfolios in a clinical department

- Weekly audits of clinical activities.
- Joint audits with other relevant disciplines.
- Journal clubs.
- Weekly lectures on currently relevant clinical topics.
- Organizing teaching sessions by trainees.
- Organizing teaching sessions by consultants.
- Organizing a consultant roster.
- Organizing the trainee roster.
- Organizing rotations and attachments.
- Coordinating clinical research.
- Coordinating laboratory research.
- Supervising individual research projects.
- Supervising PhD students.
- Supervising undergraduate projects.
- Supervising medical student attachments, teaching and assessment.
- Acting as liaison officer for visiting overseas doctors.
- Organizing social activities:
  - arranging for a pool of funds contributed by staff;
  - arranging annual dinners;
  - arranging events to mark retirements and special occasions; and
  - arranging for cards and flowers for births, deaths and significant events.
- Arranging the choice, purchase and use of disposables.
- Arranging the choice, purchase and use of equipment.
- Handling complaints.
- Lecturing in courses.
- Convening and arranging scientific meetings.

Most patients are managed by a group of people rather than by one individual, especially in large hospitals. It is highly desirable for the group to be working to some clearly documented plan. Such care plans are called *clinical pathways* and can facilitate well coordinated and timely care when the diagnosis is known and the required response is clear cut.[13] However, the situation is more difficult when it comes to patients with uncertain diagnoses and complex problems.

Clinical pathways are the equivalent of *standard operating procedures* in industry. Introducing standard operating procedures to aviation in the 1950s is thought to have been a major factor in the development of the airline industry's enviable reputation for safety. Of course, most commercial aviation lends itself to standardization, and much of healthcare does not. Nevertheless the opportunity for improving the performance of clinicians through the use of standardized approaches in healthcare is substantial, even in dealing with uncertainty. This is particularly true when time is of the essence, as in a crisis, for example.[14] The advent of affordable computers provides the opportunity to introduce complex Boolean algorithms into clinical practice, and thereby promote standardization and reduce unwarranted variation in practice (see Chapter 12). The challenge for individual clinicians will be to embrace these opportunities. This will involve additional training and the willingness to question 'the way things have been done around here' (see Appendix IX).

Managing Fatigue and Stress

Healthcare professionals traditionally work long shifts and unsociable hours. This improves continuity of care, but has been exploited by health services. The whole approach needs modulating by an understanding of human performance in the industrial setting. Moves have been made in most countries to regulate the hours of junior doctors in hospitals, but some general practitioners and specialists (often in private practice) continue to work in a manner which would be regarded as completely unacceptable in other industries. In the transport industry in Australia, for example, both drivers and line-managers are legally accountable if excessive hours are worked.[15] Working continuously for 18 hours affects performance in a manner equivalent to a blood-alcohol of 0.05 mmol per litre,[16] at which level it is an offence to drive a motor vehicle in most countries (see page 122).

At the moment, with staff shortages, it is sometimes unavoidable to ask nurses to work double shifts, and for doctors to work for similar periods of time, or even longer. The hours for hospital specialists are not regulated, and it is quite possible, and not unusual, for a senior doctor to work 24 hours or more in one stretch. Line managers must be fully aware that this is happening and the process must be actively managed to the extent possible. There is no longer any justification for a doctor to carry on with the day's routine, non urgent work after a whole night up. A number of countermeasures to fatigue may be possible, including good supervision, appropriate breaks, and leaving safety critical tasks to other people. Caffeine is effective in counteracting fatigue, up to a point. New drugs offer some promise, at least for short term use, but the long term health implications of chronic sleep disruption are also relevant.[17] Staff matter, if only because unwell or unhappy staff will simply aggravate the problem of staff shortages.

It is no longer acceptable for junior staff to 'moonlight' at a private hospital and then work their normal shift in a public hospital (see page 77). Such arrangements must be declared, and both the doctor and the line manager should be held liable for any adverse consequences of overwork. There have been legal precedents in which corporate violations of exactly this nature have been the subject of successful litigation.

Many organizations and managers are actively introducing risk-management practices to reduce tiredness and mental fatigue in the workplace. A fatigue counter-measures programme needs to be a little more comprehensive than a new roster. Fatigue arises from many sources. Domestic disputes, partying (not unknown in junior doctors and nurses), worry (over examinations or patients for example) can all contribute to lost sleep. Hangovers do not improve performance, and neither does a viral infection or a gastric upset. Even though the onus for reducing fatigue in the workplace lies heavily with the organization, practitioners must also take responsibility for their own stress and fatigue and need to be aware of the association with mistakes and the potential for adverse events. Doctors in particular tend to take great pride in never missing work, and tight rostering systems certainly create considerable pressure to pull one's weight.

The point of pride needs to shift to patient safety. Rostering needs to build in a little more flexibility, and doctors need to take time off when appropriate. The authors can testify that this is happening in their own hospitals. Things are not perfect, but a great improvement has taken place over the last two decades in attitudes to fatigue.

Getting it Right from the Bottom Up – for Teams and Organizers

Team Composition and Training

There are many examples of well established, stable teams in healthcare, in areas ranging from primary care to highly specialized tertiary care. A typical example is given on page 17. In a these teams the same people may work together for years and get to function in a very efficient, cohesive manner. Evidence shows that properly functioning multidisciplinary teams improve the quality of services and lower costs.[18,19,20]

However, there are many 'teams' in healthcare which assemble at short notice for some crucial task, which are composed of people, each of whom has to play a special role, who may not have met each other before. Moreover these people may never have been trained for their roles, but are expected to have picked up the necessary knowledge and skill on the job. They may all be experienced and competent in a general sense, but perhaps not in relation to the specific task at hand, such as resuscitating a collapsed patient. Furthermore, some members of the team may have just started in their rotation and be very inexperienced (see Box 8.3). People may be forced into this situation because of staff shortages, changes to rostering arrangements, and sudden perturbations such as sickness, or, often, simply because this is the way it has always been done.

Complex interactions are often required in healthcare, with people depending on each other to perform at a high level, but there is usually no team training. This is in marked contrast to aviation, for example, where pilots and cabin staff will have received training together as part of crew resource management. Modern aviation is built around standard operating procedures, so that each person knows his or her own job in a crisis, and can also rely on other members of the team to know theirs.

Unfortunately, many emergencies in healthcare are chaotic. It is worth examining some examples in which teams of people have to deal with acute problems at short notice. They are often notified by a 'group paging call' that there is a task to be done, told where to go, and then left to get on with the job.

Medical emergency teams In the late 1980s and early 1990s work was done which showed that patients seldom have cardiac arrests with no warning.[21] The vast majority have warning signs such a high heart rate, a low blood pressure and confusion. The notion of resuscitating people before they actually die has now gained traction.[22] If certain criteria are satisfied (see Box 10.8), any member of the nursing, medical or paramedical staff can summon a medical emergency team (MET). So far, few hospitals have implemented MET adequately. Moreover, in most hospitals there are, as yet, no crisis management algorithms for MET patients, although this is an area where algorithms are obviously required.[14] Ideally, the MET is made up of one doctor with acute care and airway skills, (usually an intensive care or anaesthesia care trainee), another with a broad knowledge of medicine and diagnostic skills (usually a physician trainee), and an intensive care nurse familiar with intubation and resuscitation drills. A study on the merits of MET was inconclusive (and found to be statistically underpowered),[23] but if a reasonable percentage of MET call patients are admitted to a high dependency or intensive care unit before actually arresting, there is considerable face validity for the efficacy of MET at that hospital.

Box 10.8 Typical MET call-out criteria

Airway	- threatened
Breathing	- rate <5/minute (or arrest)
	- rate >36/minute
Circulation	- pulse<40/minute (or arrest)
	- pulse >140/minute
	- systolic blood pressure <90 mmlg
Neurological	- sudden fall in level of consciousness
	- repeated or prolonged seizures
General	- any patient you are seriously worried about

Cardiac arrest teams In many hospitals the MET will also respond to cardiac arrests. In the absence of a MET in a hospital, there will usually be a team with a composition similar to that described above for a MET. This is one of the few areas in which there are recognized standard operating procedures and formalized training courses accredited by national resuscitation councils.[24] Hospitals, supported by medical registration boards, are increasingly recognizing the importance of requiring such certification of their staff.

Trauma teams In designated trauma hospitals, there are criteria for calling a trauma team to assemble, usually in the minutes before a trauma patient arrives at the hospital. This is another area in which protocols exist for systematically assessing and resuscitating patients. The best established approach is known as the early management of severe trauma (EMST),[25] or advanced trauma life support (ATLS),[26] essentially different names for the same process.

This approach was originally developed by a practitioner whose relatives were poorly managed after suffering multiple trauma at a remote location, and has now been widely adopted. Some hospitals have aligned the documentation of the assessment and early management of trauma with the EMST or ATLS protocol. There is no doubt that certain aspects of the management of trauma have been improved by this approach, such as the diagnosis and appropriate management of spinal injuries. There is a two day course by which people can be accredited and certificated as EMST or ATLS competent. In these courses certain important procedures may be practised, such as percutaneous cricothyroidotomy (in anaesthetized sheep, usually). However, although nurses play a major role in the resuscitation of trauma patients, they are not usually part of the training process. The concept of training people in the professional groups in which they will work rather than the groups in which they received their tertiary education is still novel in healthcare, although a few initiatives to promote inter-professional training have emerged recently.[27,28]

Airway management teams Patients may lose their airways and need tracheal intubation for a variety of reasons, including becoming comatose, or suffering infection, malignancy and trauma. This can produce a terrifying and truly dangerous situation with sudden death as an imminent possibility. They may also need tracheal intubation as part of managing more generalized illnesses, because of a requirement to protect and/or ventilate their lungs, or because they need an anaesthetic for a surgical procedure. Tracheal intubation is technically difficult and can easily go wrong. The emergency management of airway problems is associated with considerable morbidity and mortality.[29] Ideally, airways should be secured in an environment, such as an operating suite, where all the equipment which might possibly be required is immediately to hand, including back up equipment, and where many trained, experienced personnel are available. However, emergency airway management often takes place in the emergency department, intensive care unit or anywhere else in the hospital where a patient has suddenly decompensated. It may also have to take place at remote locations, sometimes at the roadside, when retrieval teams are called to critically ill or injured patients.

If a patient's trachea cannot easily be intubated, ventilation must be maintained using a self-inflating bag and a mask. This may also require considerable skill and close co-ordination, potentially with one person having to hold the mask with both hands to maintain a patent airway, and another person having to squeeze the bag.[30] It is not adequate for staff who may have to perform these tasks to be expected to pick up the required skills on the job. Formal training in the basic skills of resuscitation has become relatively common, and certification of staff in cardiopulmonary resuscitation (CPR) is a requirement in many institutions. However, the real need is for the staff who will have to work together as a team to train together in similarly constructed teams. For example, a resuscitation team may include nurses, technicians and doctors from more than one specialty. Simulation provides a way of practising the team interactions inherent in this work (see pages 242–243).

Teams in Healthcare

It is clear that there is a long way to go before properly trained teams, working to well established standard operating procedures, are the rule rather than the exception. Ideally, equipment, checklists and a syllabus should be standardized, multi-disciplinary training in teams should take place according to agreed protocols, and people should be regularly credentialled to play specified roles in these teams.

What Healthcare Professionals and Workers Need to Know about Safety and Quality

Healthcare professionals and workers need to have a common understanding of the basic elements of quality, patient safety, and ethics. To meet this need, a patient safety education framework has been developed in Australia.[31] This involved identifying the current body of knowledge by reviewing the available information and then grouping this into categories termed 'learning areas' and 'learning topics' (see Table 10.1). Information relevant to 'knowledge', 'skills', and 'behaviours and attitudes' was then identified for each learning topic and listed for each of four levels of healthcare worker (see Figure 10.2)

Level one is the foundation level and identifies the information that every healthcare worker needs to have. *Level two* is designed for those who provide direct clinical care to patients, including those who work under supervision. *Level three* is for healthcare workers or senior clinicians who have managerial, supervisory or advanced clinical responsibilities. *Level four* identifies the information required for clinical and administrative leaders with organizational responsibilities. This level does not form part of the continuum for progressive learning that is represented by the first three levels.

Area 1 Topic 1	Level 1	Level 2	Level 3	Level 4
Knowledge				
Skills				
Behaviours & attitudes				

Figure 10.2 A structured grid for the learning objectives for four levels of healthcare workers[31]

Although the literature is biased towards the hospital workforce, the framework uses generic descriptors suitable for all locations and types of health service. Progress has been made in developing a shared language based on common concepts and preferred terms (see Appendix I). The World Alliance for Patient Safety, under the auspices of the World Health Organization, is developing an international patient safety classification which will provide the basis for the universal classification at the centre of Figure 1.5.[32,33] This will facilitate inter-professional learning and teamwork.

The core competencies described relate to and are important to patients. The literature review undertaken in developing the framework revealed little information about educating health workers about patient safety. The most relevant source was the Institute of Medicine 2003 report *Health Professions Education: A Bridge to Quality*, which sets out a number of areas of essential learning for healthcare professionals.[34] All of these are covered in Table 10.1.

Strategies for Learning about Safety, Quality and Ethics in Healthcare

There has been little emphasis on educating doctors or nurses in safety, quality and ethics in the past. Although opportunistic teaching and learning can play a role, there is a need for strategies for teaching directed specifically towards these areas (see page 227).

First, there is a need for systematic teaching at undergraduate level. A start can be made by courses for nursing, medical and other healthcare students with some lectures on these subjects and by incorporating some of the topics in Table 10.1 into problem based learning sessions, tutorials and case presentations. However, a more systematic and comprehensive approach is needed, with dedicated courses of one or two days duration..

The postgraduate level is also important. Few administrators and clinicians in any discipline will have had systematic teaching in these areas, which should therefore be a prime target of CPD. There is an argument for all healthcare professionals and workers to be exposed to some systematic teaching on the topics listed in Table 10.1. In some countries, there has been a national effort to train as many healthcare professionals and workers as possible in the theory and practice of RCA (see Chapter 9), using programmes based on the three day course developed by the VA in the United States.[35] These have been truncated in some centres to two days, although there is a good argument that as many as possible of the topics in Table 10.1 should be dealt with in courses of this sort, which provide a good opportunity for multidisciplinary learning. There is evidence that training and participation in RCA has a powerful effect in recruiting people to systems thinking, promoting a just culture, and empowering healthcare workers to have a real influence in areas they know well from years of experience.[36] RCA can be a powerful antidote to the feelings of helplessness described on page 60. Those who institute and take part in RCA also end up with a strong and legitimate interest in monitoring the implementation of the measures that emerge from the process.

Table 10.1 The seven learning areas and 22 topics of the patient safety education framework (and where they are dealt with in this book)[31]

---

1. Communicating effectively
- Involving patients and carers as partners in healthcare (pages 165 and 166)
- Communicating risk (pages 30–37)
- Communicating honestly with patients after an adverse event (open disclosure) (pages 179–189)
- Obtaining consent (pages 149-152 and 166–169)
- Being culturally respectful and knowledgeable (pages 162–163)

2. Identifying, preventing and managing adverse events and near misses
- Recognizing and managing adverse events and near misses (Chapter 9)
- Managing risk (pages 256–261)
- Understanding healthcare errors (pages 111–131)
- Managing complaints (page 195)

3. Using evidence and information
- Employing best available evidence-based practice (Chapter 6)
- Using information technology to enhance safety (Chapter 12)

4. Working safely
- Being a team player and showing leadership (pages 233–240)
- Understanding human factors (Chapter 5)
- Understanding complex organizations (Chapter 5)
- Providing continuity of care (page 11)
- Managing fatigue and stress (pages 236–237)

5. Being ethical
- Maintaining fitness to work or practise (pages 172–173)
- Ethical behaviour and practice (pages 160–171)

6. Continuing learning
- Being a workplace learner (pages 225–227)
- Being a workplace teacher (pages 225–227)

7. Specific issues
- Preventing wrong site, wrong procedure and wrong patient treatment
- Medicating safely

Simulation, Multidisciplinary Training and Teamwork

The tradition of learning invasive procedures on real patients and about crisis management during real crises is evidently undesirable. Similar risks in aviation led to the development of flight simulators and their adoption as essential tools in training and the maintenance of professional skills.

Simulation has been extended to healthcare, using sophisticated computerized dummies with physiological models that replicate the body's responses to medical interventions. These are placed in simulated operating or ward rooms to recreate realistic clinical situations. Individual and group performance can be observed and video-taped for debriefing and research. Simulation is becoming increasingly important internationally in the training of those who undertake the care of patients involved in trauma or acute medical emergencies.

Gaba emphasizes that the key element of simulation is not a piece of technology but a technique that replaces or amplifies real experiences with guided artificially created experiences that evoke substantial aspects of the real world in a fully interactive manner.[37] Technological advances have now resulted in devices and equipment that permit a diverse range of clinical skills to be learned without putting patients at risk. Examples include intubation of the trachea, insertion of intravenous lines and epidural needles, suturing, colonoscopy and bronchoscopy.

Simulation allows clinicians to learn new skills; to practise existing skills and to demonstrate knowledge in a controlled environment in scenarios that mirror real life as closely as possible. This brings teamwork and crisis management into the mix. It is possible to expose students to the aftermath of a simulated crisis and take them through the issues of dealing with a patient death through realistic role-playing, followed by structured debriefing. Simulation can even be applied to the promotion of organizational change.

The main draw-back of simulation is that it is expensive. This expense is offset by a complete lack of risk to patients at the time teaching occurs. The value of this is predicated on the notion that the teaching is effective, and that the harm is not simply delayed until the patient is put back into the frame. There are strong reasons to believe from first principles that this assumption is true, and considerable anecdotal evidence to support this contention, but as with so many initiatives to promote safety and quality, there is little formal research to prove the point. In reality the merits of practising on dummies or training devices before attempting a new procedure on patients are obvious. The main changes in recent times have related to the extension of what is possible with the available technology and what is taught to include human factors and team work. Arguments for standard operating procedures and training in multidisciplinary teams were advanced on pages 237–240. The logistical difficulties of bringing clinicians from a variety of disciplines together for training in standardized approaches to clinical problems are substantial, but the potential advantages are great.[34]

There is merit in promoting greater sharing of educational resources and activities between the various clinical 'silos'. This may apply particularly to the development of a common patient safety curriculum. The development of a collaborative model for curriculum development would facilitate cooperation across all education sectors and professional disciplines.[38] This would lead to a greater appreciation of other people's roles by everyone on the team, and a common view of the underlying aims and objectives in healthcare.

Conclusion

The people in healthcare are by far its greatest resource. Patients can and should play a far greater role in ensuring that the care they receive is appropriate and meets their needs, and is safe and going to plan. Front-line clinicians represent a huge financial investment – as much as two thirds of all that is spent on hospital care, and most likely as much as 80 per cent or more of all that is spent on healthcare overall. It makes sense to look after this massive investment and take all reasonable steps to ensure that we all get the maximum dividend possible, by facilitating and directing the powerful innate desires of all healthcare professionals to do the right thing.

Notes

1   Australian Council for Safety and Quality in Health Care (2003), *10 Tips for Safer Health Care* (Canberra: Australian Council for Safety Health Care), available at: <http://www.safetyandquality.org/articles/Publications/10tipsbwnobox.pdf> accessed 27 Jun 2006.
2   Australian Council for Safety and Quality in Health Care (2003), *Open Disclosure Standard: A National Standard for Open Communication in Public and Private Hospitals, Following An Adverse Event in Health Care* (Canberra: Australian Council for Safety and Quality in Health Care), available at: http://www.safetyandquality.org/OpenDisclosure_web.pdf accessed 27 Jun 2006.
3   The Quality Use of Medicines (QUM) program in Australia was driven by consumers [web-page], <http://www.health.gov.au/internet/wcms/publishing.nsf/Content/nmp-quality.htm> accessed 29 May 2006.
4   The World Federation for Medical Education, based in the University of Copenhagen, Denmark, has produced a set of global standards for quality improvement. In Australia, the Learning, Education and Professionalism (LEAP) framework offers a related approach to CPD. In each case the broad principles are probably of greater value to most people than the fine detail. The LEAP framework is built around three main strands – clinical practice, risk management and professional values and responsibilities. CPD should cover each strand (ten domains of professionalism are identified within the three strands), and activities are classified at levels one, two or three. *Level one* activities provide information and increase knowledge and skills. *Level two* activities demonstrate that competence is being maintained, and include such things as clinical audits. *Level three* activities are in effect analogous to the PDCA cycle (see page 259), and involve evaluating the outcomes of interventions designed to address identified problems [webpage] <http://www.ranzcog.edu.au/leapframework/> accessed 27 Jun 2006.
5   Braithwaite, J., Healy, J. and Dwan, K. (2005), *The Governance of Health Safety and Quality* (Canberra: Commonwealth of Australia).
6   Australian Council for Safety and Quality in Health Care (2004), *Standard for Credentialling and Defining the Scope of Clinical Practice* (Canberra: Australian Council for Safety and Quality in Health Care), available at: <http://www.safetyandquality.org/credentl.pdf> accessed 27 Jun 2006.
7   Australian Council for Safety and Quality in Health Care (2003), *Standards Setting and Accreditation Literature Review and Report* (Canberra: Australian Council for Safety and Quality in Health Care), available at: <http://www.safetyandquality.org/articles/ACTION/ssacrfinrep.pdf> accessed 27 Jun 2006.
8   Australian Council for Safety and Quality in Health Care (2005), *Complaints Management Handbook for Health Care Services* (Canberra: Australian Council for Safety and Quality in Health Care), available at <http://www.safetyandquality.org/complntmgmthbk.pdf> accessed 27 Jun 2006.

9 The Quality and Outcomes Framework rewards general practitioners in the United Kingdom for providing quality care. Practice achievement is measured against a range of evidence-based clinical indicators and indicators of practice organization and management <http://www.ic.nhs.uk/services/qof> accessed 27 Jun 2006.

10 This is an account of what happened to the mother of one of the authors.

11 For example, an Intensive Care Manual is available on-line at: http://www.health. adelaide.edu.au/icu/rah/files/manual_icu.pdf accessed 27 Jun 2006.

12 'Graded assertiveness' is a communication technique adopted from aviation crew training to enable one team member, often a subordinate, to communicate risk of an action. It involves four stages of increasing urgency (Probe, Alert, Challenge and Emergency). It has been recommended as a process to improve medication safety: Australian Council for Safety and Quality in Health Care (2005), *National Medication Safety Breakthrough Collaborative Improvement Toolkit* (Canberra: Australian Council for Safety and Quality in Health Care). The ErroMed organization has prepared a training video: 'Communication Styles and Graded Assertiveness', available from ErroMed at https://erromed.com/x/node/1 accessed 27 June 2006.

13 For details on clinical pathways see: Agency for Healthcare Research and Quality, National Guideline Clearinghouse [webpage] <http://www.guideline.gov> accessed 27 Jun 2006.

14 Runciman, W.B. and Merry, A.F. (2005), 'Crises in Clinical Care: an Approach to Management', *Quality and Safety in Health Care* 14:3, 156–63.

15 National Transport Commission, Australia (2004), 'The Road Transport Reform (Compliance and Enforcement) Bill', *National Transport Commission Information Bulletin,* January, available at: http://www.ntc.gov.au/filemedia/bulletins/ ChainofResponsibilityFeb2004.pdf accessed 27 Jun 2006.

16 Dawson, D. and Reid, K. (1997), 'Fatigue, Alcohol and Performance Impairment', *Nature* 388:6639, 235.

17 Spiegel, K., Leproult, R. and Van Cauter, E. (1999), 'Impact of Sleep Debt on Metabolic and Endocirine Function', *Lancet* 354:9188, 1435–9.

18 Baldwin, D. (1996), 'Some Historical Notes on Interdisciplinary and Interprofessional Education and Practice in Health Care in the US', *Journal of Interprofessional Care* 10:2, 173–87.

19 Burl, J.B. et al. (1998), 'Geriatric Nurse Practitioners in Long Term Care: Demonstration of Effectiveness in Managed Care', *Journal of the American Geriatrics Society* 46:4, 506–10.

20 Wagner, E.H. et al. (2001), 'Quality Improvement in Chronic Illness Care: a Collaborative Approach', *Joint Commission Journal on Quality Improvement* 27:2, 63–80.

21 Hillman, K.M. et al. (2001), 'Antecedents to Hospital Deaths', *Internal Medicine Journal* 31:6, 343–8.

22 Buist, M.D. et al. (2002), 'Effects of a Medical Emergency Team on Reduction of Incidence and Mortality from Unexpected Cardiac Arrests in Hospital: a Preliminary Study', *British Medical Journal* 324: 7334, 387–90.

23 Hillman, K. et al. (2005), 'Introduction of the Medical Emergency Team (MET) System: a Cluster-Randomised Controlled Trial', *Lancet* 365: 9477, 2091–7.

24 Emergency Cardiac Care Committee and Subcommittees, American Heart Association (1992), 'Guidelines for Cardiopulmonary Resuscitation and Emergency Cardiac Care. Part III: Adult Advanced Cardiac Life Support. 1992 National Conference on Cardiopulmonary Resuscitation (CPR) and Emergency Cardiac Care (ECC)', *Journal of the American Medical Association* 268: 16, 2199–241.

25 Trauma Committee, Royal Australasian College of Surgeons (1992), *Early Management of Severe Trauma* (Box Hill, Victoria: Capitol Press).

26 Committee on Trauma, American College of Surgeons (1988), *Advanced Trauma Life Support* (Chicago: American College of Surgeons).

27 Buysse, D.J. et al. (2003), 'Sleep, Fatigue, and Medical Training: Setting an Agenda for Optimal Learning and Patient Care', 26:2, 218–25.

28 Sokol, P. and Cummins, D.S. (2002), 'A Needs Assessment for Patient Safety Education: Focusing on the Nursing Perspective', *Nursing Economics* 20:5, 245–8.

29 Runciman, W.B. (2005), 'Iatrogenic Harm and Anaesthesia in Australia', *Anaesthesia and Intensive Care* 33:3, 297–300.

30 Paix, A.D., Williamson, J.A. and Runciman W.B. (2005), 'Crisis Management in Anaesthesia: Difficult Intubation' *Quality and Safety in Health Care* 14:3, e5.

31 Walton, M. et al. (2005), *National Patient Safety Education Framework* (Sydney: University of Sydney), available at: http://www.patientsafety.org.au/pdfdocs/national_patient_safety_education_framework.pdf accessed 27 Jun 2006.

32 Runciman, W.B. et al. (2006), 'An Integrated Framework For Safety, Quality and Risk Management: An Information and Incident Management System Based On a Universal Classification', *Quality and Safety in Health Care* 15:Suppl I, i82-i90.

33 World Health Organization (2005), *Project to Develop the International Patient Safety Event Taxonomy. Report of the WHO World Alliance for Patient Safety Drafting Group, Vancouver, 24–25 October 2005* (Geneva: World Health Organization), available at: http://www.who.int/patientsafety/taxonomy/Final_Report_of_Drafting_Group.pdf accessed 27 Jun 2006.

34 Greiner, A.C. and Knebel, E. eds, 'Committee on the Health Professions Education Summit, Board on Health Care Services', Institute of Medicine (2003), *Health Professions Education: A Bridge to Quality* (Washington: National Academies Press). Available at: <http://www.nap.edu/books/0309087236/html/> accessed 27 May 2006.

35 Bagian, J. et al. (2002), *Root Cause Analysis Tools*, VA National Center for Patient Safety [web resource], available at: http://www.va.gov/ncps/CogAids/RCA/index.html accessed 27 Jun 2006.

36 Kaplan, H.S. and Rabin Fastman, B. (2003), 'Organization of Event Reporting Data For Sense Making and System Improvement', *Quality and Safety in Health Care* 12:Suppl.2, ii68–ii72.

37 Gaba, D.M. (2004), 'The Future Vision of Simulation in Health Care', *Quality and Safety in Health Care* 13: Suppl. 1, i2–i10.

38 Harden, R.M. (2002), 'Developments in Outcome-Based Education', *Medical Teacher* 24:2, 117–20.

Chapter 11

Getting the Best Out of the System

Introduction

Everyone would like a healthcare system that supports the provision of safe, high quality care for all who need it. In the year 2000, the Institute of Medicine produced a report which drew attention to the frequency and severity of iatrogenic harm (catalogued in Chapter 2), and set a goal of halving the rate within five years.[1] This proved to be very optimistic; most frontline healthcare professionals feel that little has changed since then. It has now been realized that changing the way in which healthcare is delivered is a much more difficult proposition than was initially imagined.[2,3] The much vaunted 'low hanging fruit' has proved to be firmly attached to the vine. Although those who occupy the upper echelons of the system have produced scores of above down edicts and guidelines, clinical practice at the level of the patient-clinician interface is proving remarkably resistant to change (see Box 11.1).

Box 11.1 Catastrophic failures – again and again and again

The anti-cancer drug vincristine has been injected by mistake into the fluid surrounding the brain and spinal cord via lumbar puncture, rather than intravenously, in over 50 cases on record.[4] This usually happens to young patients, who go on to become quadriplegic or die an agonizing death within a few weeks. Concentrated potassium chloride has been injected intravenously instead of saline or 5 per cent dextrose on many occasions causing patients to die, quite literally, on the end of the needle. Operations are performed on the wrong patient or part of the body with remarkable frequency.

There have been national initiatives in several countries to put measures into place to prevent these disasters from happening. The experience of those charged with getting the changes introduced and accepted has been frustrating and difficult, and, years after their introduction, acceptance and adherence to the new processes has been piecemeal and unsatisfactory.[5]

It is perhaps not surprising, therefore, that introducing and getting change accepted for less dramatic problems is proving difficult, and that this difficulty is a major impediment to reducing the rate of iatrogenic harm.

There has been some progress. Multidisciplinary teams are being formed, there is some real dialogue between clinicians and administrators (some prompted by root cause analyses), and collaborative efforts are moving healthcare towards the application of evidence-based medicine and the development of better systems. However, we are still a long way from where we need to be.

Action is needed across the board, informed by an understanding of what is going wrong, and of what needs changing. In Chapter 10 we focused on getting the best out of the people involved in healthcare. However, mundane events and circumstances can and do conspire together to produce tragic outcomes from well intentioned acts, even by competent, well motivated individuals. To be successful in improving patient care we also need to understand the factors and processes which influence how the system works at local organizational, regional, national and international levels, and work to change these at the same time as getting the best out of people. In this chapter we turn to getting the best out of the system at each of these levels (see Figure 1.1 and Table 11.1). Some factors are important at more than one level and individuals are part of the process at every level. We will conclude with an example of quadruple-loop learning and a discussion of how the manifestations of such learning, together with behavioural changes in the people involved in healthcare, have the potential to produce a culture change and profoundly improve healthcare at every level.

Table 11.1 The layout of this chapter

The need for action – the Red Bead Game
Collecting information
Evidence
The local organizational layer
    Dealing with individual incidents – the reactive approach
    Risk management and tools for improvement – the pro-active approach
One hill at a time
The regional or national layer
    Regulation and accreditation
    Ethics, under-funding and rationing
    Restructuring versus redesigning
    Looking after the people
    Accountability versus learning – statutory immunity
    A just culture
The international layer
    The WHO resolution on patient safety – four action areas.
    The World Alliance for Patient Safety – six initiatives
Quadruple-loop learning
Changing the culture of healthcare

The Need for Action – the Red Bead Game

William Edwards Deming[6] has described an instructive game, best played before an audience, which can be used to demonstrate the limitations of traditional approaches to improving quality. Volunteers are asked to participate in a role play of an industrial process to produce white beads. The raw material for this process is a container full of beads (most of which are white, but some of which are red). The 'plant' is a purpose-designed scoop (Figure 11.1). The 'process' is for the volunteer 'worker' to mix the beads and then procure a scoop full of 'product'. Sometimes the process will be written down to illustrate the concepts of *structure* (the employee, the scoop, and the protocol), *process* (what the participant does) and *outcome* (the beads collected) (see page 262–263). Inevitably a fair number of red beads will be collected along with white ones. At this point, the master of ceremonies (the 'employer') displays great disappointment, and then goes through a range of managerial responses. One is to measure outcome. The number of contaminating red beads is recorded on a blackboard at successive iterations of the production process and the data are used as feedback to facilitate enhanced performance. Some iterations of bead-scooping will produce a smaller number of contaminants, in which case the employer can express great satisfaction.

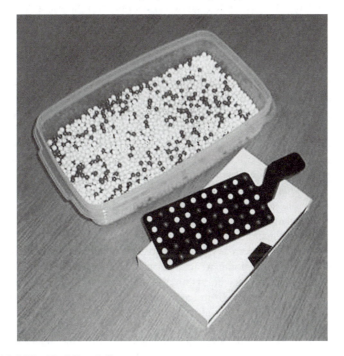

Figure 11.1 The Red Bead Game

Inevitably, any improvement will not be sustained. Another response might be the provision of incentives for better performance. One can then proceed to counseling, re-training, punishment, dismissal and replacement of the employee, and so on. Naturally, none of these approaches makes any difference. The moral of this exercise is encapsulated in a sentence attributed to Einstein and popularized by Berwick: 'Insanity is doing the same thing again and again and expecting different results.' It is also succinctly captured by Berwick's aphorism: 'Every system is perfectly designed to produce the results it does produce.'[7]

The message is clear – if we want to improve safety and quality in healthcare, we need to change the system. Our aim is improved outcomes for patients. To achieve this will require action – action informed by information and evidence, but action nevertheless. First, however, we will address the need for collecting information and assembling evidence.

Collecting Information

There is intense debate about what information should be collected in pursuit of high quality healthcare and how this should be done, with people at one end of the spectrum demanding adherence to sound epidemiological principles,[8] and those at the other arguing for the opportunistic gathering of naturalistic data from frontline activities.[9] Each has its place. For example, at the present time we do not even have an accurate estimate of anaesthetic mortality according to an agreed definition, although a superficial appraisal would conclude that the death of a patient on the table from anaesthesia would seem to be an event worth noting.[10,11,12] This makes it difficult to monitor progress over time with any confidence. On the other hand too much emphasis on the reliability and precision of evidence risks the possibility that nothing will be done about serious problems that are relatively easy to identify and remedy. We should not keep measuring while people die, when we can see obvious preventive strategies.[13] We suggest that the former approach to collecting information is desirable for defined purposes in circumscribed areas of activity, but that the latter has more to offer with respect to characterizing the myriad things that go wrong across the whole system.

There is no single source of information on iatrogenic harm. It is necessary to exploit all available sources, as each has strengths and weaknesses (Table 2.5). Progress is being made towards improving the collection of information relevant to enhancing safety in healthcare, but much more needs to be done. In order to improve the system it is necessary to know not only what aspects of healthcare are inappropriate, and what is going wrong, but also how and why these deficiencies continue to occur. The primary aim is not to count the bad things which happen in healthcare – it is to stop them from happening. For identifying why something is going wrong, simple qualitative information is much more useful than a precise count.

In relation to vincristine disasters, for example, we don't need an accurate estimate of the rate at which they occur to conclude that it is too high.[14] What we need is an effective way of eliminating a problem which is clearly preventable and obviously unacceptable. In other situations, such as nosocomial infection, accurate counting is important, and may provide a useful tool for monitoring progress over time.

Improving safety in healthcare will be greatly facilitated by a pragmatic approach that recognizes what is obvious and matches the tools of data collection and analysis to the questions that need answering.

Evidence

In Chapter 6 we discussed the importance of evidence based medicine (EBM) and the limitations of medical knowledge, and identified a number of organizations devoted to facilitating the use of EBM (see Appendix IV). There is no glib formula with respect to the generation or weighting of evidence. With respect to what treatments are effective and appropriate, there are a number of important considerations: commercial bias in the funding and interpretation of studies; poor design of studies; publication bias; research fraud; publication in a form that impedes or prevents systematic review and meta-analysis; and the ethics of subjecting patients to unnecessary risk by additional studies being carried out when the evidence is already in.

The majority of things that go wrong in healthcare occur too infrequently to be amenable to characterization or analysis using prospective quantitative methodology.[15] The insistence on a randomized controlled trial (RCT) to justify healthcare expenditure to improve safety creates a major barrier to the implementation of sensible, obviously valuable initiatives. EBM does include the lower ranked sources of evidence and expert opinion, but, until better ways are available for aggregating the rich data from the many sources listed in Table 2.5, much useful information will be inaccessible to those who wish to improve the safety and quality of healthcare. The information should feed into a safety and quality data repository (ideally a national one, as shown in Figure 1.5). Such a repository has recently been called for in the USA,[16] and a process is underway for developing an international patient safety classification.[17]

Evidence for Patients

In Chapter 10 we discussed the key role patients can play in their own care. Patients will improve the care they receive if they become better informed.[18] Improving the knowledge of individuals can also lead to improvements to the system as a whole. A better informed society will lead to better political decisions and more sensible changes in the overall direction and design of healthcare.

The provision of high quality, accessible information to patients has been neglected by the healthcare professions. The web has provided access to an extraordinary amount of information on almost any topic, but the quality of the information is variable. Some sites are reputable (Appendix X) but others may be misleading. Also, there are often difficulties in placing facts into context. A major problem is the free-for all nature of the internet and the fact that much unsubstantiated opinion and misinformation masquerade as verified fact. It is not difficult for patients to end up with incorrect views in relation to healthcare (see Box 11.2). A system for guiding patients to better quality information would be very valuable. Perhaps experts representing specialist colleges or other reputable organizations could provide websites which point to endorsed, clearly presented bodies of information on healthcare-related topics.

Box 11.2 A continent of ignorance in a sea of information[19]

Over half the Australian population used complementary or alternative medicine in the year 2003/2004. Of those that did, nearly three quarters believe that the substance or process in question had been tested and endorsed for safety and/or efficacy by an agency of the Federal Government.[19] This is a sobering thought; it means there are continents rather than islands of ignorance in a sea of information, which includes the internet.

More structured approaches to the provision of information for patients include information sheets, videos, DVDs and even educational sessions for groups of people with common conditions (such as antenatal classes for parents-to-be). These approaches are to be applauded, but the personal interaction between the patient and the clinicians involved in an episode of care must be retained and strengthened. This depends on recognizing that communication is a critically important component of healthcare, and building the cost of the necessary time into funding models.

Evidence and Healthcare Professionals

There is little point in having access to large amounts of data if practitioners are unable to interpret or apply it. Most undergraduate curricula for healthcare training now include EBM, and evidence-based practice in nursing is being widely promoted.[20] The key is to integrate the basic theory of EBM into clinical courses, demonstrate the practical application of EBM and include exercises in EBM in the assessment of health sciences students during their exposure to clinical disciplines. The degree to which this sort of educational exercise translates into improved practice is of course strongly influenced by the role-models provided by senior clinicians in their clinical practice. It remains the case that students see many examples of idiosyncratic and unsupportable practice, but the trend towards the greater application of EBM does seem to be gaining momentum.

Evidence and Safety

There is much that can be done to enhance the safety of healthcare by improving the way processes are engineered. One barrier to innovation is funding – there seems to be ongoing reluctance to spend money on safety innovations. One technique used in support of this reluctance is to point out minor imperfections in proposed innovations. The question should be 'will this innovation improve on the status quo?' rather than 'will it be a complete and perfect solution?' Another, discussed above, is an unrealistic demand for evidence. Evidence comes in many forms, and EBM implies using the best evidence available to answer clinical questions. It is simply inappropriate to insist on objective data demonstrating saved lives in RCTs before funding sensible safety initiatives. There are a number of reasons for this, not least because the size of the trials needed to obtain such data would be prohibitive. Moreover these trials are not always needed.[9] Leape, Berwick and Bates summarized the situation in respect of practices aimed at improving patient safety as follows:

'Policymakers must consider the entire experience with safety practices, both in healthcare and in other industries, when deciding which practices should be recommended for widespread use. Evidence from randomized trials is important information, but it is neither sufficient nor necessary for acceptance of a practice. For policymakers to wait for incontrovertible proof of effectiveness before recommending a practice would be a prescription for inaction and an abdication of responsibility. There will never be complete evidence for everything that must be done in medicine. The prudent alternative is to make reasonable judgments based on the best available evidence combined with successful experiences in health care. While some errors in these judgments are inevitable, we believe they will be far outweighed by the improvement in patient safety that will result.'[21]

In fact, it can be difficult to implement practices across the board even when evidence for them is strong. In the USA, a report on Patient Safety Practices was produced by the Evidence Based Practice Centre in San Francisco in response to a recommendation in the Institute of Medicine report 'To Err is Human'.[22] Information was sought for a number of safety practices with respect to: the prevalence and cost of the problem being addressed; the efficacy and risks of the practice; and the cost and other problems of implementing the practice. Eleven of 79 practices identified were judged to have very strong evidence of efficacy and a further 14 to have good evidence. These are listed in Box 11.3. Many of these practices have not been universally adopted, despite the evidence supporting them. A cynical view would be that an expensive new drug, supported by aggressive marketing from a company, will gain widespread acceptance long before a simple measure such as the use of sterile procedures for central line insertion, even if the benefit to risk ratio of the latter is far superior.

Virtually all the measures in Box 11.3 are preventive ones. However, many of the things which have the potential to cause harm to patients cannot necessarily be prevented. There are many safety measures which may not prevent problems, but do allow their early detection and/or facilitate the management of their sequelae.

Box 11.3 Safety practices with very strong or strong evidence of efficacy[22]

Very strong evidence for efficacy
- Appropriate use of venous thromboembolism prophylaxis.
- Appropriate use of perioperative beta-blockers.
- Use of maximum sterile barriers during central venous catheter insertion.
- Appropriate use of antibiotic prophylaxis for surgical patients.
- Asking patients to recall and restate what they have been told.
- Continuous aspiration of subglottic secretions to reduce VAP*.
- Use of pressure-relieving bedding materials to prevent pressure ulcers.
- Use of real-time ultrasound guidance during central line insertion.
- Patient self management of coumadin using home monitoring devices.
- Appropriate nutrition, especially enterally, for critically ill patients.
- Use of antibiotic impregnated cental venous catheters.

Strong evidence for efficacy
- Referring complicated surgery to high volume centres.
- Semi-recumbent positioning to prevent VAP*.
- Using hip protectors to prevent injury after falls.
- Use of computer monitoring for potential adverse drug events.
- Use of supplemental perioperative oxygen.
- Changing nursing staffing to reduce patient morbidity and mortality.
- Use of audio or video information to facilitate informed consent.
- Selective decontamination of the digestive tract to reduce VAP*.
- Active management of intensive care unit patients by an intensivist.
- Information transfer between inpatient and outpatient pharmacies.
- Multi-component delirium prevention.
- Use of a geriatric evaluation and management unit.
- Non-pharmacologic interventions (e.g. relaxation, distraction) for pain.

* VAP: Ventilator-associated pneumonia.

Evidence and Managers

Unfortunately there is no parallel trend towards evidence-based decision-making for managers in healthcare (although there is in public health).[23] In fact, it is not clear that there is very much of what medical scientists would consider as evidence to guide managers in their approach to the overall administration of healthcare.

Given that managers have as much or more impact on the quality of healthcare as clinicians, it does seem sensible for them to be exposed to the concepts of evidence, and to have some understanding of the dimensions of quality and of how to measure these. A good starting point would be an agreed minimal training as a prerequisite to a career in healthcare management.

A major innovative step towards getting the best out of the system would therefore be the regulation of healthcare administrators. In almost every country in the world the requirement for doctors and nurses to be registered is recognized; it is time that similar requirements were implemented for healthcare administrators.

The Local Organizational Layer

In Chapter 3 we outlined the dysfunctional nature of many healthcare organizations. Widespread confusion reigns, with some health services having patient safety officers, risk managers, quality improvement practitioners, nosocomial infection units, epidemiologists, and more, with as many as 15 different reporting and/or management systems all doing essentially the same thing, but using different paradigms.[24] We need to work towards an integrated and more standardized framework, and to ensure that lessons are learnt at all four levels of the 'quadruple-loop learning' shown in Figure 1.5 (see Box 11.9).

This framework needs to encompass both reactive and proactive responses to problems and risks. Reactive responses are represented by the top half of Figure 1.5 and pro-active responses by the bottom half. Nearly all healthcare organizations have some system in place for the reactive responses which are needed after individual incidents, although most could be improved. However, the systems for proactive risk management are far less well developed. One of the reasons for this is that everyone is so busy with everyday work and with reacting to crises that there is no time left for reflection, gathering evidence, and devising and implementing proactive strategies to prevent the very crises that are consuming so much of the time. Another reason is that the currently available tools for data collection and classification are primitive. Finally, everyone has become desensitized to the vagaries of the system and simply accepts its defects and inefficiencies. It is this that we must strive against (see the 'normalization of deviance' on page 233, a failure to respond to obvious deficiencies (see Box 3.1) and the need for a new safety culture on pages 271–273).

Dealing with Individual Incidents – the Reactive Approach

A practical approach to responding to an incident in healthcare has been outlined in Chapter 8. An ideal response when a patient has been harmed is summarized on page 100. The steps to take to prevent a recurrence have been outlined in Chapter 9, including RCA and the actions which follow. After something has gone wrong, people at all levels can put pressure on line managers and administrators to ensure that the right thing is done. The principles of open disclosure need to be properly understood and disseminated, and a transparent and explicit process used if there is any question of culpability (see pages 204–205). It is an organizational responsibility to ensure that healthcare professionals and workers are exposed to multidisciplinary teaching about the concepts covered in this book and how to respond to an incident. Ideally this should be organized at a regional or national level (see pages 240–243).

Risk Management and Tools for Improvement – the Pro-active Approach

The nature of risk and a framework for its management were discussed in Chapter 2. Figure 2.1 should be reviewed now, as it provides the basis for the discussion below.

The context The issue of culture will be discussed at the end of this chapter. There is no doubt that there are pockets of excellence throughout the healthcare system. However, a noticeable feature confirmed by the experience of accreditation organizations, backed up by indicator data, is that excellence is often found in close juxtaposition to pockets of mediocre or sub-standard practice.[25] The factors that combine to create excellence, mediocrity, or poor performance, are the subject of much speculation. Much is made of the importance of leadership, but in these days of fiscal constraint, leadership in the sense of administrative leadership from a particular individual (a CEO for example) is generally very short lived. For example, it was reported in the *Guardian* newspaper that the chief executive of the Shrewsbury and Telford NHS Trust in the UK was the fourth in 10 months. This sort of turnover clearly defeats any possibility of sustained leadership.[26]

Administrators tend to be trapped by their accountability to political masters and their responsibility for constrained budgets. Clinicians tend to stay far longer in the job, and have a primary inalienable responsibility to their patients, rather than bureaucratically dictated devotion to the 'bottom line'. In general, improvement in clinical practice is more likely to be driven and safeguarded by clinicians than by administrators. A shift in the paradigm to reflect this reality in the organizational hierarchies of healthcare would be a major step in the right direction. Other important contextual factors will be considered below.

Identify the risks. Identification of things that go wrong at the organizational level is largely dependent on capturing information after the event (see Figure 1.5, Chapter 9).[27,28] Inappropriate variation in healthcare is harder to characterize, but is also a major risk, because it means that some patients are not receiving the types of care they need, whilst resources are being wasted by exposing other patients to the avoidable risks of unnecessary treatment (see Figure 1.2).[29] The machinery for addressing both of these types of problem at a national level is poorly developed. If organizations collated all the information from the sources in Table 2.5, had a greater commitment to EBM, and better adherence to care pathways and protocols, the extent of the problem could be substantially reduced. An integrated approach is summarized in Figure 1.5.

We have discussed the use of root cause analysis (RCA) to prevent the recurrence of serious adverse events (see Chapter 9). However, only a tiny fraction of the things that go wrong will trigger an RCA. Sixty percent of the resource consumption associated with adverse events is taken up by mundane events which would be highly unlikely to trigger an RCA on their own (although they might, by way of aggregate analysis, if the system is set up to identify recurrent problems).[15] It is at least as important to subject these risks to systematic analysis and evaluation, with a view to dealing with them, as it is to tackle dramatic failures.

Lists of the general categories into which these mundane events fall are given in Chapter 2 (see Tables 2.7 and 2.8). Reporting and analyzing near misses is also important because problems can thereby be addressed before they harm patients. Also, as there are far more near misses than adverse events, they are a valuable source of information for characterizing the individually rare types of events which collectively make up the bulk of the things that go wrong, in order to facilitate the development of corrective strategies for them.[27]

Analyze and evaluate the risks There are several reasons why a particular set of incidents may be chosen for evaluation; some are idiosyncratic.[28]

First, problems are chosen because they are common or routinely consume resources. This is rational, but paradoxically, familiar risks which meet these criteria are often not properly addressed. The best example is smoking, which has a mortality, for smokers, of sixty-fold greater than vehicle accidents, and which is far more easily prevented. An example from anaesthesia is breathing circuit disconnection. This was tolerated for over 40 years after muscle relaxants were introduced, consistently causing brain damage and death, before the routine use of simple devices to detect when disconnection occurred was introduced in the late 1980s. Disconnection is difficult to prevent, but easy to detect with such a device, and easy to manage once detected.

Poor adherence to basic nursing practices[20] and protocols for common conditions also fall into this category (e.g. antenatal care, diabetes, asthma). For a useful list of areas which we now know should be targeted see Figure 1.2.[29]

Second, problems are chosen because, even if rare, they are dangerous and have an obvious solution. Examples include the elimination of concentrated potassium chloride from ward stock, and of Seldinger wires with one sharp end (rather than two floppy ends), which may perforate the heart and cause cardiac tamponade if inadvertently inserted sharp end first.[28]

Third, problems are chosen because they have a particularly abhorrent outcome. A good example in Australia was the tragic case of a young patient who contracted HIV from donor blood, which was a major factor in putting into place very expensive preventive mechanisms to reduce the chance of a recurrence of this disaster (see Box 1.2).

Fourth, issues that are topical tend to receive attention. 'Awareness' under anaesthesia is not uncommon. However, it was only after a well publicized case in a patient who was undergoing a hip replacement that the APSF analyzed their collection of incidents involving vaporizers, and made recommendations that led to the introduction Australia-wide of volatile agent monitors for anaesthetized patients.[27]

This is not a comprehensive list. The point is that a more systematic method of deciding which risks to address would lead to better use of resource.[5] We have discussed the details of RCA in Chapter 9 in relation to individual serious events and to the aggregate analysis of groups of more mundane events. It may be that the best approach would be to coordinate this type of analysis at a national level, as the information and solutions can then be applied across a whole country and, when proven to be cost effective, introduced worldwide (see Box 11.9).[22] It is worth remembering that this is how the lessons from RCA are applied within the VA hospitals in America, and that the VA system serves a population as large as that of Australia, or one third of England.

Treat the risks Some examples of strong, intermediate and weak safety interventions were listed in Table 9.1. An example of *defence in depth*, with the progressive introduction of measures over many years to prevent hypoxic brain damage and death under anaesthesia, is given in Box 11.4. These measures include equipment changes, standardization, forcing functions, crisis management algorithms and redundancy.

Where possible, it is ideal to error-proof the system by design or by a physical forcing function (see page 132).[30] This is not always easy. It is important to recognize the strengths of humans, and to understand that people are better than machines at doing certain things. The concept of 'soft engineering' involves design that combines human strengths with the strengths of machines, allocating tasks appropriately between the two (see Page 125) .[31] It is extraordinary how many entrenched practices and processes fly in the face of this concept. Relying on memory for drug doses and interactions, or expecting an anaesthetist to remain vigilant and detect gas leaks and circuit disconnections throughout their working days and nights, for decades, are both examples of expecting machine-like perfection for tasks in which human failure is absolutely guaranteed.

Box 11.4 Preventing brain damage and death from hypoxia during anaesthesia – defence in depth

Preventing hypoxic gas mixtures
- Using bulk gas supplies with alarms and reserve systems.
- Using colour coding for pipelines, hoses and backup cylinders.
- Using standard gas-specific connections to prevent misconnections.
- Installing audible alarms for failing oxygen supplies.
- Using banks of flow meters which cannot deliver less than 21 per cent oxygen.

Detecting hypoxic gas mixtures and their consequences
- Using oxygen analyzers in line in the breathing circuit.
- Using pulse oximeters for detecting inadequate oxygenation of the blood.
- Using capnographs for detecting misplaced tubes and inadequate. Ventilation.

Managing the situation after detection
- Using standard validated crisis management algorithms for systematically dealing with failures of tissue oxygenation when these do occur (because of hypoxic mixtures, misplaced tubes and inadequate ventilation and tissue oxygen delivery from a variety of causes).

Conversely, some machines are designed to fail when least expected. When 14 disconnect alarms were evaluated in the early 1990s, remarkably, nine were found to have no power failure alarm or battery backup.[32] Systems comprise humans and technology: the trick is to optimize the roles and performance of each, and, more particularly, to make sure they can function safely together.

Monitor and review – PDCA Quality improvement depends on repeating the following steps over and over again: identifying the problems, evaluating and analyzing them and then treating or managing them, followed by monitoring and reviewing the problems again. This is essentially identical to the PDCA cycle (Plan-Do-Check-Act) or PDSA cycle (with S standing for Study) (Figures 11.2 and 1.5), which was originally conceived by Walter Shewhart in the 1930s, and later adopted by W. Edwards Deming.[6] This cycle has been widely adopted as a model for quality improvement in healthcare, with the concept of a *ramp of improvement* as each turn of the cycle takes the state of quality progressively higher than the turns before (see Figure 11.2).

Getting the best out of the system

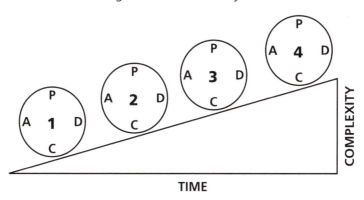

TIME

Figure 11.2   The PDCA cycle and ramp representing a process for progressive improvements of quality in organizations[33]

Consult and communicate[34] Major problems with introducing change (turning research into practice) are now well recognized (see pages 215–216). Getting people 'on board' before the implementation of a new strategy is absolutely vital. A critique of the available methods is presented in Appendix IX. The 'soft systems' approach outlined in Chapter 9 and in Appendix IX provides a structured way to gain acceptance and ownership of a change.

Risk registers[35] Problems which have been identified which are beyond the control of an organization, or which can be properly addressed only when further technology or extra funding is available, should be placed on a risk register pending a definitive solution. One example, in response to the fatal event described in Box 3.3, would be a call for a decision support system to automatically identify drug interactions as part of a computer order entry system for prescribing drugs. Such a system would flag potential interactions such as the one between coumadin and certain antibiotics, both at the time of prescribing and at the time of dispensing, and suggest safer alternatives.[36] Another example, in response to the lack of capacity to train and credential intensive care nursing staff operating complex equipment (see Box 3.1), would be to log this problem on a risk register pending the allocation of the necessary funds. Logging problems onto a risk register is a mechanism by which clinicians can formally draw attention to deficiencies, and put pressure on administrators and funders to acknowledge that there is a problem that needs addressing. Once an area of risk has been identified, there are several proactive methods for systematically prioritizing problems and identifying solutions; two are shown in Figure 1.5 and are discussed below.

Failure mode and effects analysis (FMEA)[37,38] FMEA is a proactive process aimed at predicting the nature and effect of equipment and system failures. Each component or stage is examined in turn to determine how it may fail with a view to identifying preventive or corrective measures. The Institute for Safe Medical Practice has been using FMEA to 'examine the products and the design of new services and processes to determine points of potential failure and what their effect would be – before error actually happens'.[39]

Sociotechnical-probabilistic risk analysis (ST-PRA)[40] FMEA can identify the effects or failures by working forward and considering all possibilities. Probabilistic risk analysis starts with an outcome, and works backwards by progressively constructing a fault tree. When the model includes the contributions of human error the process is known as sociotechnical probabilistic risk analysis (ST-PRA). ST-PRA starts with an undesirable outcome and then investigates and models all combinations of process and equipment failures that may lead to it. A technical description of this complex modeling tool is beyond the scope of this book. It was developed in the 1970s to improve safety in the nuclear power industry, and, using 'fault tree' software, can suggest priorities for preventive and corrective strategies such as building double checks and forcing functions into a system to ensure that certain dangerous components or stages are error proofed. An example would be introducing unique connectors for nasogastric, intravenous and intrathecal tubes or catheters to prevent misconnection, analogous to the small, matched filling nozzles and ports for unleaded petrol.

One Hill at a Time[7]

Another of Donald Berwick's aphorisms is the exhortation to 'take one hill at a time' (the analogy being to an invading army controlling one objective at a time, rather than attempting to invade an entire country at once). The tendency has been for national patient safety organizations to produce above down initiatives, such as standards for credentialling or open disclosure which, whilst commendable and necessary, do nothing to address specific problems at the level of interactions between patients and the machinery of healthcare. In fact, most of the risk in healthcare is related to thousands of specific, mostly uncommon problems, each of which need tailored solutions. Although such problems need to be identified locally and local corrective strategies are needed, the solutions should ideally be disseminated and applied nationally and internationally (see Box 11.5).

The breakthrough technique Donald Berwick and his organization, International Healthcare Improvement (IHI) pioneered and disseminated this technique. Once a problem area has been identified, a small team facilitates the PDSA cycle to as many aspects of the problem as practicable. The process emphasizes 'thinking outside the box' and involves everyone in coming up with innovative methods to solve problems. It recognizes the wealth of experience and expertise that frontline clinicians have in understanding many of the underlying problems. It taps into and changes the hidden culture and can be a very powerful force for change from passive acceptance to active intervention.[41,42]

Box 11.5 A potentially fatal dose error

One of the authors was taking methotrexate, a drug which in overdose can wipe out the bone marrow and produce a fatal depletion of white blood cells. He ran out of medication and got a prescription from a physician friend for a new supply. He was taking eight 2.5mg tablets per week. When he reached the end of his new supply of 200 tablets, he looked at the bottle for the first time, and noticed the tablets were 10mg, not 2.5mg. He had been unaware of the existence of an absolutely identical small yellow tablet which was four times the strength of the usual one. This problem has in fact been reported repeatedly, and fatalities are inevitable whilst the situation is allowed to persist. The solution is to eliminate the availability of the identical 10mg tablets, which serve no real purpose. This should ideally be done at both national and international levels, which would represent an example of quadruple-loop learning (see Box 11.9). This problem, like thousands of other specific problems, is not amenable to solution by above down exhortations.

The Regional or National Layer

The topics considered at this level are those which are not usually under the control of individual healthcare facilities or organizations. These are often problematic for healthcare administrators at the organizational level. In effect, others dictate the environment in which the organization has to operate, and in doing so often create intrinsically conflicting demands. For example, directives may come from on high that an emergency department is to continue to take all comers, whilst the hospital may be full and the emergency department understaffed or staffed with inadequately trained people. Hospitals may thus be forced to lurch from one crisis to another, with senior health administrators, often at the behest of politicians, micro-managing visible problems, without regard to the flow-on consequences to the rest of the organization. Clinicians then have to cope at the level of the individual patient in sub-optimal circumstances created by people over whom they too have no control.

These top-down edicts often consume resources allocated to and needed for other areas of practice (such as improving safety), in an environment with a fixed budget. Putting extra resources into reducing waiting lists whilst hospitals are operating at full capacity is commonplace, in spite of the fact that this can only be done at the expense of the timely management of acute cases. There is now good evidence that prolonged delays in emergency departments and full, gridlocked hospitals are associated with increased morbidity and mortality for patients[43] and high turnover of the stressed staff (see Box 11.6).[44] To improve the system, therefore, initiatives at the regional or national level should be grounded (but seldom are) in the realities of the individual and organizational levels.

Box 11.6 Going solid[45]

Going solid is a slang term in the nuclear industry for when a nuclear power plant goes into a safety critical situation (when all the water in the boiler has become steam). This is a highly volatile and very dangerous situation. A gridlocked hospital, in which patient flow is blocked by rate limiting bottlenecks, has been likened to this situation. Hospitals frequently 'go solid' when they relentlessly continue to do elective surgery because the hospital depends on the bonus money for shortening waiting lists, whilst they have insufficient staff to operate in a timely manner on the patients who are arriving at the emergency department (see Box 10.5). This is fundamentally unethical as patient welfare is being traded for political credit.

Regulation and Accreditation

Accreditation – the current state of play Accreditation is the formal process for certifying that a healthcare facility complies with agreed (ideally predefined) standards. In the USA accreditation by the Joint Commission for Accreditation of Healthcare Organizations (JCAHO) is required to obtain reimbursement from Medicare and Medicaid (healthcare funding for the elderly and poor respectively). In many other countries accreditation is currently not compulsory, and is not as comprehensive. In most systems, little can be done when facilities fail to meet agreed standards, other than putting them on notice that they will be inspected again within a shorter time than usual.

Traditionally, accreditation is considered under the headings structure, process and outcome, as originally proposed by Donabedian.[46] *Structure* includes buildings, equipment, personnel, policies and governance. *Process* describes the protocols and clinical pathways that should be in place; both administrative and clinical processes can be subject to accreditation. For example there could be a requirement that every patient undergoing surgery should be seen by the surgeon and an anaesthetist pre-operatively, and that certain records should be created and be available for audit. Formal clinical pathways (see page 235) should be used for common diseases and procedures; this allows deviations from these pathways to be identified and audited. *Outcomes* are obviously all that really matter in the end, but these are difficult to measure with the current state of documentation in healthcare. Indicators are commonly collected which may estimate the rates of compliance with certain processes and outcomes (for example the fraction of eligible patients who receive deep vein thrombosis prophylaxis, or the number of patients who get a wound infection).[47] These collections have suffered from a lack of rigor with respect to definition, risk adjustment and reliability. For example, many wound infections manifest after discharge, and are lost to follow-up. A problem with many indicators is that if the rates do fall outside certain limits, information about how or why this may be is often lacking.

Regulation and accreditation – some suggestions We indicated at the end of Chapter 7 that substandard, idiosyncratic clinical practices and regular corporate violations continue to be commonly encountered in healthcare, in part because of ineffective, piecemeal regulation. Figure 7.1 shows that at least ten organizations are involved in the regulation of healthcare, but that no organization has any real accountability at any level, and none is involved across all levels. Many of those which are influential at Levels I and II (self regulation) have little or no regulatory power. Those which have regulatory power (Level IV) are not currently involved in promoting or maintaining the standard of clinical care. Meta-regulation (checking that self-regulation is satisfactory, Level III), as indicated above, is often voluntary and the indicators collected open to gaming. Finally, a fundamental element of any regulatory system is the meaningful prospect of escalating sanctions for persistent non-compliance. This is poorly developed in healthcare, both for individuals and organizations. It is necessary not only to set standards and monitor compliance, but also to apply progressive sanctions when standards are not met.

It must not be forgotten that there is an enormous amount of goodwill, expertise, energy and altruism which, properly harnessed, could deliver far safer, better healthcare than we experience today. Indeed, these attributes of the workforce keep the 'show on the road' and safeguard and improve the prospects of many patients trapped in the sub-optimal systems of the present time. There are three major challenges if we are to move towards improving the system through regulation and accreditation – to set standards, monitor compliance and develop sanctions.

Setting standards There is information about what should be addressed.[15,22,48] Highly credible groups should be established to examine the evidence, promulgate national standards, and develop tools to validate compliance with these standards, ideally as part of routine documentation. These groups would be responsible for defining 'best practice' for each process and keeping these definitions and the tools for monitoring compliance up to date. Specialist colleges, craft groups and consumer groups should be invited to identify appropriate people to participate, and should play a major role in these processes. Overall coordination and formal endorsement would be via organizations such as the National Centre for Patient Safety in the USA,[49] the National Institute for Health and Clinical Excellence in the UK,[50] the National Institute for Clinical Studies[51] or the Australian Commission for Safety and Quality in Health Care;[52] there are candidate organizations in all countries. Many have already made a good start in improving the safety of healthcare, but most would benefit from having a more formal role for national experts in the relevant topics.

The concept of standard operating procedures (see page 235) would have to be accepted by all concerned, as it is in aviation. A randomized control trial is not necessary to require an anaesthetist to label syringes, nor is such a trial necessary to require prescribers of medications to use a standard set of abbreviations on a standard order form. Likewise, compliance with standard regimes for obtaining consent, for thromboembolism prophylaxis or for investigating and treating essential hypertension, or a host of other common problems, should be required. It is not necessary for these standard operating procedures to be perfect, so long as they are sound (a completely different concept). Compliance with them will be far more effective in promoting good outcomes for patients than the current confusion in which everyone does something different. When deviation from standard operating procedures is necessary, practitioners would simply be required to record the reasons for this. These reasons should then be audited. A start should be made at the basic end of the spectrum. Standard procedures and protocols are already being made available on desktop or bed side computers and on personal digital assistants or palm-tops; compliance tools should be incorporated into standard charts and records (see Chapter 12).

Monitoring compliance Establishing genuine meta-regulation is clearly essential.[53] Ideally the process should involve certified external accreditation organizations which should randomly select certain people, units or aspects of clinical and corporate practice to audit, arrive unannounced, and check compliance against predefined standards. JCAHO in the United States has shown that when inspections take place unannounced, demonstration of compliance with standards falls from 98 per cent to as low as 60 per cent.[54] It is therefore clearly desirable that this should be the practice.

For example, the medical records of 10 patients who have been managed by a surgeon could be randomly selected and examined for adequacy of documentation, appropriate management of prophylaxis for wound infection and thromboembolism, and evidence of a timely, adequate discharge letter. Different standards could be chosen randomly for audit on successive visits. Only small samples would be needed, given the current low levels of compliance with basic indicators.[29,55] The surveyors should, ideally, be clinicians in the relevant disciplines and surveying could be a standard component of professional life. In this way, compliance could be checked at individual, unit, department or practice levels by regular reviews of medical records by peers using tools which should be developed as integral parts of the standards.

Standards for corporate behaviour, infrastructure and administrative processes should be agreed upon and be explicit, as it is currently possible for managers to give the impression that certain standards and protocols are routinely complied with, when in fact they are not. The suggestion is made below that anyone should be able to report violations of corporate standards.

Developing sanctions Perhaps the greatest of the three challenges will be the development of sanctions which are incremental, effective and feasible, but allow the delivery of healthcare to continue. Many practitioners perform highly-valued services in an impeccable manner from the vast majority of perspectives, but we have given many examples in this book in which failures occur, often in circumscribed aspects of practice. Non-compliance with agreed standards of best practice should initiate an escalating series of responses, starting with a discussion about the reasons for the non-compliance and ending, with a referral to the relevant registration board for review. Measures taken at this stage might include retraining and counseling (see page 172-174). This would provide sufficient incentive for change in the vast majority of cases. Continuing failure to respond could result in public reporting of the individual and listing the nature of the breaches. Deregulation would be the ultimate sanction for seriously non-compliant individuals.

Corporate non-compliance should be handled in a similarly escalating way, with counseling, loss of accreditation and adverse publicity. Healthcare professionals should perhaps be given the right to log (anonymously if they wish) corporate non-compliance on a risk register. Attention would have to be paid to principles of natural justice (as indeed it would in cases of individual non-compliance). If such a complaint is validated, the response by the organization should also be logged. A risk not addressed within a timeframe defined in each relevant standard could be posted by the accreditation organization on the internet for public surveillance.

In summary, we have good evidence that there is a problem with standards in healthcare, and that trying to change clinical and corporate practices through persuasion and current conventional administrative processes produces unacceptably poor results (see Appendix IX). Experience from other areas which require behavioural change, such as drunk-driving, or violating safe rostering practices in the transport industry, indicate that the proactive use of clear standards backed by progressively escalating sanctions can be effective in overcoming inertia and producing a lasting cultural change.

Ethics, Under-funding and Rationing[56]

The amount spent on healthcare by different countries varies greatly (see Figure 1.3), as does the distribution of funds within each country. Regardless of this, however, every country faces the problem that all that is wanted is not affordable, and the gap is likely to widen progressively as more people survive for longer and seek evermore expensive (and effective) treatments.

We have discussed the massive but futile disruptions associated with restructuring, produced in the hope of increasing efficiency. The ubiquitous variability in healthcare is a manifestation of huge inefficiencies right across the system, yet, surprisingly, few resources are directed towards systematically addressing this issue. In Chapter 1 we presented a utilitarian argument for preferentially funding those interventions and improvements which are most cost effective.

To do otherwise is unethical. If a dollar is wasted on a less cost effective treatment, then it cannot be spent on a more cost effective treatment. It is testament to the institutionalized irrationality that pervades healthcare that interventions such as hip replacement and cataract removal, which are amongst the most cost effective of all procedures, are those most commonly rationed by having the longest waiting lists.

Rationing generally ends up affecting the disenfranchised, poor, elderly or infirm, and has been defined as occurring 'when anyone is denied (or simply not offered) an intervention that everyone agrees would do them some good and which they would like to have'.[56] It has been proposed that this extraordinary state of affairs persists because of powerful supply side advocacy. Much healthcare funding ends up either in the coffers of the pharmaceutical or device industries or in the bank accounts of the healthcare workforce, and these powerful vested interests continuously pursue the new, exciting or remunerative at the expense of the mundane. A 'chronic lack of transparency in decision making and accountability for actions' allows the situation to be perpetuated. The status quo continues because of 'lack of public awareness, fear of ill health and death and the political dynamics of the healthcare market-place' which 'obscure the limitations of the knowledge base and facilitate the dominance of "experts" who declare that under funding is *the* policy problem'.[56]

If explicit transparent rationing was to be put in place, the threshold for what is funded and what is not could be determined by public debate, based on best evidence (which would have to be collated and made available in an easy-to-understand format).[57] Society could then focus on whether more or less should be spent on healthcare, with a tangible basis for decision-making. The challenge is to modulate the demands of those who stand to gain from an injection of more funds. Public opinion cannot easily be mobilized whilst the problem is diffuse and mysterious. Focusing the debate will allow a collective response about how government funds should be allocated.

Maynard states: 'A health service in "political denial" stunts the development of socially agreed rationing principles that are openly discussed and accountably applied, and creates a market of special pleading on both the demand (for example, patient advocacy groups) and supply sides (for example, the pharmaceutical industry)'.[56]

In many countries there is virtually no ongoing large scale evaluation or re-evaluation of the cost effectiveness of services provided, no financial incentives for providing evidence-based care and no attention paid to trying to determine what the objectives of society are.[58] In each country the threshold for funding basic healthcare should be determined by public debate, informed by syntheses of the best available evidence.

Restructuring Versus Redesigning[59,60]

An almost reflex response of politicians and senior bureaucrats to crises in healthcare has been to restructure (see Chapter 3). The repeated disruptions damage the perceptions of job security – one of the few (now partially defunct) magnets to attract staff to the public sector. The wave of restructuring has been likened to a global epidemic starting from a single source of infection in Baltimore in 1983. Of 20 teaching hospitals in Australia surveyed over a six year period, 12 underwent restructuring once, and four twice.[59]

It has now been shown that restructuring causes considerable disruption to services[60] and does not result in any increase in efficiency, in spite of this being the stated objective in three quarters of cases.[59] Moreover, three quarters of physicians surveyed reported no improvement in patient care. It is important to distinguish restructuring from redesigning patient care. Restructuring reorganizes the hierarchical structure of organizations, usually affecting people from head of unit upwards to the highest positions in a department of health. Many of the people adversely affected are the very clinical leaders who need some stability as a platform from which to redesign the processes of healthcare. Examples of redesign are given in Boxes 11.5 and 11.9.

Looking After the People[44,61]

Much of Chapter 10 was given over to what patients, clinicians, teams and clinical managers can do to safeguard safety and provide high quality care. Their efforts can be greatly enhanced by good morale. This implies a working environment in which there are adequate numbers of qualified people, and a culture which fosters cooperation and teamwork centred around patient care. Unfortunately, many healthcare professionals feel that they are being forced to work under conditions which are unfair both to their patients and themselves (see Chapter 3). It has been shown in at least seven widely diverse countries, that hospitals with poor working environments and inadequately trained and poorly supported staff are at heightened risk for adverse events. A review of 15 studies exploring hospital attributes and medical and nursing care made recommendations to:[44]

- 'maximize the proportion of registered nurses and baccalaureate prepared registered nurses in hospital nursing staff
- develop and implement initiatives designed to strengthen collaborative relationships between nurses and physicians
- maximize the proportion of board certified medical specialist care providers in hospital medical staff
- establish and sustain clinical nursing support systems to enhance the delivery of patient care'

An editorial which accompanied the publication of this review added two more recommendations:[61]

- 'that clinicians and leaders must realize that improving safety in healthcare is not only a matter of implementing new and improved procedures and equipment (such as computerized provider order entry) but is also about fundamentally rethinking the environment in which care is delivered; and
- that stakeholders must realize that positive organizational features in hospitals and other healthcare settings … do not appear spontaneously, nor do they usually exist in isolation. They are put in place and maintained over time by skilful managers and executives who operate from a vision of patient care driven by an understanding of patient needs.'

Dissatisfaction with working conditions has led to a progressive increase in the number of doctors working only part time in the public sector (where this is possible), and a huge increase in the number of nurses working through agencies. Not only is this more expensive for the institutions who employ them, but it is also unsafe. Many agency nurses have had limited exposure to the hospitals in which they work, and are unfamiliar with local protocols and practices. Moreover, there are usually no requirements for them to become familiar with these practices and protocols. The point is often missed that measures which reduce risk for staff, or in other ways improve their working environment, are actually very much in the interests of patients. This has relevance at the organizational level, but also needs to be understood at higher levels, where many of the pressures originate which lead to poor conditions for staff.

Accountability Versus Learning – Statutory Immunity[62,63,64]

An important debate is still under way with respect to the inherent conflict between accountability and learning. On the one hand it is clearly desirable that facts and figures about the performance of clinicians, departments, units and healthcare facilities be available in a manner that provides accessible information to guide choice. On the other hand, iatrogenic harm is not always acknowledged and the true causes are often not forthcoming, because those involved feel threatened (see Boxes 3.3 and 3.8). To address this deficiency we described a two stage process for allowing the basic facts to be obtained whilst also facilitating a learning process (see Chapter 9). This learning process requires statutory immunity.

It is highly desirable for those involved in an adverse event to express their opinions early, frankly and freely. Statutory immunity provides a safe way for people to participate in identifying and correcting problems quickly, that might take years to deal with through the courts. It also protects these people from (possibly undue) criticism within their workplace. Mutual trust between healthcare professionals is as important as mutual trust between patients and healthcare professionals. The existence of penalties for disclosing any information or opinions brought into existence during quality and safety activities is a vital safeguard. Statutory immunity also generally prevents information brought into existence for these purposes from being admissible in a court of law. This is also of fundamental importance.

In Australia there are provisions for statutory immunity of one sort or another in the federal arena, and in each of the states. In the USA a bill has passed through Congress providing statutory immunity for reports which go to declared patient safety organizations.[63] Such provisions are increasingly being introduced around the world. A far reaching act was passed in Denmark by which immunity is given even for criminal offences which come to light as a result of a confidential patient safety investigation.[64] The UK is a notable exception, with no such provision. Provisions for confidentiality, and for anonymous reporting, where necessary, are also important. The administrative processes for accountability and for learning should be quite separate, but should inform each other. The generic information from each should be available to all involved in improving patient safety.

A Just Culture[65]

Leaders in the patient safety movement have emphasized the need for a 'just culture' and the importance of distinguishing between human error and morally culpable behaviour.[65,66,67] We have discussed this in Chapter 9 (see page 202–205).

The International Level

Safe, high quality healthcare should be everyone's business (see Chapters 1 and 12), not only because some issues cross international boundaries (such as control of infectious diseases), but for basic humanitarian and ethical reasons. There should be mechanisms for the lessons learnt in the more affluent countries to be applied appropriately in countries which may not have the resources to properly characterize the problems or develop solutions.

Some of the foundations for reliability in healthcare need to be established at an international level, in the same way as measures to improve airline safety have been systematically applied at an international level for decades. It is only recently that the necessity for global measures to improve patient safety has been accepted. In May 2002, the World Health Organization (WHO) Assembly passed a resolution on patient safety and set out four proposed areas for action (see Box 11.7).[68]

The WHO Resolution on Patient Safety – Four Action Areas

This resolution paves the way for international co-operation to improve patient safety in all countries, rich and poor. The potential for dissemination of educational materials, standards, guidelines and safety initiatives has been hugely enhanced by the global uptake of the internet. To provide a vehicle for these initiatives a World Alliance for Patient Safety was launched in October 2004.[69] There are six initiatives that are underway (see next section).

Box 11.7 The WHO resolution on patient safety: four action areas[68]

- Determination of global norms, standards and guidelines for the definition, measurement and reporting of adverse events and near misses in health care and the provision of support to countries in developing reporting systems, taking preventive action, and implementing measures to reduce risks.
- Promotion of framing of evidence-based policies including global standards that will improve patient care, with particular emphasis on such aspects as product safety, safe clinical practice in compliance with appropriate guidelines and safe use of medicinal products and medical devices, and creation of a culture of safety within healthcare organizations.
- Development of mechanisms, through accreditation and other means, to recognize the characteristics of healthcare providers that offer a benchmark for excellence in patient safety internationally.
- Encouragement of research into patient safety.

The World Alliance for Patient Safety – Six Initiatives

The World Alliance for Patient Safety has six initial initiatives (see Box 11.8). The first of these, a global patient safety challenge, is to be a rolling program of such challenges, with major projects open to every WHO member state. These challenges will run over two year cycles and are intended to be sustainable. The project for 2005 and 2006 was healthcare associated infection.[70] It was chosen because it is a massive problem with a huge financial burden. Data from the UK and the USA show that hospitals may lose as much as four to five thousand dollars for each nosocomial infection; also it is the second most common adverse event (see page 43). The WHO already has programmes in place of relevance to this problem. These include getting rid of unsafe injection practices, eliminating transmission of HIV through unsafe healthcare procedures and eliminating transmission of infection by blood transfusion. The program targets five action areas: clean hands; clean practices; clean products; clean environment; and clean equipment. The plan is to use evidence-based practices, to engage patients, service users and healthcare providers and to ensure the sustainability of all actions beyond the initial two year period.

Other international organizations have also recognized the importance of patient safety. For example, in 2004, the World Federation of Societies of Anaesthesiologists elevated its (formerly minor) Safety and Quality of Practice Committee to the status of a standing (or major) committee. The International

Society for Quality in Healthcare has safety as part of its brief in setting standards for accreditation.[71] This type of action provides moral support for the cause of safety and quality in healthcare, and has already led to some initiatives which may have far reaching benefits in the developing world. Organizations of this sort are often constrained financially, but have unusually good opportunities to disseminate information, identify common ground, promote discussion and inspire and motivate individuals throughout the world to contribute to enhancing the safety and quality of healthcare.

Box 11.8 The World Alliance for Patient Safety Initiatives[69]

- A global patient safety challenge.
- An ongoing project for patient and consumer involvement.
- A project to develop a world patient safety classification as part of the family of WHO international classifications.
- Research in the field of patient safety.
- Solutions to reduce the risks of healthcare and improve its safety.
- Reporting and learning to improve patient safety.

Quadruple-loop Learning

The PDCA cycle tends to be thought of as an iterative process taking place at one level (usually within an organization) over time. The cycles can, however, loop through successively higher levels of the system, with lessons first learned by individuals finally finding endorsement and being applied at the national or international levels (see Figure 1.5 and Box 11.9).

Changing the Culture of Healthcare

The great call to arms of the safety and quality movement in healthcare is a cry for a fundamental change in culture. The idea that the culture of healthcare is dysfunctional and that this lies at the root of much of what is wrong in healthcare has been widely canvassed. In Chapter 3, we pointed out that we had made huge advances in the science and technology of medicine over the last 200 years, but have not been able to realize all the potential benefits of these advances because of deficiencies in the way that individuals and organizations behave. Expressed another way, we have not developed the cultural competence to handle these advances. How then can we improve the culture of the healthcare system? This question is not easily answered. If it was, the improvement would already have happened, because, as we have intimated many times in this book, the problem is not one of mal-intent, but one of good intentions being poorly directed and executed.

Box 11.9   An example of quadruple-loop learning: oximetry and capnography in anaesthesia[24]

In the mid to late 1980s individual anaesthetists started using oximetry (which allows heartbeat-by-heartbeat monitoring of the oxygen saturation of haemoglobin) and capnography (which allows breath-by-breath monitoring of carbon dioxide). The applications and limitations of these techniques were discussed at unit or departmental level (single-loop learning). Unit and departmental managers then tried to have these devices introduced for every case. This was resisted by hospital managers on the grounds of expense, and there was only partial success in achieving double-loop learning. In Australia, a national meeting was then called and a symposium issue of the journal Anaesthesia and Intensive Care produced as a result, which called for national monitoring standards.[72,73] The Australian and New Zealand College of Anaesthetists then mandated the use of oximetry and capnography for every case (triple-loop learning).[74] All of this was supported by incident monitoring data from anaesthetists in both these countries from mid-1988. In 1993 another symposium issue was produced in which analyses of the first 2,000 incidents reported to the Australian Incident Monitoring Study (AIMS) were presented.[75] These showed that half of all incidents under anaesthesia were first detected by a monitor, and that the combination of oximetry and capnography would have detected 90 per cent of these.[76] This information had a major impact on the International Standard for Anaesthesia Safety which was endorsed by the World Federation of Societies of Anaesthesiologists (with about 100 member countries) at a meeting in the Hague in 1994 (quadruple-loop learning).[77,78,79] Feedback at subsequent meetings of this Society has confirmed that these standards had a major impact in influencing countries to purchase appropriate monitoring devices ahead of equipment which previously would have taken precedent, such as compressed gas anaesthetic machines and electrocardiographs. In a recent review of 4,000 incidents and more than 1,200 medicolegal reports there were no cases of brain damage or death due to undetected oesophageal intubation or inadequate ventilation during anaesthesia in Australia over 5 years, in marked contrast to the situation which prevailed before the introduction of oximetry and capnography.[80]

In Chapter 10 we emphasize the importance of the individual patients and clinicians in healthcare. There are a number of attributes one might identify as desirable in a clinician. These can be categorized as those related to knowledge, skill and behaviour (Figure 10.2). The need for extensive knowledge and considerable skill is self-evident, but in any department there are, amongst the cognoscenti, clinicians held out as the doctors or nurses to choose for given situations, and others perceived to be the doctors or nurses to avoid. Often this relates not to any particular differences in skill or knowledge, but to subtle attributes that might be collectively called the *X-factor*. The tangible manifestation of this X-factor is in the individuals' behaviour.

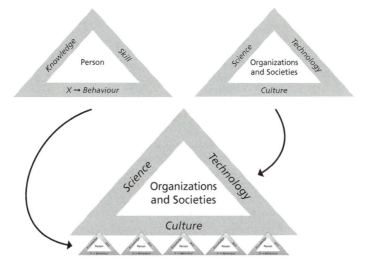

Figure 11.3 **The attributes of an individual clinician (top left) and of an organization (top right), each depicted as three sides of a safety triangle. The culture of an organization reflects the collective behavioural attributes of the individuals within it (the large triangle)**

In a similar way, there are a number of attributes one might identify as desirable in an organization. These can be categorized as those related to its empirical and scientific knowledge (its 'science'), those related to its technology, and those related to its culture (Figure 11.3). Again, amongst the cognoscenti, some organizations are considered to have a great culture and others a poor one.

The culture of an organization or system can be seen as reflecting the collective attributes of the individuals within it. The skills and knowledge of individuals are in the end closely aligned to the state of science and technology in society – the abilities of a surgeon in 2006 are different from those of one in 1750. Behaviour is influenced by skill and knowledge, but also by the behaviour of those with whom one works.

If one works in an organization in which the focus is strongly on safety, one is likely to develop a personal focus on safety and behave in safer ways. By contrast if the culture is focused on throughput and tolerates carelessness, one is more likely to tolerate carelessness in ones colleagues and to behave carelessly oneself. Behaviour is modified by the prevailing culture, but, in a cyclical way, behaviour creates and reinforces that very culture. In fact, the culture of any group is little more than a manifestation of the collective attitudes and behaviours of the individuals within it. It follows that the key to changing the culture of a system is to change the behaviour of the individuals within it. This change must begin with one's own behaviour.

Notes

1 Kohn, L.T., Corrigan, J.M. and Donaldson, M.S., eds (2000), *To Err is Human: Building a Safer Health System* (Washington: Committee on Quality of Health Care in America, Institute of Medicine, National Academies Press).

2 National Health Service Modernisation Agency (2005), *Improvement Leaders' Guide to Building and Nurturing an Improvement Culture* (London: Department of Health).

3 Brennan, T.A. et al. (2005), 'Accidental Deaths, Saved Lives, and Improved Quality', *New England Journal of Medicine* 353:13, 1405–9.

4 Australian Council for Safety and Quality in Health Care (2005), 'Medication Alert! Vincristine Can Be Fatal If Administered by the Intrathecal Route', *Alert* 2, December. Available at: http://www.safetyandquality.gov.au/council/vincristine/index.htm.

5 Personal communication from Professor Sir Liam Donaldson, Chief Medical Officer of the National Health Service in the United Kingdom, and Maureen Robinson, Christy Pirone and Dorothy Jones who have been responsible for implementing such initiatives system-wide in Australia.

6 William Edwards Deming was an electrical engineer (with a PhD in mathematics and mathematical physics from Yale) and musician who lived in Washington DC. He is renowned for his contributions to the theoretical understanding of quality control in industry. *The W. Edwards Deming Institute*, historical biography [web-page] http://www.deming.org/theman/biography.html accessed 11 April 2006.

7 Berwick, D.M. (1996), 'A Primer on Leading the Improvement of Systems', *British Medical Journal* 312:7031, 619–22.

8 Perneger, T.V. (2005), 'Investigating Safety Incidents: More Epidemiology Please', *International Journal for Quality in Health Care* 17:1, 1–3.

9 Runciman, W.B. (1993), 'Qualitative Versus Quantitative Research – Balancing Cost, Yield and Feasibility', *Anaesthesia and Intensive Care* 21:5, 502–5.

10 Lagasse, R.S. (2002), 'Anaesthesia Safety: Model or Myth? A Review of the Published Literature and Analysis of Current Original Data', *Anesthesiology* 97:6, 1609–17.

11 Mackay, P. ed. (2002), *Safety of Anaesthesia in Australia. A Review of Anaesthesia-Related Mortality 1997–1999* (Melbourne: Australian and New Zealand College of Anaesthetists).

12 Gibbs, N. and Borton, C. (2006), *Safety of Anaesthesia in Australia: A Review of Anaesthesia-Related Mortality 2000–2002* (Melbourne: Australian and New Zealand College of Anaesthetists).

13 Webster, C.W. (2004), *Implementation and Assessment of a New Integrated Drug Administration System (IDAS) as an Example of a Safety Intervention in a Complex Socio-Technological Workplace*, Ph.D. Thesis (Auckland: University of Auckland).

14 Toft, B. (2001), *External Inquiry into the Adverse Incident That Occurred at Queen's Medical Centre, Nottingham* (London: Department of Health).

15 Runciman, W.B., Edmonds, M.J. and Pradhan, M. (2002), 'Setting Priorities for Patient Safety', *Quality and Safety in Health Care* 11:3, 224–9.

16 Clinton, H.R. and Obama, B. (2006), 'Making Patient Safety the Centerpiece of Medical Liability Reform', *New England Journal of Medicine* 354:21, 2205–8.

17 World Health Organization, World Alliance for Patient Safety, *International Patient Safety Event Taxonomy* [web page]: http://www.who.int/patientsafety/taxonomy/en/ accessed 5 Jun 2006.

18 Institute of Medicine Committee on Quality of Health Care in America (2001), *Crossing the Quality Chasm: a New Health System for the 21st Century* (Washington DC: National Academies Press).

19 MacLennan, A.H., Myers, S.P. and Taylor, A.W. (2006), 'The Continuing Use of Complementary and Alternative Medicine in South Australia: Costs and Beliefs in 2004', *Medical Journal of Australia* 184:1, 27–31.

20 The *International Journal of Evidence-Based Healthcare* (formerly JBI Reports), the Joanna Briggs Institute, Blackwell Publishing. The Journal is available online at Blackwell Synergy www.blackwell-synergy.com and provides reports on systematic reviews and meta-analyses of nursing practices.

21 Leape, L.L., Berwick, D.M. and Bates D.W. (2002). 'What Practices Will Most Improve Safety? Evidence-Based Medicine Meets Patient Safety', *Journal of the American Medical Association* 288:4, 501–7.

22 Shojania, K.G. et al. (2001), *Making Health Care Safer: a Critical Analysis of Patient Safety Practices,* Evidence Report/Technology Assessment No. 43 (Rockville, Maryland: Agency for Healthcare Research and Quality).

23 Brownson, R.C. et al. (2003), *Evidence-Based Public Health* (Oxford: Oxford University Press).

24 Runciman, W.B. et al. (2006), 'An Integrated Framework for Safety, Quality and Risk Management: an Information and Incident Management System Based on a Universal Patient Safety Classification', *Quality and Safety in Health Care* 15:Suppl I, i82-i90. Also, Box 11.9 (page 272) is adapted from Box 1 in this publication.

25 Personal communication, Associate Professor Bob Gibberd, School of Medicine and Public Health, University of Newcastle, New South Wales consultant statistician for the Australian Council on Healthcare Standards, robert.gibberd@newcastle.edu.au.

26 Carvel, J. (2006), 'Blair's Mantra for Health Chiefs: No Gain Without Pain', *Guardian* 13 April.

27 Runciman, W.B. (2002), 'Lessons from the Australian Patient Safety Foundation: Setting Up a National Patient Safety Surveillance System: Is This the Right Model?', *Quality and Safety in Health Care* 11:3, 246–51.

28 Runciman, W.B. and Moller, J. (2001), *Iatrogenic Injury in Australia* (Adelaide: Australian Patient Safety Foundation).

29 McGlynn, E.A. et al. (2003), 'The Quality of Health Care Delivered to Adults in the United States', *New England Journal of Medicine* 348:26, 2635–45.

30 Norman, D.A. (1988), *The Psychology of Everyday Things* (New York: Basic Books).

31 Norman, D.A. (1993), Things That Make Us Smart: Defending Human Attributes in the Age of the Machine (Reading: Perseus).

32 Myerson, K.R., Ilsley, A.H. and Runciman, W.B. (1986), 'An Evaluation of Ventilator Monitoring Alarms' *Anaesthesia and Intensive Care* 14:2, 174–85.

33 Modified from *The Clinician's Black Bag of Quality Improvement Tools*, at http://www.dartmouth.edu/~ogehome/CQI/index.html accessed 5 Jun 2006.

34 Braithwaite, J. et al. 'Introducing Soft Systems Methodology Plus (SSM+): Why We Need It and What It Can Contribute', *Australian Health Review* 25:2, 191–8.

35 Standards Australia International Ltd. and Standards New Zealand (2004), *Risk Management AS/NZS 4360:2004* (Sydney and Wellington: SAI Global).

36 Bates, D.W. (2005), 'Computerized Physician Order Entry and Medication Errors: Finding a Balance', *Journal of Biomedical Informatics* 38:4, 259–61.

37 Bagian, J. et al. (2006), *Healthcare Failure Mode Effects Analysis^{TM} Process,* VA National Center for Patient Safety [web resource]. Available at: http://www.va.gov/ncps/CogAids/HFMEA/index.html accessed 30 Jun 2006.

38 Senders, J.W. (2004), 'FMEA and RCA: the Mantras of Modern Risk Management', *Quality and Safety in Health Care* 13:4, 249–50.

39 Institute for Safe Medical Practices (ISMP) (2001), 'Failure Mode and Effects Analysis Can Help Guide Error Prevention Efforts', *ISMP Safety Alert* 17 October. Available at: http://www.ismp.org/newsletters/acutecare/articles/20011017.asp accessed 5 Jun 2006.

40 Marx, D.A. and Slonim, A.D. (2003), 'Assessing Patient Safety Risk Before the Injury Occurs: an Introduction to Sociotechnical Probabilistic Modelling in Health Care', *Quality and Safety in Health Care* 12:Suppl.2, ii33–8.

41 Institute for Healthcare Improvement (2003), *The Breakthrough Series: IHI's Collaborative Model for Achieving Breakthrough Improvement* (Boston, Massachusetts: Institute for Healthcare Improvement) [Web document], available at http://www.ihi.org/IHI/Results/WhitePapers/ accessed 30 Jun 2006.

42 Reinertsen, J.L., Pugh, M.D, and Bisognano, M. (2005), *Seven Leadership Leverage Points for Organization-Level Improvement in Health Care* (Cambridge, Massachusetts: Institute for Healthcare Improvement), available at: http://www.ihi.org/IHI/Results/WhitePapers/ accessed 30 Jun 2006.

43 Sprivulis, P.C. et al. (2006), 'The Association Between Hospital Overcrowding and Mortality Among Patients Admitted Via Western Australian Emergency Departments', *Medical Journal of Australia* 184:5, 208–12.

44 Tourangeau, A.E., Cranley, L.A. and Jeffs, L. (2006), 'Impact of Nursing on Hospital Patient Mortality: a Focused Review and Related Policy Implications', *Quality and Safety in Health Care* 15:1, 4–8.

45 Cook, R. and Rasmussen, J. (2005), '"Going Solid": a Model of System Dynamics and Consequences for Patient Safety', *Quality and Safety in Health Care* 14:2, 130–4.

46 Donabedian, A. (1966), 'Evaluating the Quality of Medical Care', *Milbank Memorial Fund Quarterly* 44:3 Suppl, 166–206.

47 Australian Council on Healthcare Standards (2004), *ACHS Clinical Indicator Summary Guide* (Ultimo, New South Wales).

48 Australian Council for Safety and Quality in Health Care (2003), *Standards Setting and Accreditation Literature Review and Report* (Canberra: Australian Council for Safety and Quality in Health Care), available at: <http://www.safetyandquality.org/articles/ACTION/ssacrfinrep.pdf> accessed 29 May 2006.

49 VA National Center for Patient Safety [web site]: http://www.va.gov/ncps/.

50 National Institute for Health and Clinical Excellence (United Kingdom): http://www.nice.org.uk/.

51 National Institute for Clinical Studies (Australia): http://www.nicsl.com.au/.

52 Australian Commission for Safety and Quality in Health Care [web page]: http://www.safetyandquality.org/.

53 Braithwaite, J., Healy, J. and Dwan, K. (2005), *The Governance of Health Safety and Quality* (Canberra: Commonwealth of Australia).

54 Joint Commission on Accreditation of Healthcare Organizations (JCAHO), in the United States, approved a proposal to conduct all accreditation surveys on an unannounced basis from January 2006 [web document]. Further details are available at: http://www.jointcommission.org/AccreditationPrograms/SVNP/qa_uannounced.htm accessed 5 Jun 2006.

55 'The Joint Commission's accreditation process should create an impetus for each organization to be in compliance with 100 percent of the standards 100 percent of the time', says Dennis S. O'Leary, M.D., president, Joint Commission. 'Making on-site evaluations less predictable and more focused on potential performance issues is intended to satisfy both public demand for greater organization accountability and organization demand for greater value in undergoing these outside evaluations': Media

Release: Joint Commission on Accreditation of Healthcare Organizations, 'Commission Shifts to Unannounced Surveys and Certification Reviews', 17 April 2006. Available at: http://www.jointcommission.org/NewsRoom/NewsReleases/jc_041706.htm accessed 5 Jun 2006.

56 Maynard, A. (2001), 'Ethics and Health Care "Under-Funding"', *Journal of Medical Ethics* 27:4, 223–7.

57 Eddy, D.N. (1996), *Clinical Decision Making: from Theory to Practice* (Sudbury, Massachusetts: Jones and Bartlett).

58 Richardson, J.R.J. (2005), 'Priorities of Health Policy: Cost Shifting or Population Health', *Australian and New Zealand Health Policy* 2:1, 1. Available from: http://www.anzhealthpolicy.com/content/2/1/1 accessed 5 Jun 2006.

59 Braithwaite, J. et al. (2006), 'Does Restructuring Hospitals Result in Greater Efficiency? – An Empirical Test', *Health Services Management Research* 19:1, 1–12.

60 Fulop, N. et al. (2002), 'Process and Impact of Mergers of NHS Trusts: Multicentre Case Study and Management Cost Analysis', *British Medical Journal* 325:7358, 246–9.

61 Clarke, S.P. and Aiken, L.H. (2006), 'More Nursing, Fewer Deaths', *Quality and Safety in Health Care* 15:1, 2–3.

62 Australian legislation prevents disclosure of factual information received through a declared quality assurance activity unless the conduct involves a serious offence against the law. Commonwealth of Australia, *Health Insurance Act of 1973*, Part VC: 'Quality Assurance Confidentiality'. Searchable web document version available at: http://www.austlii.edu.au/au/legis/cth/consol_act/hia1973164/ accessed 5 Jun 2006.

63 Certain protections from liability within the context of the error disclosure program are in proposed legislation in the United States: National Medical Error Disclosure and Compensation (MEDiC) Bill (S. 1784). See: Clinton and Obama (2006) cited above.

64 The Danish system is a "learning" system. 'A healthcare professional reporting an adverse event shall not as a result of such reporting be subject to disciplinary investigations or measures by the employing authority, supervisory reactions by the National Board of Health or criminal sanctions by the courts', part 3, item 6 of: Parliament of Denmark (2003) *Act on Patient Safety in the Danish Health Care System, Act No. 429 of 10/06/2003* [English translation web document], available at: http://www.patientsikkerhed.dk/admin/media/pdf/133907d0940e4d5f751852ec8f6b1795 .pdf accessed 5 Jun 2006.

65 David Marx (USA); Marx, D. (2001), *Patient Safety and the "Just Culture": a Primer for Health Care Executives* (New York: Columbia University). Available at: www.mers-tm.net/support/marx_primer.pdf accessed 5 Jun 2006.

66 James Bagian (USA); VA National Center for Patient Safety (2002), *VHA National Patient Safety Improvement Handbook* (Washington DC: Department of Veterans Affairs, Veterans Health Administration, United States) [Web document], available at: <http://www.va.gov/ncps/Pubs/NCPShb.pdf> accessed 26 Jun 2006.

67 James Reason (USA); National Patient Safety Agency (2004), *Incident Decision Tree* National Patient Safety Agency, United Kingdom, web resource. Available at: http://www.npsa.nhs.uk/health/resources/incident_decision_tree accessed 26 Jun 2006.

68 World Health Assembly (2002), 'Quality of Care: Patient Safety', Resolution WHA55.18, 55th World Health Assembly, 18 May 2002. Available at: http://www.who.int/gb/ebwha/pdf_files/WHA55/ewha5518.pdf accessed 5 Jun 2006.

69 World Health Organization (2004), *World Alliance for Patient Safety: Forward Programme* (Geneva: World Health Organization), available at: www.who.int/ patientsafety/en/brochure_final.pdf accessed 5 Jun 2006.

70 World Alliance for Patient Safety (2005), *The Global Patient Safety Challenge 2005-6: Clean Care is Safer Care* (Geneva: World Health Organization). Available at: http://www.who.int/patientsafety/challenge/en/ accessed 30 Jun 2006.
71 International Society for Quality in Health Care (ISQua): http://www.isqua.org.au/.
72 Symposium (1988), 'Monitoring and Patient Safety', *Anaesthesia and Intensive Care* 16:5–116.
73 Cass, N.M., Crosby, W.M. and Holland, R.B. (1988), 'Minimal Monitoring Standards', *Anaesthesia and Intensive Care* 16:1, 110–3.
74 Australian and New Zealand College of Anaesthetists (2000), *Policy Statement 18: Recommendations on Monitoring During Anaesthesia* (Melbourne: Australian and New Zealand College of Anaesthetists) [web document], available from: http://www.anzca.edu.au/publications/profdocs/profstandards/ps18_2000.htm (accessed Nov 2005).
75 Symposium (1993), 'The Australian Incident Monitoring Study', Anaesthesia and Intensive Care 21:5, 501–695.
76 Webb R.K., et al. (1993), 'The Australian Incident Monitoring Study. Which Monitor?' An Analysis of 2000 Incident Reports', *Anaesthesia and Intensive Care* 21:5, 529–42.
77 International Task Force on Anaesthesia Safety (Australia, Runciman; Canada, Duncan; Finland, Tammisto; France, Desmonts; Germany, Stoeckel; Japan, Ikeda; Netherlands, Booi; UK, Hanning; USA, Eichhorn & Gravenstein) (1993), 'International Standards for A Safe Practice of Anaesthesia', *European Journal of Anaesthesiology* 10: Suppl. 7, 12–5.
78 International Task Force on Anaesthesia Safety (Australia, Runciman; Canada, Duncan; Finland, Tammisto; France, Desmonts; Germany, Stoeckel; Japan, Ikeda; Netherlands, Booi; UK, Hanning; USA, Eichhorn and Gravenstein) (1993), 'Commentary on Equipment Recommendations', *European Journal of Anaesthesiology* 10: Suppl. 7, 16–8.
79 Runciman, W.B. (1993), 'Risk Assessment in the Formulation of Anaesthesia Safety Standards', *European Journal of Anaesthesiology* 10: Suppl. 7, 26–32.
80 Runciman, W.B. (2005), 'Iatrogenic Harm and Anaesthesia in Australia', *Anaesthesia and Intensive Care* 33:3, 297–300.

Chapter 12

Where to Now?

The Destination

At the beginning of this book we cited the 1948 World Health Organization (WHO) definition of health – 'a state of complete physical, mental and social well-being and not merely the absence of disease or infirmity'.[1] One might imagine a future Utopia[2] in which the quality of health was uniformly high, the risk of iatrogenic harm remote, and publicly funded universal healthcare was regarded world-wide as 'a right of all and the duty of each state'.[3] Into this imagined future one might place the following elements:

- National policies to ensure the provision of clean water, shelter, adequate food, a basic education and security for all.
- A clearly articulated comprehensive programme for immunization and the promotion and monitoring of preventive health measures.
- Nationally and internationally standardized indications and structured care-plans for the evidence-based management of medical and surgical conditions.
- A transparent and explicit basis for the rationing of the healthcare services provided by the public purse, taking into account the likely cost-benefit for individual patients after allowing for their specific mix of demographic variables and co-morbidities.
- Effective coordination of the healthcare provided to each patient by a designated case manager, utilizing a universal electronic medical record accessible by all concerned at any reasonable point of care (e.g. a general practitioner's office, a hospital, or an ambulance at the roadside).
- Electronically accessible and easily assimilated information in relation to options for investigations and surgical or medical treatments, so that patients can make informed choices and know what to expect.
- High levels of system-engineering underpinned by electronic, mechanical and procedural support systems to promote safety and reduce the risk of avoidable errors and failures in the provision of healthcare.
- Evidence-based decision support at the point of care for investigations and treatments (particularly in relation to the choice, administration and monitoring of drug therapy).
- Financial incentives for practitioners who provide healthcare in line with national guidelines and standards.

- Tools which structure care plans and also document their implementation to provide evidence of compliance which can be securely stored and audited electronically.
- Freely available online information about these tools (with how and why they were developed) for all patients, practitioners, units, practices and healthcare facilities.
- A national system for credentialling clinicians and accrediting healthcare facilities.
- Representation of and input from patients and consumer groups at all levels of healthcare.
- Representation of and input from senior clinicians specifically charged with responsibility for the clinical risk register and with setting priorities for healthcare expenditure at the highest system and organizational levels.
- A national reporting system for things that go wrong which can be used by patients, other consumers and healthcare professionals.
- National and international repositories of data relevant to patient safety and the quality of healthcare fed by information from all available sources (including reporting systems), collated using agreed terminology and an international patient safety classification.
- A culture of open disclosure underpinned by a system of no-fault compensation and adequate provision for an appropriate and just social, medical and legal response when things go wrong.

What Would this Look Like?

What would this look like from the perspectives of the various layers of healthcare depicted in Figure 1.1? In Utopia, poverty would no longer exist. We are acutely aware that the realities of the foreseeable future are in stark contrast to this assumption, but much of this book has been about the substantial deficiencies in the delivery of healthcare that exist today even in wealthy countries. The following comments could perhaps be seen as applying primarily to those parts of the world where affluence is the norm. In the second part of this chapter we will place them into a more sober perspective, which takes into account the global priorities for healthcare.

The Patient

All citizens would have access to their own universal and comprehensive medical record. Key phrases in this record would be 'hot linked' to succinct, up to date information about the relevant aspects of healthcare. This information would be arranged in layers of increasing complexity and would be endorsed by national and international bodies of accredited experts in the relevant fields, who would keep it up to date. Users would be able to drill down to progressively more detailed information and even to the sources of this information. The record would automatically generate reminders, some for all, such as reminders for scheduled vaccinations, and others tailored to each patient's individual needs.

The Individual Clinician

Individual clinicians would, with the patients' authority, have access to the universal medical records from anywhere in the world. These records would start with a top level summary, but would allow access to any level of detail required, including explanations of why a patient chose one option over another at a particular time, and a record of who authorized and who carried out various aspects of patient care. This would allow automatic electronic audit of the practices and complications of individual clinicians, teams, units, or organizations. Selected aspects could be called up and the performance of the practitioner or unit in question compared to risk adjusted figures from similar practitioners or units. This could be used to guide CPD; all practitioners would have structured time to attend update sessions and reviews of aspects of their practice. Financial incentives would promote compliance with best practice.

The Team Level

The knowledge, skills and training required for each role in any particular team would be explicitly documented and regular credentialling of each team member would be required, using training devices and simulators. Team activities which take place in relatively controlled environments, such as the resuscitation of trauma victims and establishing emergency airways in intensive care, would be recorded on video from time to time, for teaching and debriefing purposes.

The Level of the Organization, Healthcare Facility or Practice

Regulation would be structured around profiles individualized to each practice or healthcare facility, and would incorporate effective methods of monitoring and ensuring compliance, including compliance with recommendations arising from incident reports and root cause analyses. Each healthcare facility would provide time for all staff to undertake continuous professional development and for selected practitioners to contribute to the development and updating of clinical standards and standard operating procedures at a national or international level.

The State or National Layer

Each country would have one body to coordinate the development and maintenance of clinical standards and officially endorsed information related to healthcare. This body would be responsible for identifying priorities, gathering and tasking groups of volunteer (paid) experts, documenting and structuring their findings and recommendations, and providing support in the way of statistical and epidemiological expertise. It would be responsible for identifying the particular country's priorities in healthcare, and would be expected to consult with consumers in doing so.

The International Layer

The World Alliance for Patient Safety (WAPS) of the WHO would act to collate and co-ordinate these national activities so that agreed best practices and the tools for achieving these could be disseminated world-wide. The current aims of the WHO and WAPS are listed on pages 270 and 271.

In addition, some degree of collective responsibility for the world as a whole would be very important, and could be coordinated at this level. This would include an improved United Nations Security Council, able to deal effectively with groups or countries which threaten the security of others; it would include effective measures to preserve our global environment, and it would include a major drive to eliminate poverty from the world.

How Can we Get There?

The Patient

The key to achieving greater input into healthcare by the general public lies in improving the overall level of understanding within the community of the issues at stake. Ready access to succinct, authoritative information about healthcare must be ensured. Insufficient attention has been paid to ensuring that people of low literacy can properly understand and assimilate information. At the moment there is a bewildering variety of information of variable quality. A few of the many organizations operating in this area have been listed in Appendices IV and X, but there is much room for improvement with respect to having a few very well presented sets of information for lay people, rather than a plethora of sets of information of varying complexity, quality and clarity.

Patients should have much more input into how healthcare is organized and delivered. In Sweden, for example, there is a patients' advisory committee, independent of healthcare, in every county council, with elected representatives and full time staff with experience in education, health sciences, behavioural science, psychology, psychiatry, economics and law.[4] Problems are dealt with quickly and efficiently and all problems are registered in a database in categories such as attitude, access, care, administration, treatment, co-operation, and information and advice giving. Analysis of the database is reported yearly to the National Board of Health and the statistics are widely disseminated.

There should be a toll free-number so that patients can report incidents (not just complaints) and make suggestions as to how the healthcare system can be improved. This system could also be used for post-marketing drug surveillance, which is currently poorly addressed.

The Individual Clinician

As outlined in Chapter 6, no individual clinician has the time and few have the expertise to assemble the best evidence. The emphasis must move from knowing what to do to knowing how to find out what to do. The move from traditional authority-based decision making to evidence-based medicine in partnership with other clinicians and with patients must continue to gain momentum. Much more emphasis must be placed on developing decision support tools tailored to individual patients, and on the co-ordination of care. Case managers should be appointed for significant health interventions and for the management of chronic conditions.

Greater emphasis is needed on the principles of quality in healthcare, and particularly on patient safety, in undergraduate, postgraduate and continuous professional development programmes.

The Team Layer

Again, the key here is to continue the movement away from an emphasis on the individual in healthcare to a recognition of the importance of teamwork. In many countries root cause analyses are being conducted and simulators have been purchased. Although multidisciplinary team training and formal accreditation for activities such as medical emergency teams are poorly developed at the moment, the basic ingredients for proper systems are slowly being put into place. It will fall to clinicians and people involved in these activities to start to develop the curricula, training programmes and certification and credentialling processes. Credentialling team members for specific roles should become a requirement for accreditation of healthcare facilities.

The Level of the Organization, Healthcare Facility or Practice

Proposals for developing clinical and corporate standards, and for building compliance checks into tools for meeting these standards, have been made on pages 263–264. The emphasis must be on organizations providing time and infrastructure to facilitate self-regulation and professionally-led regulation at the level of the individual clinician and of departments and units. This implies the education of administrators as well as clinicians and other healthcare workers in the topics listed in Table 10.1.

Many safety and quality initiatives fail to gain traction because a conventional business case cannot be mounted. The fallacy of this requirement in relation to patient safety is that it is often impossible to quantify the risks of iatrogenic harm which could potentially arise from human error in a given situation, and also impossible to quantify precisely the reduction in risk likely to be achieved by a given intervention. Few safety interventions will eliminate a particular risk altogether, and it is usually not possible to confidently attribute a change to an intervention, as there is almost invariably a host of other uncontrolled variables which can impact on what is being measured.

Box 12.1 The fallacy of the business case – an example

The widespread introduction of pulse oximetry and capnography into anaesthesia has been associated with a dramatic reduction in the number of patients killed or brain damaged by circuit disconnections or other causes of hypoxia in anaesthesia (Box 2.5). However, this evidence is only emerging now, 15 years after the widespread adoption of this technology. Attempts to demonstrate definitive safety benefits of oximetry through RCTs were predictably unsuccessful, because of the large size of trial that would be needed. Although compensation for hypoxic brain damage and death can run to millions of dollars, in most systems the hospital does not even pay the insurance premium, let alone the compensation. There is no immediate financial incentive, therefore, to invest in technology purely for safety reasons. Pulse oximetry and capnography were introduced because of strong leadership by the professional bodies representing anaesthetists.

   Today pulse oximetry is much cheaper than when it first became available. It is highly likely that the overall financial impact to society of its introduction has been a net saving, and few anaesthetists would doubt that there has been a substantial gain in the human costs of hypoxic brain damage. Putting a dollar value on this is a different matter altogether.

Although the most cost effective healthcare at a societal level is usually achieved by doing the right thing, the first time, safely, the difficulty is to demonstrate this, particularly ahead of time. This creates major problems for those who want to gain access to new technology, and for those to have to allocate limited funds between competing groups within an organization. One reasonable approach seems to be to establish interprofessional groups of respected senior staff to assess new technologies and decide which ones to introduce. It is of course also important to ensure that existing technologies are being used safely and properly (see Box 3.1).

The State or National Layer

Many countries now have at least one organization set up to enhance patient safety and/or other elements of quality in healthcare. Quite large sums of money have been made available for this purpose in some countries, particularly in the years since some national reports on iatrogenic harm were published at the turn of the last century.[5,6,7] Several organization are now devoted to the advancement of evidence-based medicine and the production and dissemination of clinical guidelines and pathways. However, national initiatives to change clinical practice have been quite idiosyncratic and have tended to focus on rare and dramatic incidents (exemplified by sentinel events) (Table 2.9). Instead, attention should be focused on the more common things that are going wrong, particularly those that are consuming the most resources.[8,9]

At the national level, the task is one of identifying priorities and coordinating activities to address the problems identified. Iatrogenic harm is not homogenous, but is made up of multiple problems, each with its own profile and each requiring its own tailored solution. There are experts in each of the problem areas in most countries. These should be engaged in reviewing the state of play in their problem area, and then setting evidence-based standards and developing tools for their implementation. Wherever possible, the problem should be designed out of the system (see Box 11.5). Where process-based solutions are required, mere guidelines should be avoided and actual tools developed. These tools should serve the triple purpose of outlining what should be done, confirming that it has been done and facilitating coding that it has.

The introduction of responsive regulation is required. The emphasis should be on self-regulation and professionally-led regulation, backed up by compulsory meta-regulation based on random inspections[10] (page 264). As electronic records gain traction it should become easier to audit compliance with standards. Public reporting of the practice profiles of individuals, units, departments, practices and organizations should become the norm. However, there is a long way to go before the science catches up with the philosophy, and attention must be directed towards presenting risk-adjusted information in a manner that is comprehensible to administrators, politicians and the public at large. Crude 'league tables' which may be exploited for local political purposes should not be produced. More will be gained to improve standards by harnessing the goodwill and facilitating the willing efforts of those who work in healthcare than by heavy-handed top-down measures.

A particular challenge at this level relates to the provision of services which are patient-centred. National surveys similar to that conducted by the RAND organization[11] would be of great value in engaging the public in the process of improving healthcare. Interviewing a randomly selected sample of the population and reviewing their medical records from the proceeding year or two would provide a guide to the degree of success achieved over that time in delivering appropriate and acceptable evidence-based healthcare to the population. This information could be integrated with other indicators of quality in healthcare, and used to guide regular adjustments to overall strategy and funding priorities. In this way an ongoing cycle of patient-centred continuous improvement could be established.

The International Layer

With the passing of the WHO resolution on patient safety and the formation of the WAPS,[12,13] machinery was put into place to standardize taxonomy, measurement and reporting, evidence-based policies, clinical standards and tools for their implementation and audit. This machinery should also facilitate the sharing and dissemination of lessons learnt in one country with other countries.

Six initiatives of the WAPS were listed in Box 11.8. An important one is the global patient safety challenge which will consist of two-yearly rolling cycles, in which attention will be directed towards a particular problem which requires sustained change. As part of this process, it will be necessary to set evidence-based priorities for patient safety.

Appropriately, the first challenge chosen was that of healthcare-associated infection.[14] A formal statement has been developed for countries to pledge their support to the implementation of actions to reduce these infections and to share results and learnings internationally. This initiative is particularly appropriate because it covers areas as diverse as hand hygiene, blood safety, injection and immunization safety, clinical procedures' safety and water, sanitation and waste management safety. These are issues of importance to all countries, whatever their financial status. Also, it is consistent with a key message of this book: safety and quality in healthcare is not only about preventing and managing things that go wrong, but also about ensuring the health and wellbeing of all.

The question arises as to what the next global challenges should be. Problems with devices and medications have been suggested as candidate areas; we think it is also worthwhile to examine priorities identified by the WHO.

Global priorities What are the priorities for healthcare at the beginning of the new millennium? The Global Burden of Disease study was a landmark study in which not only mortality but disability from major illnesses was studied.[9,15,16,17] It was initiated in 1992 at the request of the World Bank, was supported by the WHO, and involved over 100 scientists from more than 20 countries. For each disease and its sequelae, estimates of incidence, prevalence, remission, duration and mortality were developed for different populations of the world.

Over 50 million people died worldwide in 1990. Ischaemic heart disease (IHD) caused more deaths than any other disease or injury; 2.7 million of the 6.3 million who died of IHD were in the developed world. Cerebrovascular disease (stroke) caused the deaths of 4.4 million people, of which 1.4 million were in developed world. Next on the list were diseases of the developing world: pneumonia (4.3 million people) and diarrhoeal diseases (2.9 million).

Disability was measured in this study using DALYs (see page 12). Taking disability into account in this way led to recognition of the profound impact of mental illness on society. Neuropsychiatric conditions accounted for 22 per cent of the DALYs in developed countries.

Depression was ranked fourth in the estimate of disease burden in 1990, ahead of IHD, cerebrovascular disease and tuberculosis,[16] and other mental health problems also ranked highly. With the demographic, social and epidemiological changes thought likely to occur, depression was projected to be second as a cause of disability by the year 2020.[17,18] The original study has been repeated and in 2002 unipolar depressive disorders ranked second in developed countries, first in developing countries with low mortality and seventh in developing countries with high mortality.[19] The need for studies of interventions aimed at risk factor modification, treatment and prevention of mental health conditions was one of the policy implications listed in reports from the Global Burden of Disease Study.[15] Many countries including Australia, Britain, the United States and others have now conducted large campaigns to try to reduce levels of depression in the community. This effort is well directed and could be extended worldwide as a future global patient safety challenge. Suicide is a leading cause of death, for women, as well as for men.

Overall, about 5 million people died of injuries of all types, and most of these were young adults (i.e., 15–44 years old). Road traffic accidents were the leading cause of death for men and the 5th for women. The most important cause of injury deaths in Sub-Saharan Africa is war, for both women and men.

We have already noted that expenditure on the military in the USA rivals that on health (US$450 billion versus US$500 billion).[20] One third of this would meet the total WHO recommendation for aid around the globe.[21] A global strategy to reduce the money wasted on wars would be highly desirable and the funds saved could be redirected to the alleviation of poverty by investing in infrastructure in the countries which most need it

Poverty Overall, poverty is a massive problem in healthcare. In 1997 Indonesia hosted the United Nations 4th International Conference on Health Promotion. The Jakarta Declaration (1997) made it clear that health and mental health are inextricably linked with the environment within which individuals live (see Table 12.1).[22]

Table 12.1 Prerequisites or determinants for health as defined by the Jakarta declaration

1.	peace	7.	income
2.	shelter	8.	the empowerment of women
3.	education	9.	a stable eco-system
4.	social security	10.	sustainable resource use
5.	social relations	11.	social justice
6.	food	12.	and respect for human rights, and equity

Thirty thousand deaths a year, mostly in children, are attributable to a lack of clean water and basic health facilities. These would not be identified in this way in the Global Burden of Disease study, because the methods used depend on coding, and lack of clean water is not a code in the International Classification of Diseases. In the same way, most cases of iatrogenic harm are identified by retrospective review of case records, and are not captured by coding (see page 43). Clearly there is still a pressing need to bring information from multiple sources into a single pool, and from this to place the obvious priorities in healthcare into a common perspective.[23]

The allocation of resources – a question of politics Perhaps the most disappointing aspect of the state of healthcare today lies in the obvious examples of misapplied investment and effort, from the perspective of the common good of society, both locally and globally. Gains have certainly been made in our understanding of pathology, of therapeutics, of evidence-based medicine, of effective surgery, and of the priorities for public health. A huge shift has occurred towards recognizing the autonomy of patients, although there is still a long way to go in achieving the right balance between the competing interests of all concerned with healthcare (consumers, funders, providers and society as a whole).

The capitalist approach, based substantially on competition within a free market, has produced gains, but has also produced obscene distortions of common sense in the allocation of resource and effort. We have seen (in Chapters 1 and 3) that healthcare is characterized everywhere by astonishing degrees of unwarranted variation. Practitioner preference, not the needs of patients, or even the availability of resource, seems often to be the determining factor in the allocation of healthcare services.

Within the predominantly capitalist societies of the world, much investment in healthcare is self-evidently self-serving. Would a more socialist approach do any better, on balance? One can find examples, such as Cuba, in which the national provision of appropriate healthcare services seems in many ways to be ahead of richer countries in the so-called free world, but one can find others (such as Zimbabwe) in which it does not (on any measurement). In the end (as with many other aspects of the organization of healthcare) one finds oneself grappling with political theory rather than the principles of quality in healthcare.

What is clear is that enormous gains can be made if politics can be put to one side, and rational decisions made with respect to implementing policies at both national and international levels. An example of a striking success at a national level is the anti-AIDS programme in Brazil.[3] In the early 1990s both Brazil and South Africa had HIV rates of 1.5 per cent. Brazil made some hard decisions about providing anti-retroviral drugs free to all who needed them, which greatly enhanced their aggressive AIDS prevention programme, whereas South Africa took the soft option of 'looking the other way'. Areas of Southern Africa now have HIV rates of over 30 per cent in young adults, whereas the rate is 0.6 per cent in Brazil. The AIDS problem is crippling healthcare in Southern Africa, whereas the cost of hospital admissions due to HIV has fallen progressively in Brazil since these measures where introduced.[3]

Examples of major successes at the international level are the eradication of small pox in the past and the current highly successful anti-measles programme.[24] Death from measles worldwide has almost halved over five years through a concerted vaccination campaign focusing on Africa. The numbers of measles deaths were cut from 870,000 in 1999 to 450,000 in 2004.

It seems that in healthcare, as in other aspects of the affairs of mankind, patches of rational, constructive, extremely successful activity are found in close juxtaposition to *laissez faire*, ineffective approaches.

Lessons we Should Heed

Progress is Possible

Throughout healthcare, from small groups of individuals to major national campaigns, there are examples of extraordinary progress and success, such as those outlined above. The first thing, with respect to the safety and quality of healthcare, is to accept there are problems which are unacceptable. The next thing is to believe that something can be done to alter this state of affairs. The final thing is to try to *ensure* that something *is* done. This will require an effort from everyone involved in healthcare.

Insisting on Being Different

There seems to be a deep seated desire (need?) on the part of many healthcare professionals to believe that they and/or their patients and/or the institutions in which they work are different from their colleagues, other peoples' patients and other institutions. This, coupled with a desire for 'clinical freedom' contributes to the huge variability in clinical practice which characterizes healthcare. As argued earlier, this is intrinsically unethical with respect to the equitable distribution of the finite resources available for healthcare.

Perhaps one of the greatest contributions individual healthcare professionals could make would be to systematically suppress the ubiquitous manifestations of dysfunctional territorial behaviour, in the interests of the common good.

The Limitations of Above-Down Edicts

In most countries national bodies have been involved in developing documents which constitute generic exhortations to improve practice in one area or another. Whilst these are commendable and necessary, it is important that their generation and dissemination does not divert resources and attention from the myriad specific problems that contribute to risk and harm in healthcare.

All Things Great and Small

There has been a marked tendency for considerable effort to go into addressing dramatic problems which, whilst important to eliminate, make up a tiny fraction of 1 per cent of the things that harm patients.[8] More systematic effort should be put into addressing the mundane problems which consume most of the resources. Also, healthcare is characterized by hundreds, even thousands, of similar small projects, all over the world, being carried out simultaneously. Most of these are underpowered and are doomed to Type II errors. There would be an enormous increase in efficiency if these efforts could be coordinated nationally and internationally to design and conduct studies to provide definitive answers to important questions.

The Desire to Use Administrative Data

It is evident that there is a powerful urge to use administrative data (coded using the ICD system) to attempt to 'benchmark' and track trends in patient safety. Whilst some useful studies have been done,[25] the data are not sufficiently robust to provide a reasonable measure or picture of what is going on, as the medical records upon which the codes are based often fail to identify adverse events explicitly, and contain virtually no information about contextual or contributing factors, an understanding of which is essential if appropriate corrective strategies are to be developed.[26]

Difficulties in Transferring the Findings of Research into Clinical Practice

In Chapter 6 we discussed the long delays that characteristically occur between the establishment of evidence in relation to practice, and its implementation. There are many reasons for this. One, which we discussed, relates to the synthesis of data from multiple trials and the dissemination of the information from such synthesis to practitioners for use in their day-to-day practice. A second problem relates to unrealistic expectations about the efficacy of traditional ways of introducing change in healthcare. Methods which take into account the complex socio-political environment of healthcare are necessary to get change accepted by the many people in the system who traditionally oppose it (see pages 215–216 and Appendix IX). Another relates to cost – new drugs and techniques are typically expensive, particularly when first developed. Their adoption may be seriously inhibited by economic realities, particularly in less wealthy countries. Many of the initiatives discussed above fall into this category, and it will be a long while before they become part of the way of life in much of Sub-Saharan Africa, for example.

Limitations of Information Technology

Although it has been shown that clinicians will use on-line information and decision support, and that these can improve their decision-making,[27,28,29,30] evidence is emerging that there are major problems with most commercially available information technology systems.[31] Many have been developed with little regard for how they will impact on the work flow of clinicians, and many new types of error are emerging ('automation bias'). An argument has been put that there is an urgent need to regulate software and information technology systems which impact on patient care, as the potential for serious harm is great.[32]

   Even for those countries that can afford computers and all that goes with information technology (IT), there are many disappointments along the path to Utopia. The potential for revenge effects is considerable, and there are those who would argue that the IT revolution has created as many problems as it has solved (thus far, at any rate); certainly, objective evidence of widespread benefits is not yet evident.[33] For example, the advent of relatively cheap computing power has created the illusion that massive databases will provide answers to all the important questions in healthcare. In reality, the answers depend not only on the capacity to store data, but also on the quality of the data collected, its relevance, the sophistication with which it is analyzed, and the degree to which the whole process is grounded in the reality of clinical practice. Only too often, at the national and institutional level, decisions are made on the basis of data that are simply not recognized as meaningful by those at the workface.

In the design of support systems for the clinical environment there is much to be learned from the concept of soft engineering promoted by Norman (see pages 125 and 258).[34] The fact is that machines (including computers) are better than humans at doing some things, but less good at others. The best solutions to problems are obtained by combining the strengths of each.

Summing Up

In this book our aim has been to identify major challenges to quality in healthcare, with an emphasis on the element of safety and a bias towards ethics as the key to doing the right thing. The age of healthcare directed on the basis of medical authority, originating in the days in which it was a cottage-industry (captured in A.J. Cronin's stories of Dr Finlay),[35] needs to give way to one in which evidence will inform the activities of teams of heath-care professionals working in concert with their patients.

This does not mean that the role of clinicians will be diminished. Healthcare is one of the most challenging domains of modern society, and it will certainly be essential to maintain a group of professionals with the highest possible levels of ability, expertise and commitment in the pursuit of the WHO definition of health. In the future, many of these professionals will still be doctors and nurses, although the scope for those whose background lies elsewhere has already increased and will continue to do so.[36]

Whatever the future brings in re-arranging the roles and scope of the traditional guilds of healthcare, all who work in healthcare will need to have a common understanding of the issues around ethics, safety and quality. We suggest that there has been too great an emphasis on knowledge of the technical aspects of healthcare, and too little on the principles by which this technical knowledge should be applied. If healthcare professionals are to do the right thing in the future, an immediate priority is to expose them to the concepts outlined in this book and summarized in Table 10.1. These concepts need to be incorporated more comprehensively into the undergraduate curricula and continuing professional development programmes of all who work in healthcare. Our hope is that this book will contribute to the growing number of publications promoting a re-evaluation of priorities in healthcare, and that it (and books like it) will influence those who can make a difference today.

High quality in healthcare is not easily achieved. Its pursuit requires an understanding of all the elements which contribute to quality. From the preceding paragraphs it is obvious that safety is not by any means the only issue demanding attention in healthcare. However, for many of the practitioners who might be expected to read a book of this sort, it is certainly one of the priorities, and one that lends itself to the attention of every individual who has the privilege of looking after patients, be that individual a doctor, a nurse, an orderly, an administrator or a minister of health. Given the extent of ill-health and injury already in the world, Hippocrates was right: in our efforts to reduce this burden we should, as an over-riding objective, at least not add to it. That is why this book is primarily about safety.

The challenge for all who work in healthcare is to recognize and to exploit the strengths we have as human beings – our humanity, sense of justice and capacity for compassion, and our enormous abilities in pattern recognition (which manifest as clinical acumen) and in learning and performing highly skilled tasks. However, at the same time we must devise and implement systems to prevent, detect and manage the problems that arise from things we are bad at – routine tasks, repetitive tasks, tasks requiring vigilance for prolonged periods, and crises, when our limited cognitive capacity becomes overloaded. It is in all of these areas that we need to harness the tools developed in other industries such as bar-coding, computerized order entry, standard operating procedures and team training. We need to match these initiatives to the economic and social realities of each particular region. Counter-intuitively, ensuring that all care offered to patients is actually appropriate care is probably the single initiative most likely to enhance patient safety. The challenge is to ensure that the system of healthcare genuinely addresses the real needs of patients, and that the technology employed in doing this complements the strengths of healthcare professionals whilst safeguarding patients against human frailties. As human beings we cannot get rid of error. As healthcare professionals, we have a duty to do the right thing by our patients: we must ensure that they receive the care they need and only the care they need, and we must do everything possible to prevent them from being harmed in the process.

For the foreseeable future, the safety and wellbeing of our patients will continue to depend on the goodwill, patience, dedication and skill of individual healthcare professionals striving, every day, to get it right. We are still a long way from being able to rely on 'the system' and we will continue to have to interrupt what we are doing, frequently, to react to and counter its deficiencies. This book will, we hope, provide insight into the environment in which we work, and into the principles of safeguarding our patients and improving the quality of their care.

Notes

1   World Health Organization, Preamble to the Constitution of the World Health Organization as adopted by the International Health Conference, New York, 19–22 June 1946: signed on 22 July 1946 by the representatives of 61 States (*Official Records of the World Health Organization*, no. 2, p.100) and entered into force on 7 April 1948.
2   The term 'Utopia' was used by Sir Thomas More for a fictional island where society and government live in harmony and there is no poverty, tyranny or war: More, T. (1515), *De Optimo Reipublicae Statu deque Nova Insula Utopia*. A web-copy based on the 1901

Cassell and Company edition is available from Project Gutenberg [web page]: http://www.gutenberg.org/etext/2130 accessed 5 Jul 2006.

3   Okie, S. (2006), 'Fighting HIV – Lessons from Brazil', *New England Journal of Medicine* 354:19, 1977–1981.

4   For example: Stockholm County Council (2005), *Stockholm County Council in brief.* (Stockholm, Sweden: Stockholm County Council) p. 15 [Web document], available at: http://www.sll.se/docs/w_sll2/engelskinfobroschyr2005.pdf accessed 5 Jul 2006.

5   Kohn, L.T., Corrigan, J.M. and Donaldson, M.S. (2000), *To Err is Human: Building a Safer Health System* (Washington DC: National Academies Press).

6   United Kingdom Department of Health (2000), *An Organisation with a Memory – Report of an Expert Group on Learning from Adverse Events in the NHS Chaired by the Chief Medical Officer* (London: The Stationery Office).

7   Runciman, W.B. and Moller, J. (2001), *Iatrogenic Injury in Australia* (Adelaide: Australian Patient Safety Foundation). Available at <http://www.apsf.net.au>.

8   Runciman, W.B., Edmonds, M. and Pradhan, M. (2002), 'Setting Priorities for Patient Safety', *Quality and Safety in Health Care* 11:3, 224–9.

9   Murray, C.J., Lopez, A.D. and Jamison, D.T. (1994), 'The Global Burden of Disease in 1990: Summary Results, Sensitivity Analysis and Future Directions', *Bulletin of the World Health Organization* 72:3; 495–509.

10 Braithwaite, J., Healy, J. and Dwan, K. (2005), *The Governance of Health Safety and Quality* (Canberra: Commonwealth of Australia).

11 McGlynn, E.A. et al. (2003), 'The Quality of Health Care Delivered to Adults in the United States', *New England Journal of Medicine* 348:26, 2635–45.

12 World Health Assembly (2002), 'Quality of Care: Patient Safety', Resolution WHA55.18, 55th World Health Assembly, 18 May 2002. Available at: http://www.who.int/gb/ebwha/pdf_files/WHA55/ewha5518.pdf accessed 5 Jul 2006.

13 World Health Organization (2004), *World Alliance for Patient Safety: Forward Programme* (Geneva: World Health Organization). Available at: www.who.int/ patientsafety/en/brochure_final.pdf accessed 5 Jul 2006.

14 Pittet, D. and Donaldson, L. (2006), 'Challenging the World: Patient Safety and Health Care–Associated Infection', *International Journal for Quality in Health Care* 18:1, 4–8.

15 Murray, C.J.L. and Lopez, A.D. (1996), 'Evidence-Based Health Policy: Lessons from the Global Burden of Disease Study', *Science* 274:5288, 740–3.

16 Murray, C.J. and Lopez, A.D. (1997), 'Global Mortality, Disability, and the Contribution of Risk Factors: Global Burden of Disease Study', *Lancet* 349:9063, 1436–42.

17 Murray, C.J.L. and Lopez, A.D.(1997), 'Alternative Projections of Mortality and Disability by Cause 1990–2020: Global Burden of Disease Study', *Lancet* 349:9064, 1498–504.

18 Ustun, T.B. (1999), 'The Global Burden of Mental Disorders', *American Journal of Public Health* 89:9, 1315–8.

19 Mathers C.D. et al. (2004), *Global Burden of Disease in 2002: Data Sources, Methods and Results. Global Programme on Evidence for Health Policy Discussion Paper No. 54* (Geneva: World Health Organization) [Web document], available at: http://www3.who.int/whosis/burden/gbd2000docs/paper54.pdf accessed 5 Jul 2006.

20 In 2004, the United States of America spent US$456 billion on military defence compared to US$240 billion on health and US$269 billion on Medicare. Office of Management and Budget, United States of America (2005), *Mid-Session Review: Budget of the U.S. Government, Fiscal Year 2006* (Washington D.C: Office of Management and Budget, Executive Office of the President of the United States) p. 39.

Available at: <http://www.whitehouse.gov/omb/budget/fy2006/pdf/06msr.pdf> accessed 17 May 2006.

21 Sachs, J.D. (2005), 'Can Extreme Poverty Be Eliminated?', *Scientific American* 293:3, 56–65.

22 United Nations (1997), *Jakarta Declaration on Leading Health Promotion into the 21ˢᵗ Century.* 4ᵗʰ International Conference on Health Promotion, Jakarta. Available at: http://www.who.int/hpr/NPH/docs/jakarta_declaration_en.pdf.

23 Runciman, W.B. (2002), 'Lessons from the Australian Patient Safety Foundation: Setting Up a National Patient Safety Surveillance System – Is This the Right Model?', *Quality and Safety in Health Care* 11:3, 246–51.

24 Anonymous (2006), 'Africa Leads Measles Purge', *New Scientist* 18ᵗʰ March, p. 7.

25 Sprivulis, P.C. et al. (2006), 'The Association Between Hospital Overcrowding and Mortality Among Patients Admitted Via Western Australian Emergency Departments', *Medical Journal of Australia* 184:5, 208–12.

26 Wilson, R.M. et al (1995), 'The Quality in Australian Health Care Study', *Medical Journal of Australia* 163:9, 458–71.

27 Westbrook, J.I., Coiera, E.W. and Gosling, A.S. (2005) 'Do Online Information Retrieval Systems Help Experienced Clinicians Answer Clinical Questions?', *Journal of the American Medical Informatics Association* 12:3, 315–321.

28 Coiera, E., Westbrook, J.I. and Wyatt, J.C. (2006), 'The Safety and Quality of Decision Support Systems', *Methods of Information in Medicine* 2006; 45 suppl.1, forthcoming.

29 Bates, D.W. et al. (1998), 'Effect of Computerized Physician Order Entry and a Team Intervention on Prevention of Serious Medication Errors', *Journal of the American Medical Association* 280:15, 1311–6.

30 Bates, D.W. et al. (1999), 'The Impact of Computerized Physician Order Entry on Medication Error Prevention', *Journal of the American Medical Informatics Association* 6:4, 313–21.

31 Wachter, R.M. (2006), 'Expected and Unanticipated Consequences of the Quality and Information Technology Revolutions', *Journal of the American Medical Association* 295:23, 2780–3.

32 Coiera, E.W. and Westbrook, J.I. (2006), 'Should Clinical Software Be Regulated?', *Medical Journal of Australia* 184:12, 601–2.

33 Chaudhry, B. et al. (2006), 'Systematic Review: Impact of Health Information Technology on Quality, Efficiency and Costs of Medical Care', *Annals of Internal Medicine* 144:10, 742–52.

34 Norman, D.A. (1988), *The Psychology of Everyday Things* (New York: Basic Books).

35 Cronin, A.J. (1979), wrote *Short Stories From Dr. Finlay's Casebook*, which was adapted into a popular television series.

36 Various authors (2006) *Medical Journal of Australia* 185:1, entire issue on Task Transfer.

Appendix I

Preferred Terms and Definitions for Key Safety and Quality Concepts*

A group was formed under the auspices of the Australian Council for Safety and Quality in Health Care and a series of meetings was held to decide on some preferred terms and their definitions. It was decided to avoid long definitions with several 'qualifiers', but instead to start with simple, basic definitions, and then 'build' by defining the key terms used in these definitions. It is therefore necessary to read the terms and their definitions in the sequence provided below:

1. Incident	17. Safety	33. Accountable
2. Health care incident	18. Hazard	34. Blame
3. Health	19. Outcome	35. Negligence
4. Health care	20. Health care outcome	36. Monitor
5. Event	21. Preventable	37. Benchmark
6. Circumstance	22. Adverse reaction	38. Standard
7. Agent	23. Side effect	39. Accreditation
8. Harm	24. Error	40. Credentialling
9. Complaint	25. Root cause analysis	41. Iatrogenic
10. Loss	26. System failure	42. Nosocomial
11. Disease	27. System improvement	43. Stakeholder
12. Injury	28. Quality	44. Standard
13. Suffering	29. Quality of health care	45. Suffering
14. Disability	30. Risk	46. System failure
15. Adverse event	31. Risk management	47. System improvement
16. Near miss	32. Liability	48. Violation

An alphabetically arranged list of preferred terms with their agreed definitions is provided on the next two pages. In this list, an asterisk (*) indicates that there are further terms within that definition which are also defined. For example, the term "**incident***" contains the additional terms (in **bold**) "**event**", "**circumstance**", "**harm**", "**complaint**" and "**loss**", which are themselves defined. The definition for "**harm***", in turn, contains the terms "**disease**", "**injury**", "**suffering**" and "**disability**", each of which are also defined.

This list has been submitted to the World Alliance for Patient Safety of the World Health Organization for consideration for its concepts and preferred terms to be included in the proposed International Patient Safety Classification.

---

*   Adapted from Runciman, W.B. (2006), 'Shared Meanings: Preferred Terms and Definitions for Safety and Quality Concepts', *Medical Journal of Australia* 184:10, S41–3.

Table A.1 Alphabetical list of preferred terms and definitions

---

*Accountable***:** Being held responsible.

Accreditation*: Being granted recognition for meeting designated **standards** for structure, process and **outcome**.

Adverse Event* An **incident** in which **harm** resulted to a person receiving **health care**.

Adverse Reaction* An adverse reaction describes an **adverse event** where the correct process was followed for the context in which the event occurred but unexpected and unpreventable **harm** resulted.

Agent One who, or that which, acts to produce a change.

Benchmark A criterion against which something is measured.

Blame To hold at fault (implies culpability).

Circumstance* All the factors connected with or influencing an **event**, **agent** or person/s.

Complaint An expression of dissatisfaction with something.

Credentialling* The process of assessing and conferring approval on a person's suitability to provide a defined type of **health care**. (Can be synonymous with clinical privileging).

Disability* Any type of impairment of body structure or function, activity limitation and/or restriction of participation in society, associated with past or present **harm**.

Disease A physiological or psychological dysfunction.

Error Unintentionally being wrong in conduct or judgement. (Error may occur by doing the wrong thing (commission) or by failing to do the right thing (omission).

Event Something that happens to or with a person.

Harm* Harm includes **disease, injury, suffering, disability** and death.

Hazard* A **circumstance** or **agent** that can lead to **harm**, damage or **loss.**

Health* A state of complete physical, mental and social well-being and not merely the absence of **disease** or infirmity.

Health Care* Services provided to individuals or communities to promote, maintain, monitor, or restore **health**. Healthcare is not limited to medical care and includes self care.

Iatrogenic* Arising from or associated with **health care** rather than an underlying **disease** or **injury**.

Incident* An **event** or **circumstance** which could have, or did result, in unintended or unnecessary **harm** to a person and/or a **complaint, loss** or damage.

Health Care Incident* An **event** or **circumstance** during **health care** which could have, or did result in unintended or unnecessary **harm** to a person and/or a **complaint, loss** or damage.

Health Care Outcome* The **health** status of an individual, a group of people, or a population which is wholly or partially attributable to an **action, agent** or **circumstance**.

Injury* Damage to tissues caused by an **agent** or **circumstance**.

Liability Responsible for an action according to the law or in a legal sense.

Loss Any negative consequence, including financial.

Monitor To check, supervise, observe critically, or record the progress of an activity, action or system on a regular basis in order to identify and/or track change.

Near Miss* An **incident** that did not cause **harm.**

Negligence* (civil or criminal) An incident causing **harm,** damage or **loss** as the result of doing something wrong or failing to provide a reasonable level of care in a **circumstance** in which one has a duty of care.

Nosocomial Pertaining to or originating in a hospital. (synonymous with "hospital acquired").

Outcome* The status of an individual, a group of people or a population which is wholly or partially attributable to an action, **agent** or **circumstance.**

Preventable* Accepted by the community as potentially avoidable in the particular set of **circumstances.**

Quality (degree of)* The extent to which a service or product produces a desired **outcome/s.**

Quality of Health Care (degree of)* The extent to which a **health care** service or product produces a desired **outcome/s.**

Risk The chance of something happening that will have a (negative) impact. It is measured in terms of consequences and likelihood.

Risk Management* In **health care,** designing and implementing a program of activities to identify and avoid or minimize **risks** to patients, employees, visitors and the institution; to minimize financial **losses** (including legal **liability**) that might arise consequentially; and to transfer **risk** to others through payment of premiums (insurance).

Root Cause Analysis* A systematic process whereby the factors which contributed to an **incident** are identified.

Safety* Freedom from **hazard.**

Side effect* An effect, other than that intended, produced by an **agent.** (see also 'adverse reaction').

Stakeholder Those people and organizations who may affect, be affected by, or perceive themselves to be affected by, a decision or activity.

Standard Agreed attributes and processes designed to ensure that a product, service or method will perform consistently at a designated level.

Suffering* Experiencing anything subjectively unpleasant. This may include pain, malaise, nausea and/or vomiting, **loss,** depression, agitation, alarm, fear or grief.

System failure A fault, breakdown or dysfunction within an organization's operational methods, processes or infrastructure.

System improvement* The result or outcome of the culture, processes and structures that are directed towards the prevention of **system failure** and the improvement in **safety** and **quality.**

Violation A violation is a deliberate, but not necessarily reprehensible, deviation from safe operating procedures, standards or rules.

Appendix II

Public Expenditure on Healthcare in Selected Countries

Table A.2 Public Expenditure as a Percentage of Total Expenditure (Health)*

Czech Republic	91	New Zealand	78	Austria	70
Slovak Republic	89	Finland	76	Canada	70
Sweden	85	France	76	Australia	68
Norway	83	Italy	75	Netherlands	63
United Kingdom	83	Ireland	75	Switzerland	58
Iceland	83	Poland	72	Greece	52
Denmark	83	Spain	71	Korea	50
Japan	82	Portugal	71	Mexico	45
Germany	79	Hungary	70	United States	45

*   Organization for Economic Co-operation and Development (2005). *OECD Health Data 2005: Statistics and Indicators for 30 Countries*. (Paris: Organization for Economic Co-operation and Development). Copyright: OECD HEALTH DATA June 2005.

Appendix III

Risk Matrix*

The risk matrix for the safety assessment codes. See Appendix VII for examples of healthcare incidents which fall into the various 'likelihood' and 'consequences' categories.

	Consequences			
Likelihood	Minor	Moderate	Major	Catastrophic
Frequent	2	2	3	3
Occasional	1	2	3	3
Uncommon	1	1	2	3
Remote	1	1	2	2

Figure A.1 Risk Matrix for Safety Assessment Codes

* Adapted from the Safety Assessment Code (SAC) Matrix developed by the VA National Center for Patient Safety, see http://www.va.gov/ncps/matrix.html

Appendix IV

Evidence-Based Medicine: Sources of Information

Examples of organizations promoting evidence based medicine:

Agency for Healthcare Research and Quality (AHRQ), USA, http://www.ahrq.gov/ is a Federal agency for research on health care quality, costs, outcomes, and patient safety. Its functions include the establishment of evidence based practice centres whose role is to produce reports on particular aspects of practice or technology

The Cochrane Library, Britain, http://www.cochrane.org/docs/descrip.htm contains the following (regularly updated) evidence based healthcare databases: Cochrane Database of Systematic Reviews (CDSR); Database of Abstracts and Reviews of Effectiveness (DARE); Cochrane Central Register of Controlled Trials (Central-CCTR); NHS Economic Evaluation Database (NHSEED); Cochrane Database of Methodological Reviews (CDMR). The Cochrane library is coordinated by the Cochrane Collaboration (an international not-for-profit organization) and the UK's National Health Service Centre for Reviews and Dissemination (below).

The Guidelines International Network, International, http://www.g-i-n.net/ is an international initiative to improve the quality of health care by promoting systematic development of clinical practice guidelines and their application into practice.

The Joanna Briggs Institute (JBI), Australia, evidence based nursing website at http://www.joannabriggs.edu.au/about/home.php has an evidence library. The International Journal of Evidence-Based Healthcare (formerly JBI reports) is available online at www.blackwell-synergy.com and contains reports on systematic reviews and meta-analyses of nursing practices.

The National Health Service Centre for Reviews and Dissemination (CRD), University of York, United Kingdom, http://www.york.ac.uk/inst/crd/index.htm was established in 1994 to promote the use of research based information. The centre has three databases: Database of abstracts of reviews of effectiveness (DARE); NHS economic evaluation database (NHSEED); health technology assessment (HTA) database.

National Institute for Clinical Studies, Australia: http://www.nicsl.com.au/ aims to close the gaps between evidence and clinical practice.

National Institute for Health and Clinical Excellence (NICE), Britain, http://www.nice.org.uk/page.aspx?o=home is described on its webpage as 'the independent organization responsible for providing national guidance on the promotion of good health and the prevention and treatment of ill health'. It provides guidelines and systematic reviews on a wide range of clinical topics, and numerous appraisals of medical technology.

Appendix V

International Code of Medical Ethics*

Duties of Physicians in general. A Physician shall:

- always maintain the highest standards of professional conduct
- not permit motives of profit to influence the free and independent exercise of professional judgement on behalf of patients
- in all types of medical practice, be dedicated to providing competent medical service in full technical and moral independence, with compassion and respect for human dignity
- deal honestly with patients and colleagues, and strive to expose those physicians deficient in character or competence, or who engage in fraud or deception

The following practices are deemed to be unethical conduct:

- Self advertising by physicians, unless permitted by the laws of the country and the Code of Ethics of the National Medical Association
- Paying or receiving any fee or any other consideration solely to procure the referral of a patient or for prescribing or referring a patient to any source

A Physician shall:

- respect the rights of patients, of colleagues, and of other health professionals and shall safeguard patient confidences
- act only in the patient's interest when providing medical care which might have the effect of weakening the physical and mental condition of the patient
- use great caution in divulging discoveries or new techniques or treatment through non-professional channels
- certify only that which he has personally verified

Duties of Physicians to the sick. A Physician shall:

- always bear in mind the obligation of preserving human life
- owe his patients complete loyalty and all the resources of his science. Whenever an examination or treatment is beyond the physician's capacity he should summon another physician who has the necessary ability
- preserve absolute confidentiality on all he knows about his patient even after the patient has died

- give emergency care as a humanitarian duty unless he is assured that others are willing and able to give such care

Duties of Physicians to each other. A Physician shall:

- behave towards his colleagues as he would have them behave towards him.
- not entice patients from his colleagues
- observe the principles of the "Declaration of Geneva" approved by the World Medical Association

---

*   Adapted from World Medical Association (adopted 1949, amended 1968, 1983). *International Code of Medical Ethics:* http://www.wma.net/e/policy/c8.htm

Appendix VI

Jonsen's Ethics Framework*

Medical factors – beneficence and non-maleficence

1. Is the problem acute? chronic? critical? reversible?
2. What are the goals of treatment?
3. What are the probabilities of success?
4. What are the plans in case of therapeutic failure?
5. In sum, what are the risks, benefits and contingency plans?

Patient preferences (autonomy)

1. Is the patient mentally capable and legally competent?
2. If competent – what are the patient's preferences?
3. Has the patient been fully informed, understood, and given consent?
4. If incapacitated, who is the appropriate surrogate? Is the surrogate using appropriate standards for decision making?
5. Has the patient expressed prior preferences?
6. Can the patient cooperate with medical treatment? If not, why not?
7. In sum, is the patient's right to choose being respected in ethics and law?

Quality of life (beneficence and non-maleficence, autonomy)

1. What are the prospects, with or without treatment, for a return to an acceptable life?
2. What physical, mental and social deficits is the patient likely to experience if treatment succeeds?
3. Are there biases that might prejudice the provider's evaluation of the patient's quality of life?
4. Is the patient's present or future condition such that his or her continued life might be judged undesirable?
5. Is there any plan and rationale to forego treatment?
6. Are there plans for comfort and palliative care?

Contextual features (loyalty and fairness)

1. Are there family issues that might influence treatment decisions?
2. Are there provider issues that might influence treatment decisions?
3. Are there financial and economic factors?

4.   Are there religious or cultural factors?
5.   Are there limits on confidentiality?
6.   Are there problems of allocation of resources?
7.   How does the law affect treatment decisions?
8.   Is clinical research or teaching involved?
9.   Is there any conflict of interest for the providers or the institution?

---

*   Adapted from Jonsen, A.R., Siegler, M. and Winslade, W.J. (1992), *Clinical Ethics: a Practical Approach to Ethical Decisions in Clinical Medicine* (New York: McGraw-Hill).

Appendix VII

Severity Assessment Code (SAC)

The Veterans Administration has developed criteria for grading the severity of an event and the probability of its recurrence.[1] Together, these criteria can be used in a matrix to develop a SAC score of 1 (low risk), 2 (intermediate risk) or 3 (high risk) (see Appendix 3).[2] A SAC score of 3 should trigger a root cause analysis. Some incidents (notably falls and drug administration errors) are too frequent for RCA, even if their SAC is 3. Data on these incidents should be collected and reviewed periodically (quarterly for example). RCA can then be undertaken, if appropriate, on the aggregated information for the period.

Categories for Probability

Frequent Likely to occur immediately or within a short period of time.
Occasional Probably will occur several times in 1–2 years.
Uncommon May happen sometime in 2–5 years.
Remote May happen sometime in 5–30 years.

Categories for Consequences

Catastrophic Iatrogenic death or major permanent loss of function due to a sentinel event (see pages 48 and 49); a death or hospitalization of three or more *visitors* or *staff*; a *fire* that grows larger than a burning waste paper basket.

Major Impairment of function or disfigurement of a *patient*; a need for surgical intervention or an increased length of stay or level of care for three of more *patients;* hospitalization of one or two *visitors* or *staff;* three or more *staff* experiencing lost time or restricted duty; damage equal to or more than USD100,000 to equipment or healthcare facilities.

Moderate Increased length or stay or level of care for one or two *patients*; evaluation and treatment for one or two *visitors;* medical expenses, lost time or restricted duty, injuries or illness for one or two *staff*; physical damage costing USD10,000 to USD 100,000; a *fire* smaller than a waste paper basket.

Minor No injury, increased length of stay or increased level of care for *patients*; no treatment, lost time or restricted duty for *visitors* or *staff*; physical damage of less that USD 10,000 or loss of utility without harm to patients (eg power, water, communications or transport).

---

1   A Safety Assessment Code (SAC) Matrix was developed by the VA National Center for Patient Safety, see http://www.va.gov/ncps/matrix.html
2   In certain jurisdictions in Australia, such as NSW and SA, the SAC has been reversed, with SAC 1 representing the highest risk, and SAC 3 the lowest.

Appendix VIII

The Advanced Incident Management System (AIMS)[*]

AIMS provides tools to facilitate the management of incidents and to elicit information about things that go wrong in healthcare. It is based on the framework shown in Figure 1.6, which defines the relationships between the components of the classification system (classes) and the terms used to describe their attributes (concepts). There are five levels of information: information sources, incident types, components (classes), attributes (concepts) and terms.

Information Sources

These are listed in Table 2.5 (page 39).

Healthcare Incident Types (HITs)

There are 17 '*generic*' and 5 specialty HITs so far: medication and intravenous fluids; oxygen, gases and vapours; blood and blood products; nutrition; medical devices, equipment and property; buildings, fittings, fixtures and surrounds; falls; pressure ulcers; accidents and occupational health and safety; clinical management; pathology/laboratory; documentation; healthcare associated infections; organization, management and services; security; aggression – victim; aggression – aggressor. Specialty types include: anaesthesia; intensive care; hyperbaric medicine; obstetrics. Each incident may be classified using one or more HITs. For example, an overdose of morphine in an intensive care patient, because of malfunction of an infusion pump, would be classified using *medication, therapeutic device* and *intensive care* HITs.

Components (classes)

Each HIT is made up of the *components* of the GRM. Some components have attributes specific to each incident type, such as 'what happened?'.

Attributes (concepts)

To characterize the attributes of the components of the GRM, each represented by a concept, the classification process prompts classifiers to respond to cascades of relevant and intuitively arranged 'plain language' questions. The answers (concepts) are labelled by preferred 'terms'. These can vary from area to area or from country to country, but always refer to the same underlying concepts.

Terms

The *terms* (representing concepts) are presented to the classifier as possible answers to classification questions. There are over 20,000, including lists from 'controlled vocabularies' such as lists for drugs, equipment and devices. These terms may be reviewed, revised and expanded as necessary.

---

*   Runciman, W.B. (1999), 'Lessons from the Australian Patient Safety Foundation: Setting Up a National Patient Safety Surveillance System – Is This The Right Model?' *Quality and Safety in Health Care* 11:3, 246–51.

Appendix IX

Soft Systems Methodology (SSM)[*]

Healthcare is replete with complex problems. Resolution is often unsuccessful because the complex sociotechnical systems in which the problems are embedded are not taken account of.[1] There are four common approaches.

The first is the *political imperative*. The main goal is to promote one's own interests at the expense of others by positioning and advancing one's own group, acquiring and mobilizing resources, and exercising influence to further one's own objectives. 'Much of this behaviour is unseen: withholding information; guilefully influencing agendas, lobbying behind closed doors, negotiating for financial resources, securing authority and subtly reinforcing warranted or public punishing of unwarranted behaviour in others'.[*]

The second approach is based on *economic reasoning* by which almost anything valuable or useful is reduced to dollars, throughput, productivity and efficiency, ignoring any consideration of what drives behaviour and behaviour change in professionals. This has spawned case mix funding, managed care and purchaser-provider separation, all of which have induced 'an emphasis on volume over quality, adverse consequences, gaming responses, a reduced level of collaboration amongst stake holders and increased levels of divisiveness'.

The third approach is the *biomedical or scientific* one (whatever the problem, it can be reduced to a formal study, preferably an RCT). However, the reductionist and positivist thinking inherent in this approach discounts the complicated nature of healthcare systems and the fact that most problems are not amenable to solutions which artificially isolate them from the ecological and social weave.

The fourth response is the *managerialist or business oriented* approach. 'A smart young thing…working for a consulting company, comes to an identified problem with a brief case full of tools' (TQM, restructuring, change measurement, business process re-engineering, and decentralization (or centralization) of services; clinicians remain unimpressed by this approach).[*]

However, 'there remain widespread problems of policy implementation, poorly integrated services across organization/institutional settings, too few examples of successful multi-disciplinary teams and a deal of professional and patient dissatisfaction with individual services'.[*]

SSM provides a framework for solving complex problems using a staged, transparent process – 'the aim is to explain the complexities and allow space for conflicts …, rather than to pretend they do not exist (or decide to ignore them because they are not easily addressed)'.[*] The focus is not on the problems themselves, or on simple abstract solutions, but on the experiences of the stake holders and the social and organizational circumstances in which the problems

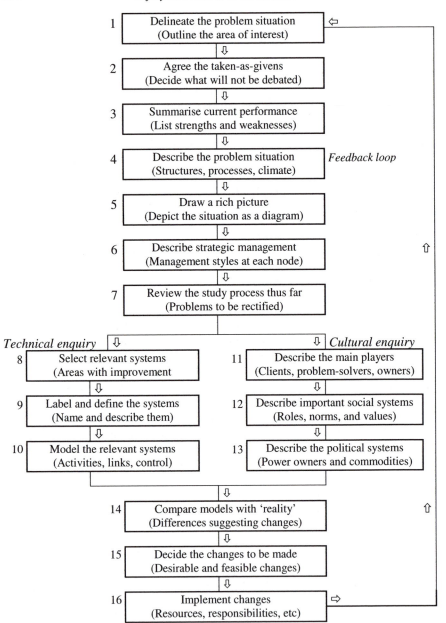

Figure A.1 Soft Systems Methodology Flowchart[*]

Braithwaite, J. (2006), personal communication. Reprinted with permission.

exist. A detailed discussion is beyond the scope of this brief summary. The 16 stages of SSM plus are shown in Figure A.2.

Braithwaite, J. et al. (2002), 'Introducing Soft Systems Methodology Plus (SSM+): Why We Need It and What It Can Contribute', *Australian Health Review* 25(2), 191–208.

Appendix X

Sources of Information for Patients

The following web-sites are examples of health-related information provided for consumers on the internet:

Agency for Healthcare Research and Quality consumer site: http://www.ahrq.gov/consumer/

American Association of Retired Persons health site http://www.aarp.org/health/

Australian Government, *Health Insite*: http://www.healthinsite.gov.au/

Food and Drug Administration consumer site: http://www.fda.gov/opacom/morecons.html

Institute for Clinical Systems Improvement http://www.icsi.org/patients/index.asp

Institute for Safe Medication Practices consumer site: http://www.ismp.org/consumers/default.asp

National Institute for Clinical Studies (Australia): http://www.nicsl.com.au/

National Institute for Health and Clinical Excellence (United Kingdom): http://www.nice.org.uk/

National Institutes of Health (United States): http://health.nih.gov/

National Library of Medicine (United States): http://www.nlm.nih.gov/

National Prescribing Service (Australia): http://www.nps.org.au/

Safe Medication (United States), a website of the American Society of Health-System Pharmacists: http://www.safemedication.com/

An excellent book for patients is: *You* Roizen, M.F. and Oz, M.C. (2006), *You: The Smart Patient: An Insider's Handbook for Getting the Best Treatment* (New York: Free Press).

Index